Troublesome disguises
Managing challenging disorders in psychiatry

Troublesome disguises

Managing challenging disorders in psychiatry

EDITED BY

Dinesh Bhugra

Professor of Mental Health and Cultural Diversity
Institute of Psychiatry, King's College London
London, UK

Gin S. Malhi

Professor and Chair
Department of Psychiatry
Sydney Medical School
University of Sydney
Sydney, Australia

SECOND EDITION

WILEY Blackwell

This edition first published 1997 © 2015 by John Wiley & Sons, Ltd.

Registered Office
John Wiley & Sons, Ltd, The Atrium, Southern Gate, Chichester, West Sussex, PO19 8SQ, UK

Editorial Offices
9600 Garsington Road, Oxford, OX4 2DQ, UK
The Atrium, Southern Gate, Chichester, West Sussex, PO19 8SQ, UK
1606 Golden Aspen Drive, Suites 103 and 104, Ames, Iowa 50010, USA

For details of our global editorial offices, for customer services and for information about
how to apply for permission to reuse the copyright material in this book please see our website at
www.wiley.com/wiley-blackwell

The right of the author to be identified as the author of this work has been asserted in accordance with
the UK Copyright, Designs and Patents Act 1988.

Library of Congress Cataloging-in-Publication Data
Troublesome disguises : managing challenging disorders in psychiatry / edited by Dinesh Bhugra,
Gin S. Malhi. – Second edition.
       p. ; cm.
    Includes bibliographical references and index.
    ISBN 978-1-119-99314-8 (cloth)
I. Bhugra, Dinesh, editor.   II. Malhi, Gin S., editor.
[DNLM: 1. Mental Disorders–diagnosis.   WM 141]
    RC469
    616.89'075–dc23
                                              2014029376
A catalogue record for this book is available from the British Library.

Wiley also publishes its books in a variety of electronic formats. Some content that appears in print may
not be available in electronic books.

Cover image: Giuseppe Arcimboldo [Public domain], via Wikimedia Commons

Set in 9.5/13pt Meridien by SPi Publisher Services, Pondicherry, India

Printed in Singapore by C.O.S. Printers Pte Ltd

1   2015

Contents

Contributors

Richard Atkinson
Consultant Old Age Psychiatrist, Lancashire Care NHS Foundation Trust, Preston, UK

Oyedeji Ayonrinde
Consultant Psychiatrist, South London and Maudsley NHS Foundation Trust, London, UK

David S. Baldwin
Professor of Psychiatry and Head of Mental Health Group, Clinical and Experimental Sciences Academic Unit, Faculty of Medicine, University of Southampton, UK

Michael Berk
IMPACT Strategic Research Centre, Deakin University, Department of Psychiatry, Orygen Research Centre, and The Florey Institute for Neuroscience and Mental Health, University of Melbourne, Australia

German E. Berrios
Emeritus Chair of the Epistemology of Psychiatry, Emeritus Consultant Neuropsychiatrist, Department of Psychiatry, University of Cambridge, Cambridge, UK

Dinesh Bhugra
Professor of Mental Health and Cultural Diversity, Institute of Psychiatry, King's College London, London, UK

Rohan Borschmann
Clinical Psychologist, Institute of Psychiatry, King's College London, London, UK

Lise Bouchard
Director of Research, Runajambi Institute for the Study of Quichua Culture and Health, Otavalo, Ecuador

Richard A. Bryant
School of Psychology, University of New South Wales, Sydney, Australia

Alistair Burns
Professor of Old Age Psychiatry, Vice Dean for the Faculty of Medical and
Human Sciences, National Clinical Director for Dementia in England,
University of Manchester, Manchester, UK

Santosh K. Chaturvedi
Department of Psychiatry, National Institute of Mental Health and Neurosciences,
Bangalore, India

Max Coltheart
ARC Centre of Excellence in Cognition and Its Disorders, and Department
of Cognitive Science, Macquarie University, Sydney, Australia

Michael H. Connors
Dementia Collaborative Research Centre, School of Psychiatry,
University of New South Wales, Sydney, Australia

Peter Falkai
Department of Psychiatry and Psychotherapy, Ludwig-Maximilians-University,
Munich, Germany

Wolfgang Gaebel
Department of Psychiatry and Psychotherapy, Medical Faculty,
Heinrich Heine University, LVR-Clinics Düsseldorf, Düsseldorf, Germany

Alkomiet Hasan
Department of Psychiatry and Psychotherapy, Ludwig-Maximilians-University,
Munich, Germany

Sean P. Heffernan
Schweizer Fellow in Affective Disorders, Johns Hopkins Hospital,
Baltimore, Maryland, U.S.

Mario Incayawar
Director, Runajambi Institute for the Study of Quichua Culture and Health,
Otavalo, Ecuador

David Jolley
Honorary Reader in Psychiatry of Old Age, Personal Social Services Research Unit,
University of Manchester, UK

Robyn Langdon
ARC Centre of Excellence in Cognition and Its Disorders, and Department
of Cognitive Science, Macquarie University, Sydney, Australia

Florence Levy
School of Psychiatry, University of New South Wales and Prince of Wales Hospital, Sydney, Australia

Constantine Lyketsos
Elizabeth Plank Althouse Professor and Chair of Psychiatry, Johns Hopkins Bayview Professor of Psychiatry and Behavioral Sciences, Baltimore, Maryland, U.S.

Berend Malchow
Department of Psychiatry and Psychotherapy, Ludwig-Maximilians-University, Munich, Germany

Sioui Maldonado-Bouchard
Research Associate, Runajambi Institute for the Study of Quichua Culture and Health, Otavalo, Ecuador

Gin S. Malhi
Professor and Chair, Department of Psychiatry, Sydney Medical School, University of Sydney, Sydney, Australia

Ivana S. Marková
Reader/Honorary Consultant in Psychiatry, Centre for Health and Population Sciences, Hull York Medical School, University of Hull, Hull, UK

Paul Moran
Reader/Honorary Consultant Psychiatrist, Institute of Psychiatry, King's College London, London, UK

Karin Neufeld
Clinical Director of Psychiatry, Johns Hopkins Bayview Associate Professor of Psychiatry and Behavioral Science, Baltimore, Maryland, U.S.

Esther Oh
Assistant Professor, Division of Geriatric Medicine and Gerontology, Johns Hopkins School of Medicine, Associate Director, the Johns Hopkins Memory and Alzheimer's Treatment Center, Baltimore, Maryland, U.S.

John M. Oldham
Senior Vice President and Chief of Staff, The Menninger Clinic, Barbara and Corbin Robertson Jr. Endowed Chair for Personality Disorders, Professor and Executive Vice Chair, Menninger Department of Psychiatry and Behavioral Sciences, Baylor College of Medicine, Houston, Texas, U.S.

Soumya Parameshwaran
Department of Psychiatry, Kasturba Medical College, Mangalore, India

Andrea Schmitt
Department of Psychiatry and Psychotherapy, Ludwig-Maximilians-University, Munich, Germany

Julia M. Sinclair
Senior Lecturer in Psychiatry, Clinical and Experimental Sciences Academic Unit, Faculty of Medicine, University of Southampton, UK

Holly Tabernik
Department of Psychiatry and Health Behavior, Georgia Regents University, Augusta, Georgia, U.S.

Julio Torales
Professor of Psychiatry and Medical Psychology and Head of the Psychodermatology Unit, Department of Psychiatry, School of Medical Sciences, National University of Asunción, Paraguay

Michael J. Vitacco
Department of Psychiatry and Health Behavior, Georgia Regents University, Augusta, Georgia, U.S.

Jüergen Zielasek
Department of Psychiatry and Psychotherapy, *Medical Faculty*, Heinrich Heine University, LVR-Clinics Düsseldorf, Düsseldorf, Germany

Preface

As a profession, psychiatry is often seen as a specialty where the classification of symptoms into syndromes is both arbitrary and varied. This perception belies the fact that clinical diagnosis is difficult per se, and especially so when considering perturbations of the mind. With an increased demand for services for people with mental health problems, and ever increasing numbers of diagnoses and subtypes, it is inevitable that clinicians may find the process challenging and may sometimes struggle to assign diagnoses with precision. Consequently, many psychiatric illnesses remain underdiagnosed, whereas others are overdiagnosed or misdiagnosed altogether. As with all rare diagnoses in medicine, unusual psychiatric illnesses remain rare, which makes them not only exotic but much more difficult to recognise. But these are not solely taxonomic or epidemiological considerations. They exact a considerable clinical cost: following misdiagnosis or missed diagnosis, patients, their families, and their caregivers continue to suffer, and the burden of disease continues to mount. Clinical experience has shown quite clearly that the longer a diagnosis is missed and remains inadequately treated, the greater the likelihood that the condition will become refractory and cause ongoing distress to those affected. The diagnosis of disease is the responsibility of physicians, whereas patients want treatment for their ailments and illnesses and lessening of their suffering. Hence there is an inherent tension within the therapeutic encounter and alliance, a theme revisited in many of the chapters in this book.

The first edition of this volume, with Professor Alistair Munro as co-editor, appeared in 1997. In the intervening period, psychiatry as a profession as well as psychiatric diagnoses have evolved considerably, highlighted most notably perhaps by the recent publication of DSM-5 and the impending arrival of ICD-11. This second edition is testament to the success of the first edition but at the same time has been completely rewritten so as to detail further some of the older conditions and provide important updates; in addition, it includes many new conditions that appear for the first time. The rates of these psychiatric diagnoses range from commonplace to rare, but all are essential knowledge for practising clinicians, who need to be aware of both frequent and extraordinary conditions that pose diagnostic conundrums and can be difficult to define. We hope that this combination of theoretical and practical considerations of various psychiatric conditions will prove useful to clinicians and researchers alike, and hence many of the clinical conditions described herein are not unusual, but are simply conditions that are often overlooked or difficult to delineate.

We envisage that readers will benefit by using the contributions to enhance their clinical awareness of these potentially troublesome diagnoses and exercise caution in blindly following any classificatory system and its unsophisticated application across populations, contexts, and cultures. In practice, the errors both of commission and omission need to be revisited on a regular basis and we hope that this volume will facilitate critical consideration of diagnosis and thereby diminish the likelihood of misdiagnosis and missed diagnoses.

We are indebted to the many contributors who have selflessly shared their expertise, experience, knowledge, and skills. In addition to thanking them, we would also like to express our gratitude to Dr Joan Marsh, formerly at Wiley-Blackwell, and her team. Finally, our thanks would not be complete without acknowledging the sterling efforts of Andrea Livingstone, who guided this project with sage diplomacy and delightful spirit.

Dinesh Bhugra and Gin S. Malhi

PART I
Challenging psychiatric conditions

CHAPTER 1

Shared pathologies

German E. Berrios[1] and Ivana S. Marková[2]

[1] Emeritus Chair of the Epistemology of Psychiatry, Emeritus Consultant Neuropsychiatrist, Department of Psychiatry, University of Cambridge, Cambridge, UK
[2] Reader/Honorary Consultant in Psychiatry, Centre for Health and Population Sciences, Hull York Medical School, University of Hull, Hull, UK

Definition

Until recently "Shared Pathologies" was the official DSM-IV-T [1] name for clinical phenomena having in common the fact that persons, through their socio-emotional relationships, may share mental symptoms or disorders similar in form and/or content. Such temporal concurrence has led clinicians to calling such complaints shared, communicated, transferred, or passed on. Although the A+B combination (*folie à deux*) is the commonest form of the disorder, this can also occur in families (*folie à famille*) or even larger social groups (schools or other institutions). This, together with the fact that the terms *shared* and *communicated* are (covertly) explanatory, has impeded the formulation of an adequate operational definition.

Both clinically and historically, folie à deux remains the core clinical phenomenon. Recently, in U.S. psychiatry, the category "297.3 Shared Psychotic Disorder (Folie à Deux)" [1] has been replaced by "298.8 (F28) 4. Delusional symptoms in partner of individual with delusional disorder" [2].

A similar concept appears in the blue (descriptive) World Health Organization (WHO) book [3]: "F24 Induced delusional disorder: A delusional disorder shared by two or more people with close emotional links. Only one of the people suffers from a genuine psychotic disorder; the delusions are induced in the other(s) and usually disappear when the people are separated. Includes: folie à deux; induced paranoid or psychotic disorder."

And in the green (research criteria) WHO book [4]: "F24 Induced delusional disorder":

(A) The individual(s) must develop a delusion or delusional system originally held by someone else with a disorder classified in F20—F23.

Troublesome Disguises: Managing Challenging Disorders in Psychiatry, Second Edition.
Edited by Dinesh Bhugra and Gin S. Malhi.

(B) The people concerned must have an unusually close relationship with one another, and be relatively isolated from other people.

(C) The individual(s) must not have held the belief in question before contact with the other person, and must not have suffered from any other disorder classified in F20—F23 in the past.

However, clinical experience suggests the existence of other presentations. For example, cases have also been reported of "contagious" obsessionality and hypochondriacal and suicidal behavior. Furthermore, if "communication" or "transfer" is to be considered as a definitional criterion, then phenomena such as the transfer of anesthesia or motor paralysis from one side of the body to the other (with the help of magnets) or indeed from one patient to another have to be included.

Lack of an adequate operational definition has precluded meaningful epidemiological research. It would be hasty, however, to conclude that the shared pathologies are clinical curiosities. Indeed, their peculiar multi-subject structure calls into question the individualistic metaphysics on which the definition of mental disorder is currently based, and challenges the plausibility of current neurobiological models of mental disorders (more on this below).

History

It is now about 150 years since folie à deux entered the nosological catalogue. Historians disagree on who reported it first. For example, Lazarus [5] states, "it was originally described by Lasègue and Falret" but Gralnick [6] and Cousin and Trémine [7] have shown that it all depends on how "locus classicus" is defined. The latter is a notion that can be characterized as resulting from the historical convergence of a name, a concept or mechanism, and a behavior [8]. Thus, if "contagion" [9] is considered as the concept involved in the convergence then Hoffbauer should be considered as the initiator; if "induction" were to be considered instead then it would be Lehmann. If the emphasis was to be on the behavior involved then the first to report the phenomenon would have to be Baillarger or Dagron. Finally, if the term *folie à deux* itself is to be used as a criterion then Lasègue & Falret should claim the accolade.

Deciding on priority has bedeviled the history of folie à deux since its inception. The official story goes that although some earlier alienists may have noticed folie à deux it was Lasègue and Falret who, in presenting a case to the *Société Médico Psychologique* in 1873, rounded it off as a new clinical phenomenon [6, 10]. Lasègue & Falret went on to publish the same paper in 1877 in two Journals: *Archives Générales de Médecine* [11] and *Annales Médico-Psychologiques* [12].

The historical reality is more complex. In his "Rectificatory note concerning the history of communicated insanity—folie à deux," Régis [13] noticed that Lehmann had identified Baillarger as the "first" who had reported cases suffering from this disorder in 1857. Régis went on to confirm this claim and stated that in his "Quelques exemples de folie communiquée" [14] Baillarger had not only reported four cases but also provided the very diagnostic criteria that were to reappear in the work by Lasègue and Falret [11, 12]. In the debate that followed Arnaud [15] tried to redefine the *locus classicus* in favor of Lasègue and Falret: "the scientific era in the study of folie à deux only starts in 1873"; and Halberstadt agreed [9]. But what did Arnaud mean by "scientific era"? Why did he dismiss Baillarger's report as "non-scientific"? It must be concluded that in Arnaud's hands the term *scientific* was little more than a rhetorical device used to resolve an ongoing rivalry between two psychiatric coteries.

Soon enough a small industry developed around folie à deux. According to the phenomenology of the cases found and the transmission mechanisms proposed, four types were described: folie *imposée* (as described by Lasègue and Falret [11, 12]; folie *simultanée* (reported by Régis in his doctoral thesis of 1880) [16]; folie *communiquée* (reported by Marandon de Montyel in 1881) [17] and folie *induite* [18]. By the turn of the century, the main risk factors had also been listed: association, dominance, lack of blood relationship, premorbid-personality, gender, and type of delusion [9].

The concept of folie à deux crossed the English Channel swiftly. Savage wrote on it in the *Journal of Mental Science* [19], Tuke in the *British Medical Journal* [20] and in *Brain* [21], and Ireland [22] included a discussion in his book *The Blot upon the Brain*. By the end of the 19th century, all that could realistically be said on the subject had been summarized by Tuke [23]:

(a) The influence of the insane upon the sane is very rare, except under certain conditions, which can he laid down with tolerable accuracy;

(b) As an almost universal rule, those who become insane in consequence of association with the insane, are neurotic or somewhat feebleminded;

(c) More women become affected than men;

(d) It is more likely that an insane person able to pass muster, as being in the possession of his intellect, should influence another in the direction of his delusion, than if he is outrageously insane. There must be some method in his madness;

(e) The most common form which cases of communicated insanity assume is that of delusion, and specially delusion of persecution, or of being entitled to property of which they are defrauded by their enemies. Acute mania, profound melancholia, and dementia, are not likely to communicate themselves. If they exert a prejudicial effect, it is by the distress these conditions cause in the minds of near relatives;

(f) A young person is more likely to adopt the delusion, of an old person than vice versa, specially if the latter be a relative with whom he or she has grown up from infancy;

(g) It simplifies the comprehension of this affection, to start from the acknowledged influence which a sane person may exert upon another sane person. It is not a long road from this to the acceptance of a plausible delusion, impressed upon the hearer with all the force of connection and the vividness of a vital truth;

(h) It is not easy to determine to what extent the person who is the second to become insane , affects in his turn the mental condition of the primary agent. Our own cases do not clearly point to this action, but there have been instances in which this has occurred, the result being that the first lunatic has modified his delusions in some measure, and the co-partnership, so to speak, in mental disorder, presents a more plausible aspect of the original delusion (Vol. 1, p. 241).

Current publications do little more than repeat what has been said in the classic texts.

Clinical phenomena

According to the received view, the clinical categories *folie à deux* and *folie communiquée* were first constructed in France by Lasègue & Falret [11, 12], and soon enough they surfaced in English as "communicated insanity" [22, 23] and in German as "induced insanity" [18]. However, equally important in Germany were the publications by Wollenberg on psychical infection [24] and the magnificent doctoral thesis by Max Schönfeldt on induced Insanity [25, 26]. Interestingly, in the German literature the term *induction* included the additional meaning that the psychosis seen in B (the "inducee") might result from stress caused by living with A, a psychosis sufferer [27].

In the event, the French expression *folie à deux* was to predominate [6, 10, 27–36] and the disorder it names has since been reported in different cultures and clinical settings [37–41]. A number of explanatory mechanisms have been suggested [5, 7, 35]. For example, based on a review of 103 cases, Gralnick [6] identified four sub-types: folie *imposée, simultanée, communiquée,* and *induite*. As we have seen above, this classification is little more than a medley of 19th-century French and German views on putative etiological mechanisms. In addition to folie à deux, clinical phenomena such as suicidal behavior (the Werther effect) [42, 43], hysterical symptoms [44], and obsessions [45, 46] should also be included in the group of shared pathologies. In this short chapter, there will only be space to deal with folie à deux.

So that the reader forms a concrete idea, a case of shared pathology from Tuke [21] is reproduced:

> The father, William Cairn, admitted Feb. 26, 1886, was 70 years of age, a farmer, and believed himself to be pursued and persecuted by the whole House of Keys; that he was the owner of extensive property, out of which he had been kept by that House and the high bailiff. He asserted that mobs had been raised to destroy his houses and cut down his trees. He had, he said, been assaulted by the men who had robbed him, with crowbars and pickaxes; when he endeavoured to obtain redress of these grievances, he had been prevented by telegrams and ghosts. His wife, ten years younger, asserted that her property had been sold against her will; that she had telegrams from invisible wires to say she must hang herself in consequence; and that her neighbours had put blood on the door and over the house. The daughter of these people, admitted on the same day, was 26 years of age; was silent and morose, with the exception of saying "first-rate" to enquiries about her health. Her mind, in fact, was too demented to allow of her entertaining the delusions of her parents. How long she had been affected is not stated, but Dr. Richardson informs me that she had returned home from service some time previously, and he is of opinion that the insane ways of her parents had much to do with inducing her present condition of mind. As to the man and his wife, the first symptoms arose about sixteen years ago after the loss of a little farm. They began to think they were entitled to property of great value, and eight years ago they went to London to Somerset House, to establish their claim, and have, their relatives say, spend "many a bright pound" in their search after the imaginary wealth (p. 413).

Epistemology

To understand why after the 1850s alienists thought it possible for insanity to be "communicated," two themes need exploring: (1) changes affecting the concept of insanity, and (2) theories and mechanisms of human communication (e.g., mimesis, imitation, contagion, infection, sympathy, etc.) [9].

Concept of insanity and the individualistic metaphysics of disease

Since the 18th century, "medical nosography" (that is, the description of disease) has been based on John Locke's notion of Individualism [47]. Like property, human rights, thoughts and selves, disease was also considered as an exclusive "personal" event. Reaffirmed as a unit of analysis, the individual and his skin became the absolute, natural boundary. By the same token society was modeled upon the Newtonian atomic paradigm and conceived as a mere collection of atoms (individuals). To get the latter to communication a theory of interaction was needed and Locke's solution was associationism, an epistemological (and later psychological) theory that set the rules as to how information might pass from one individual to the other. Because disease was a very personal event, its transmission from one person to the other needed explanation. To this effect mechanisms such as epidemics, contagion, mimesis, imitation, sympathy, empathy, and others were put forward. Constructed during the 19th century, alienism (now called psychiatry) fully adopted this individualistic notion of madness (disease).

Within this epistemological framework, the idea that madness could be "shared" or "passed on" was in principle unintelligible. This is why when clinical observation suggested that such sharing did actually occur, alienists had to resort to metaphors borrowed from physics and biology. It is in this sense that they claimed that mental disorders could be communicated, induced, caught (via contagion), and so on. In other words, a person A (the inducer) could pass on his madness to person B (the induced). The flow and direction of transmission between A and B was made in terms of features attributed to each that in practice reflected the social prejudices of the time. For example, A was said to be strong, male, superior, older, and the like, whereas B was claimed to be weak, a female, neurotic, dependent, younger, and so on. In general, metaphors taken from physics and mechanics were preferred to social accounts already available at the time such as empathy, sympathy, and imitation.

However, the idea that diseases (like selves) [48] may be shared by groups becomes less unintelligible if: (1) ontological individualism is set aside, and (2) diseases themselves are not fully reduced to their organic substratum. In this sense, the latter become processes or concatenations of events that as such can exist in multiple times and spaces (e.g., a cluster of persons) [49]. In the long term, whether this latter view is to become popular will depend more upon its usefulness in managing disease than upon some theoretical need to preserve the individualistic ontology of disease.

Theories and mechanisms of human communication

The central meaning of "to share" is "to cut into parts" [50], hence *oratio recta,* "shared pathology," should mean that parts of one symptom or disorder are being given out to different individuals. In practice, however, shared pathology means that although A + B exhibit similar symptoms or disorders, A has developed them first and passed them onto B. For completion's sake, it could be said that the clinical phenomenon is open to three theoretical interpretations: (1) one disorder is apportioned in shares to A + B; (2) one disorder is passed on (transmitted, communicated, etc.) from A to B; or (3) A + B show the same disorder but this fact is aleatory.

As currently defined, shared pathology refers to the second interpretation, that is, the situation or process whereby a disorder moves from one individual to the other. This situation, in turn, is open to three interpretations: (1) A *passes* it onto B (either intentionally or not); (2) B *imitates* or copies A, regardless of A's views or actions; or (3) a hidden (third) agent occasions the disorder to pass on from A to B.

Interestingly enough, all three options were discussed during the 19th century:

1 A→B concerned the old view that certain behaviors could be imposed or induced onto others (regardless of their will); indeed, this possibility was also reflected in the popular 19th-century pedagogical philosophy that supported the view that a teacher was able to shape the behavior of a pupil regardless of the latter's conscious wishes.

2 B could also "imitate": A; indeed, by the end of the century imitation had been proposed as a general mechanism of socialization, for example by Tarde [51]. In this regard, notions such as sympathy, empathy, imitation, mimesis, emulation, and the like were included in the process.

3 This mechanism concerned the old medical notion of contagion (i.e., the view that miasmas, spirits, microbes, and so on could facilitate the transfer of a disorder from A to B) [52]. The fact that no such agents were known to exist in regards to mental disorder led 19th century alienists to talk about psychological or moral contagion. Indeed this was a common explanation for suicide epidemics, folie à deux, addiction to opium, and other conditions. It is also possible to include under this rubric clinical situations where the transmission of symptoms from A to B is effected by another person. For example, in experiments using a magnet carried out by Babinski, symptoms such as paralysis and anesthesia were moved either from one to the other side of A or from A to B [44]. Conceptually, these cases seem to belong in the shared pathologies category even if ordinarily they are not included.

Prosper lucas and his 19th-century classification

The analysis of how certain mental disorders can be transmitted from A to B proposed by Prosper Lucas (1808–1885) remains unsurpassed to this day. In his doctoral thesis, "*De la Imitation Contagieuse. Ou de la propagation sympathique des névroses et des monomanies*" [53], he proposed a three-fold etiological classification:

1 Phenomena resulting from voluntary mimicking
   • Physiological
   • Pathological
2 Phenomena resulting from involuntary imitation (sympathetic)
   • Physiological
   • Pathological
      ○ Neurosis of movement or sensation
   • Neuroses of mental faculties
   • Complex neuroses
3 Phenomena that start as voluntary mimicking and become involuntary

Lucas's model is based on the combination of two polar dimensions: voluntary versus involuntary and physiological versus pathological. At the beginning of the 19th century, Bichat had explained the first dimension on the basis of differences in muscle type and innervation. This distinction was soon transferred to the mind and "voluntary" and "involuntary" thoughts started to be differentiated. The dimension physiological-pathological developed in the wake of the construction of the discipline of physiology itself, based on the distinction between structure and function. Like structure, function could also range from the "normal" to the "pathological."

Lucas introduced two additional concepts: imitation and sympathy. At the time, medical science still conceptualized imitation as a faculty of the mind (something similar to what is happening now in regard to the function of mirror neurons). Sympathy, in turn, was defined as a functional interdependence between the organs of the body, and by extension, between separate individuals [54]. Among the pathological phenomena Lucas included a variety of "neuroses," which he still defined in William Cullen's sense (imported into French medicine by means of the translations of Pinel and Bosquillon) [55]. There is no space in this chapter to analyze Lucas's work in more detail.

Conceptual mechanisms

The names used in the past to refer to the various shared pathologies reported in the literature reflect not only descriptive but also explanatory biases. Terms such as *induced* or *communicated* seem to be referring to hypothetical mechanisms that the authors very rarely make clear. Other concepts such as imitation, empathy, sympathy, and transfer are also mentioned in this context and some have interesting conceptual histories. Only imitation will be briefly explored in this chapter.

Imitation

Together with mimicry and mimesis, imitation constitutes a family of notions that refer to the copying the behavior (overt and subjective) of others. This action can be conscious or unconscious and its motivation varies from mere jest to admirative emulation. Known since classical times, these three notions have been put to a variety of uses. For example, mimesis plays a central role in the theories of art and the representation of nature proposed by Plato and Aristotle [56, 57].

Likewise, since early in Christianity, imitation (of God and Christ) became a principle of ethical behavior and a religious path toward the acquisition of grace. It can be found at the very basis of the concept of *theosis* or deification, that is, of the process whereby by his actions man emulates God [58]. On account of its importance, imitation is discussed by all the fathers of the

Church (from St. Augustine on) culminating in "Imitation of Christ," a classical work by Thomas à Kempis where it is enjoined that the mere "copying" of Christ (that is, of his holy behavior and preaching) should be replaced by an emulation of his interior life and withdrawal from the world [59, 60]. Luther disliked the concept of imitation and sought to replace it by passive conformism with the divine rule [61]. During the 19th century imitation returned as a pedagogic device, as something that children should do in order to become socialized and educated [61]. By the end of this period Tarde [51] proposed imitation as the central element in social development and cohesion and used it to explain all manner of social processes such as fashion, acculturation, national feelings, patriotism, and so on. Imitation has therefore been variously conceptualized. Originally considered as a power or capacity, by the 19th century it had become an instinct, something that animals and human beings did naturally. A difference was also introduced between mimicry, imitation, and mimesis and it was claimed that mimesis was an exclusively human function [62, 63, 64].

Until the end of the 20th century, writers conceived of imitation as a function of the mind. This changed when in the 1980s, neuronal clusters were reported that seemed to fire in response to imitative behavior [65]. Much debate has since been had on whether mirror neurons constitute the imitative brain engine par excellence or whether they fall short from explaining social imitation. All told, it remains unclear whether mirror neurons can discharge all the explanatory responsibilities that have been attributed to them [66]. For example, attributing to neurons full functional autonomy and agency leads to the obvious danger of a regression *ad infinitum*, that is, of the need to postulate another controlling neuronal cluster, and so on.

Part of this problem relates to the ambiguous use of the term *mirror*. Mirrors reflect passively images flashed onto them but do not start any imitative activity. By a semantic sleight of hand, mirror neurons are now used to explain imitation, that is, to start imitational behavior on the part of agent [67]. In this sense, they are no different from the old accounts that used psychological powers or faculties of the imitating agent such as sympathy, emulation, and so on.

Conclusion

The clinical phenomenon now known as shared pathologies has been well known and discussed since the 19th century. Indeed, discussion in the 20th century (and later) has contributed little to its explanation. Difficulties with providing an adequate operational definition explained the limited epidemiological information available on its incidence, prevalence, and cultural distribution. This notwithstanding, the shared pathologies are interesting both clinically and conceptually, the former because they draw the attention of the clinician toward the family setting in which mental disorders occur. There is a tendency these days to neglect such context due to the overemphasis on the individualism of disease encouraged by the neurobiological model. The latter is of interest because a proper analysis of the shared pathologies will make the clinician call into question some cherished assumptions as to the individual-istic nature of mental disorder and will encourage her to explore new con-cepts and ways of explaining the complaints expressed by sufferer.

How then can the shared pathologies be explained? The old concept of imitation could be a useful start. It might be said that for a variety of reasons human beings copy (whether consciously or not) the behaviors (including the symptoms) of relevant others. Imitation could be driven by solidarity, a wish to identify with others, and so on. Exploration of these psychological and social mechanisms has not yet been exhausted and should be pursued, not by reducing it to mechanistic neurobiological language (such as mirror neurons) but by keeping the discussion within the semantic space, the space of meaning where much of the drama of mental illness occurs.

One of the interesting issues arising from the existence of these phe-nomena concerns questions around how humans form and maintain their mental symptoms and disorders. On this nothing has been so far said in this chapter but it is, as far as we are concerned, the most promising option to understand the shared pathologies. For, irrespective of the underlying mech-anisms that the clinician may want to postulate for, say, the psychosis in A, it is unlikely that it can be explained to account for B's.

According to the Cambridge model of symptom-formation, this process starts when new information enters awareness and causes emotional dis-tress, encouraging the sufferer to want to share it with an interlocutor. The information can be of biological origin (generated by a neural net-work in distress) or symbolic in nature (originating in a social interaction). Like all other material entering awareness, this information is in an inchoate state, that is, pre-conceptual and pre-linguistic (ineffable). Because it is often novel it cannot manage in the usual way (like, say per-ceptions) by means of conventional templates that are applied to it in a habitual, non-conscious manner. Upon becoming aware of the novel information, the sufferer is forced to choose a configurator (from his or her bank of personal, familial, social, and cultural templates). Once con-figured into a speech act, the information is communicable and can be passed onto an interlocutor with whom a further negotiation can take place. A crystalized and recordable (in the case notes) mental symptom emerges at the end of this process [68].

This could explain how a shared pathology takes place. One option is that in A, the symptoms are formed as configurations of a biological signal. A and

B have a social relationship and share an intersubjective space. In the regular exchanges that follow, symbolic material is transferred into the awareness of B, who must handle it accordingly. In the ordinary state of affairs, B will configure it as what it is: a worry about A. On rare occasions, however, B may choose a configurator that expresses sympathy, identification, or imitation with A and this could lead to B's introjecting the symbol and configuring it as a mental symptom that would then be similar to that of A. The point here is simply to explicate how mental symptoms that may have the similar phenomenological presentation are the result of different configuratory mechanisms and hence have different etiology. Interestingly enough, one of the 19th-century explanatory models of shared pathologies lists as a cause of disorder in B the stress caused by living with A [27]. An explanation of this nature should carry important implications not just for understanding mental symptoms but also for approaches taken to their research and to their clinical management [69, 70].

References

1 American Psychiatric Association (1994) *Diagnostic and Statistical Manual of Mental Disorders*, 4th ed. Washington, DC, American Psychiatric Association.
2 American Psychiatric Association (2013) *Diagnostic and Statistical Manual of Mental Disorders*, 5th ed. Arlington, VA, American Psychiatric Association.
3 ICD-10 (1992) *Classification of Mental and Behavioural Disorders*. Geneva, World Health Organization.
4 ICD-10 (1993) *Classification of Mental and Behavioural Disorders, Diagnostic Criteria for Research*. Geneva, World Health Organization.
5 Lazarus A (1985) Folie à deux: psychosis by association or genetic determinism. *Comprehensive Psychiatry* 26: 129–135.
6 Gralnick A (1942) Folie à deux. *Psychiatric Quarterly* 16: 230–263.
7 Cousin F, Trémine T (1987) Folie à deux: Trajet historique, naissance d'un doute. *L'Information Psychiatrique* 63: 861–868.
8 Berrios GE (1996) *The History of Mental Symptoms: Descriptive Psychopathology since the 19th Century*. Cambridge, Cambridge University Press.
9 Halberstadt G (1906) *La Folie par Contagion Mentale*. Paris, Ballière.
10 Faguet RA, Faguet KF (1982) La Folie à Deux. In Friedmann CTH, Faguet RA (eds.) *Extraordinary Disorders of Human Behaviour*. New York, Plenum Press, pp. 1–14.
11 Lasègue C, Falret J (1877) La Folie à deux. *Archives Générales de Médecine* 30: 257–297.
12 Lasègue C, Falret J (1877) La Folie à deux ou folie communiquée. *Annales Médico-Psychologiques* 35: 321–355.
13 Régis E (1885) Note Rectificative a propos de l'historique de la folie communiquée (folie à deux). *Annales Médico-Psychologique* 43: 42–45.
14 Baillarger JGF (1885) Quelques exemples de folie communiquée. *Annales Médico-Psychologiques* 43: 212–214.
15 Arnaud FL (1893) La folie à deux. Ses diverses formes cliniques. *Annales Médico-Psychologiques* 17: 337–347.
16 Régis E (1880) *La folie à deux*. Thèse de Paris.

17 Marandon de Montyel E (1881) Contribution a l'étude de la folie à deux. *Annales Médico-Psychologiques* 39: 28–52.

18 Lehmann G (1885) Zur Casuistik des inducirten Irreseins (Folie à deux). *Archive für Psychiatrie und Nervenkrankheiten* 14: 145–154.

19 Savage G (1881) Cases of contagiousness of delusions. *Journal of Mental Science* 26: 563–566.

20 Tuke DH (1887) Folie à deux. *British Medical Journal* 2: 505–506.

21 Tuke DH (1888) Folie à deux. *Brain* 10: 408–421.

22 Ireland WW (1885) Folie à deux - a mad family. In *The Blot upon the Brain*. Edinburgh, Bell & Bradfute, pp. 201–208.

23 Tuke DH (1892) *A Dictionary of Psychological Medicine.* 2 vols. London, Churchill.

24 Wollenberg R (1889) Ueber psychische Infection. *Archiv für Psychiatrie und Nervenkrankheiten* 20: 62–88.

25 Schönfeldt M (1893) *Ueber das inducirte Irresein (folie communiquée).* Jurjew. Lankmann.

26 Schönfeldt M (1894) Ueber das inducirte Irresein (folie communiquée). *Archiv für Psychiatrie und Nervenkrankheiten* 26: 202–266.

27 Arenz D Stippel A (1999) Induziertes Irresein, Folie à deux und gemeinsame psychotische Störung. *Fortschrift für Neurologie und Psychiatrie* 67: 249–255.

28 Dewhurst K, Todd J (1956) The psychosis of association: Folie à deux. *Journal of Nervous and Mental Disease* 124: 451–459.

29 Franzini LR, Grossberg JM (1995) *Eccentric and Bizarre Behaviors.* New York, John Wiley.

30 Caduff F, Hubschmid T (1995) Folie à deux. *Nervenarzt* 66: 73–77.

31 Kashiwase H, Kato M (1997) Folie à deux in Japan: Analysis of 97 cases in the Japanese literature. *Acta Psychiatrica Scandinavica* 96: 231–234.

32 Silveira JM, Seeman MV (1995) Shared psychotic disorder: A critical review of the literature. *Canadian Journal of Psychiatry* 40: 389–395.

33 Shimizu M, Kubota Y, Toichi M, Baba H (2007) Folie à deux and shared psychotic disorder. *Current Psychiatry Reports* 9: 200–205.

34 Teixeira J, Mota T, Fernandes JC (2012) Folie à deux A case report. *Clinical Schizophrenia & Related Psychoses* 14: 1–9.

35 White TG (1995) Folie simultanée in monozygotic twins. *Canadian Journal of Psychiatry* 40: 418–420.

36 Berrios GE (1998) Folie à deux: A mad family as reported by WW Ireland. *History of Psychiatry*. Classic Text 35, 9: 383–395.

37 Kraya NA, Patrick C (1997) Folie à deux in forensic setting. *Australia and New Zealand Journal of Psychiatry* 31: 883–888.

38 Burke D., Dolan D, Schwartz R (1997) Folie à deux: Three cases in the elderly. *International Psychogeriatrics* 9: 207–212.

39 Lawal RA, Orija OB, Malomo IO, Ladapo HT, Oluwatayo OG (1997) Folie à deux: Report of two incidents. *East African Medical Journal* 74: 56–58.

40 Lerner V, Greenberg D, Bergman J (1996) Daughter-mother folie à deux: Immigration as a trigger for role reversal and the development of folie à deux. *Israel Journal of Psychiatry and Related Sciences* 33: 260–264.

41 Torch EM (1996) Shared obsessive-compulsive disorder in a married couple. *Journal of Clinical Psychiatry* 57: 489.

42 Aubry P (1894) *La contagion du muertre.* Paris, Alcan.

43 Moreau (de Tours) fils (1875) *De la Contagion du Suicide.* Paris, Parent.

44 Babinski (1886) *Recherches servant a établir que certaines manifestations hystériques peuvent être transférées d'un sujet à autre sujet sous l'influence de l'aimant.* Paris, Delahaye.

45 Grover S, Gupta N (2006) 25. Shared obsessive-compulsive disorder. *Psychopathology* 39: 99–101.

46 Mergui J, Jaworowski S, Greenberg D, Lerner V (2010) Shared obsessive-compulsive disorder: Broadening the concept of shared psychotic disorder. *Australian and New Zealand Journal of Psychiatry* 44: 859–862.

47 Locke J (1988/1690) *Two Treatises of Government*. Laslett P (ed.). Cambridge, Cambridge University Press.

48 Berrios GE, Marková IS (2003) The self in psychiatry. In Kircher T, David A (eds.) *The Self in Neuroscience and Psychiatry*. Cambridge, Cambridge University Press, pp. 9–39.

49 Madden RR (1857) *Phantasmata*. Vol. 1. London, Newby.

50 OED (2009) *Oxford English Dictionary*, 2nd ed. Oxford, Oxford University Press.

51 Tarde G (1890) *Les Lois de l'imitation*. Étude Sociologique. Paris, Alcan.

52 Nacquart J-B (1813) Contagion. In *Dictionaire des sciences médicales*. Vol. 6. Paris, Panckoucke, pp. 304–338.

53 Lucas P (1833) *De l'imitation contagieuse*. Paris, Didot le Jeune.

54 Mérat FV (1821) Sympathie. In *Dictionaire des sciences médicales*. Vol. 53. Paris, Panckoucke, pp. 537–624.

55 López Piñero JM (1983) *Historical Origins of the Concept of Neuroses*. Cambridge, Cambridge University Press.

56 Halliwell S (2002) *The Aesthetics of Mimesis: Ancient Texts and Modern Problems*. Princeton, Princeton University Press.

57 Auerbach E (1953) *Mimesis: The Representation of Reality in Western Literature*. Princeton: Princeton University Press.

58 Cross FL, Livingston EA (eds.) (1997) *Deification, The Oxford Dictionary of the Christian Church*. Oxford, Oxford University Press.

59 Kettlewell S (1877) *The Authorship of the de Imitatione Christi*. London, Rivingtons.

60 Burridge RA (2007) *Imitating Jesus: An Inclusive Approach to New Testament Ethics*. Grand Rapids, William B. Eerdmans Publishing Co.

61 Marquart K (2000) Luther and theosis. *Concordia Theological Quarterly* 64: 182–205.

62 Berthier P (1861) *De la Imitation*. Bourg, Millier-Bottier.

63 Baldwin JM (1894) Imitation: A chapter in the natural history of consciousness. *Mind* 3: 26–55.

64 Faris E (1926) The Concept of imitation. *American Journal of Sociology* 32: 367–378.

65 Di Pellegrino G, Fadiga L, Fogassi L, Gallese V, Rizzolatti G (1992) Understanding motor events: A neurophysiological study. *Experimental Brain Research* 91: 176–180.

66 Gallese V, Gernsbacher MA, Heyes C, Hickok G, Iacoboni M (2011) Mirror neuron forum. *Perspectives in Psychological Science* 6: 369–407.

67 Keysers C (2011) *The Empathic Brain*. New York, Social Brain Press.

68 Berrios GE (2011) Psychiatry and its objects. *Revista de Psiquiatria y Salud Mental (Barc.)* 4: 179–182.

69 Berrios GE, Marková IS (2002) Biological psychiatry: Conceptual issues. In D'Haenen H, den Boer JA, Willner P (eds.) *Biological Psychiatry*. New York, John Wiley & Sons, pp. 3–24.

70 Marková IS, Berrios GE (2012) Epistemology of mental symptoms. *Psychopathology* 45: 220–227.

CHAPTER 2

Paraphrenia

Richard Atkinson[1], David Jolley[2], and Alistair Burns[3]

[1] Consultant Old Age Psychiatrist, Lancashire Care NHS Foundation Trust, Preston, UK
[2] Honorary Reader in Psychiatry of Old Age, Personal Social Services Research Unit, University of Manchester, Manchester, UK
[3] Professor of Old Age Psychiatry, Vice Dean for the Faculty of Medical and Human Sciences, National Clinical Director for Dementia in England, University of Manchester, Manchester, UK

Introduction

The term *paraphrenia* was first introduced by Karl Kahlbaum in 1863 [1]. He referred to two types of paraphrenia: "Paraphrenia Hebetica," which was the insanity of adolescence, and "Paraphrenia Senilis," the insanity of the elderly. Kahlbaum did not use these terms to describe specific clinical entities but rather as a means of recognizing that particular mental disorders could arise at certain points in a person's life [2, 3]. Emil Kraepelin adopted the word *paraphrenia* in his *Textbook of Psychiatry* (published in 1913). He felt that disorders of emotions and volitions dominated the morbid state in dementia praecox (schizophrenia) due to the disintegration of the psychic personality and that paraphrenia was a separate disorder, which lacked this disturbance of emotion and volition [4]. Paraphrenia's journey through the subsequent century has led it to be discredited, adopted by later-life psychiatry, and then cast aside by international consensus. There still remains an argument for the validity of paraphrenia as a distinct diagnosis, lying somewhere on the paranoid spectrum between paranoia or delusional disorder and paranoid schizophrenia [5]. While modern treatments have meant that patients now receive antipsychotic medications that ameliorate the course of their illness, this also means that distinguishing between psychotic illnesses may have become more difficult. This is particularly true for the diagnosis of paraphrenia, which has, as one of its main distinguishing features, a lack of intellectual deterioration and degradation of personality. In itself that does not mean that functional, nonaffective psychotic illnesses should all be considered together under the title of schizophrenia. In this chapter the development of the concept of paraphrenia, since its inception, is outlined and it will be considered whether there is still validity for the diagnosis.

Kraepelin's paraphrenia

Kraepelin used Kahlbaum's term *paraphrenia* to identify a group of patients who had many similarities to people with dementia praecox but were differentiated because of "the far slighter development of the disorders of emotion and volition" and "the inner harmony of the psychic life is considerably less involved" [4, p. 283]. Kraepelin recognized that in paraphrenia, paranoid delusions were still a prominent feature along with hallucinations and that abnormalities in disposition were seen late in the illness as opposed to the early "dulness and indifference" [4, p. 283] that is seen as an early manifestation in dementia praecox. He also described how in paraphrenia behavioral abnormalities were understandable in terms of the person's delusional belief system rather than an independent disorder. Kraepelin felt that paraphrenia was a progressive illness that developed over time and caused significant morbidity.

Kraepelin described four subtypes of paraphrenia.

Paraphrenia Systemica: "the extremely insidious development of a continuously progressive delusion of persecution, to which are added later ideas of exaltation without the decay of personality" [4, p. 284].

Kraepelin believed this to be the most common subtype. He described the occurrence of persecutory delusions that developed from simple suspiciousness to complex delusional systems, which ultimately occupied the person's life totally. The person would go on to develop hallucinations, typically auditory in nature, and passivity phenomena. This group would then develop ideas of exaltation almost as a response to their negative paranoid delusions that were so dominant in their psyche. Apart from misinterpretations secondary to delusions, perception was never affected and patients remained fully orientated. Patients' moods could be described as anxious and depressed with suspiciousness and hostility later due to the ongoing negative delusional beliefs. Kraepelin described the course of this illness as being slowly progressive with only minimal fluctuations. The main differentiating factor from dementia praecox was the preservation of the psychic personality. Kraepelin found that 60 percent of patients in this group were male.

Paraphrenia Expansiva: "the development of exuberant megalomania with predominantly exalted mood and slight excitement" [4, p. 302].

Kraepelin felt that this subtype affected only women and the clinical picture was dominated by ideas and delusions of exaltation, often erotic, that involved the person being in an affair that was widely talked about in high circles or that people believed them to be saintly or close to God. There was invariably the presence of persecutory delusions; however, they did not dominate the clinical picture and hallucinations were common and were typically visual. Patients would commonly develop delusional memories. Mood was described as self-conscious cheerful and often irresponsible but with the potential for patients to fall into "violent excitement" [4, p. 306]. Again behavioral abnormalities were understandable in the context of the person's delusions.

Paraphrenia Confabulans: "distinguished by the dominant role of pseudo-memories" [4, p. 309].

This subtype only consisted of a small number of the patients Kraeplin studied and he felt that there was an equal sex distribution. Patients would have delusions of persecution along with delusions of grandeur; however, the prominent feature would be pseudo-memories and so for the patients everything would seem familiar.

Paraphrenia Phantastica: "luxuriant growth of highly extraordinary, disconnected, changing delusions" [4, p. 315].

In this subtype persecutory delusions are prominent. Patients develop auditory hallucinations and rarely visual hallucinations. They may also experience delusions of passivity and impairment of sensation, leading them to believe they are being tortured. The delusions would become ever more extraordinary and sudden in nature. In this subgroup, 60–70 percent of Kraepelin's cases were male.

Kraepelin was unable to comment on the heritability of paraphrenia; however, he did consider there to be evidence of abnormal premorbid personality traits in some patients. He also felt that this illness was due to internal causes rather than the predominant external causes of mental disorder at that time—alcohol and syphilis—and the majority of patients developed the illness between the ages of 25 and 50.

Kraepelin himself acknowledged that it was often difficult to delineate the paraphrenias that he observed from other, more accepted diagnoses. In particular he highlighted the similarities between paraphrenia confabulans and mania and paraphrenia phantastica and paranoid forms of dementia praecox. However, he maintained that his observations of these patients over many years (often over 10 years or more) indicated that there were subtle differences, particularly the preservation of emotion, volition, and intellect, that justified the separate description of these disorders.

A follow-up study of the 78 patients that Kraepelin had diagnosed as having paraphrenia cast doubt on the validity of paraphrenia as a diagnosis [6]. It was felt that only 28 of the original 78 patients still had a diagnosis of paraphrenia following 10 years of observation and 32 patients had progressed to dementia praecox. Other diagnoses were thought to be mainly affective or organic psychoses. The study also found little evidence that enabled differentiation between the subtypes proposed by Kraepelin [7] or that it was possible to differentiate between those who would go on to develop dementia praecox [8]. Mayer's findings that the majority of the patients, whom Kraepelin had identified as having paraphrenia, actually progressed to other identifiable psychiatric diagnoses and had a significant and understandably negative impact on the standing of paraphrenia within the psychiatric community. It is interesting to note, however, that a significant minority of the patients did retain a diagnosis of paraphrenia. Clearly there were some understandable reservations about Kraepelin's proposal particularly with regard to the validity of the four subtypes of paraphrenia and the delineation between paraphrenia and dementia praecox. However, what has not been satisfactorily reconciled in the literature is what should be done with the 36 percent of patients whose clinical condition seemed to retain the features of paraphrenia as proposed by Kraepelin.

The delineation between paraphrenia and dementia praecox at this time seemed questionable although Leonhard published his findings from a study of 530 people with chronic schizophrenia [9] and used the term paraphrenia to describe all paranoid schizophrenia, which was the prevailing wisdom in German psychiatry at the time [10]. Fish then related Leonhard's findings to his series of 111 female patients with chronic schizophrenia, with an age of onset of illness ranging from 14 to 56 years. He found that it was possible to use this classification system, which also included the diagnoses of catatonia and hebephrenia, to diagnose the patients in his study [10]. Whilst Fish did make use of the diagnosis of paraphrenia to describe a number of patients from his case series it could be concluded that in doing so he was simply using it as a proxy for paranoid schizophrenia. In doing this it would appear that Fish was in agreement with Mayer's theory that paraphrenia, as a distinct entity from dementia praecox, was not necessarily a valid diagnosis. More recently Leonhard's category of systematic paraphrenia was found to have only moderate validity and diagnostic stability in comparison to hebephrenia, schizophrenia and no mental illness [11]. Developments in research techniques may also lead to interesting work based on earlier studies. One area could be in molecular genetic research into subtypes of schizophrenia due to previous findings by Fish [12], that Leonhard's nonsystematic affect laden paraphrenia seemed to be the treatment sensitive subtype of schizophrenia [13].

Late paraphrenia

In a study of 150 elderly people admitted to Graylingwell Hospital in 1948, 12 patients were found to have schizophrenia. All of these patients developed the illness after the age of 60 and the description of these patients given by the authors was that their disorders were paraphrenic in nature. This was in reference to Kraepelin's description with symptoms of paraphrenic delusions occurring in "the setting of a well-preserved intellect and personality, were often 'primary' in character, and were usually associated with the passivity failings or other volitional disturbances and hallucinations in clear consciousness pathognomic of schizophrenia" [14]. In a later paper, Roth proposed the term *late paraphrenia* for the group of patients previously described as having schizophrenia. He defined late paraphrenia as being a disorder that consisted of "a well-organised system of paranoid delusions with or without auditory hallucinations in the setting of a well-preserved personality and affective response." Age of onset was thought to be after the age of 60 [15].

This idea of late paraphrenia seemed to resemble more closely Kahlbaum's descriptions of a schizophrenia-like illness that could be differentiated by the age of onset. Kraepelin's more comprehensive description of paraphrenia did not specify late age at onset but instead recognized that it could occur throughout adult life.

Kay and Roth recognized that there was a distinction between functional late paraphrenia and organic psychosis, with particular reference to the significantly higher mortality rate in the organic group. However, they did accept that there may be early or mild degrees of cerebral change in the group they designated as late paraphrenia. They studied a total of 99 patients and after consideration of environmental and hereditary factors they concluded that in their opinion late paraphrenia should be regarded as a manifestation of schizophrenia in old age. It therefore seems that Kay and Roth were aligned with the biggest critics of late paraphrenia [8, 16, 17].

An important addition to the discussion surrounding late paraphrenia was a study by Felix Post. He wrote that while there was general agreement that late-onset psychosis may fit into Kraepelin's group of paraphrenias, he did not feel that paraphrenia's reinstitution as late paraphrenia would help to further understanding in the field of schizophrenia in later life [18]. His study examined 93 people with psychosis in later life and he identified three groups of patients. Post felt that these three groups of paranoid patients lay on a continuum from schizophrenia through paranoid hallucinosis, with a schizophreniform group in between. Those in the paranoid hallucinosis group were seen to have usually auditory hallucinations that were understandable in terms of the older person's social situation and associated persecutory fears. The schizophreniform group had these symptoms in addition to more abnormal experiences and preoccupations, which would still be understandable in terms of the patient's cultural background. The schizophrenia group consisted of people who would be usually diagnosed as paranoid schizophrenia or paraphrenia. He cited difficulties in clearly differentiating between the three groups and so suggested that late schizophrenic illnesses could be viewed as a graduated expression of schizophrenia in later life. Another important finding from this study was to show that schizophrenic-like illnesses in later life did respond to treatment with phenothiazine medications.

Despite late paraphrenia suffering a similar fall from favor as the original Kraepelian concept of paraphrenia, the idea of late paraphrenia seemed to have been maintained within the consciousness of old-age psychiatrists, particularly in the UK. It was the subject of numerous studies, as opposed to paraphrenia, which has not retained a similar position in the research literature. In addition to the symptoms described above there has been general agreement that in patients identified as having late-life paraphrenia, there are common features that make the onset of psychosis in later life distinct. Risk factors that have been identified are female gender, sensory impairments, and social isolation [19]. Other notable findings have been the significant association between visual hallucinations and visual impairment but the lack of association between auditory hallucinations and deafness [20]. Almeida and colleagues conducted a comprehensive assessment of 47 patients with late paraphrenia. Their findings were consistent with previous studies with a preponderance of delusions and hallucinations with relatively uncommon incidences of thought disorder, cata-tonia and inappropriate affect [21]. Their sample also showed a preponderance of women, increased risk of hearing loss, and increased social isolation [22]. When they applied a series of diagnostic classification systems, which excluded late paraphrenia, to their group of patients there was some consistency with the diagnoses of schizophrenia, delusional disorder, and schizoaffective dis-order; however, they felt that there was sufficient disagreement between the systems to conclude that current classification systems are inadequate for the purposes of diagnosing late paraphrenia. Therefore, they felt that retaining the diagnosis of late paraphrenia was "still the best option" [21].

Central to the diagnosis of paraphrenia and subsequently late paraphrenia was the absence of changes in emotion and volition. A further assumption regarding late paraphrenia was that there should be an absence of significant organic cerebral change [15, 16]. Early studies found evidence of electroen-cephalographic changes in late paraphrenics [23]. The development of CT scanning as a means of brain imaging allowed further advances to be made. A series of studies comparing a group of patients with late paraphrenia and age-matched controls found that in paraphrenia there were neuropsycholog-ical deficits along with cerebral ventricular enlargement without cortical atrophy [24, 25]. A further study looking at 24 patients with late-life psy-chosis found that when compared to healthy controls there were more clinical abnormalities on magnetic resonance imaging and neuropsychological defi-cits were also evident [26]. As brain imaging technology advanced, more observations were brought forward and Rob Howard and his colleagues showed that the CT brain scans of 14 patients diagnosed with late paraphre-nia did not differ significantly from those of controls. However, they were able to show that people with late paraphrenia who had Schneiderian first-rank symptoms had greater cerebral atrophy than those who didn't [27]. It has also been shown that when late paraphrenia is separated from paranoia (based on Kraepelin's description where paranoia lacks hallucinations) there is a higher likelihood of incidental CT findings of cerebrovascular disease in paranoia, a finding that may further support the view that paraphrenia is a distinct entity [28]. While these findings may lead to questions about whether late-onset psychosis is a prodrome to dementia or occurs as a result of cerebrovascular disease, it would appear that it is very unlikely that late onset psychosis is a prodrome to Alzheimer's disease. However, it seems that the cortical tracts affected in early-onset schizophrenia are different from those that are implicated in late-onset schizophrenia like illnesses, which could explain the clinical differences between these groups [29].

When these findings are compared with studies of early-onset schizophrenia there seem to be sufficient differences to suggest that further studies in this area might be rewarding [30].

Late-onset schizophrenia and very-late-onset schizophrenia-like psychosis

A meeting of the International Late-Onset Schizophrenia group in 1998 produced a consensus report in order to address the uncertainty surrounding late paraphrenia and late-onset schizophrenia. They recognized two distinct illness classifications: late-onset schizophrenia (onset after the age of 40) and very-late-onset schizophrenia-like psychosis (onset after the age of 60). They concluded that schizophrenia-like illnesses not attributable to affective disorder or structural brain abnormality could arise at any time of life. There is an association with later age at onset for women and that formal thought disorder and affective blunting are less common when onset is over 60 years, whereas visual hallucinations are more common [19]. This consensus statement has seemed to bring together the opposing sides in the argument over late-life psychosis and has provided a platform from which research can proceed with clearly defined groups. It has also effectively ended the argument supporting the use of late paraphrenia. However, the issue of whether the diagnosis of paraphrenia, as a disorder occurring throughout adult life as originally described by Kraepelin, is still valid.

Paraphrenia revisited

The debate surrounding late paraphrenia does appear to have been resolved with an international consensus. There are still proponents of the separate idea that paraphrenia is a distinct entity from schizophrenia. It has been argued that the prevailing influence of the DSM and ICD classifications systems to subsume paraphrenia under schizophrenia is wrong and simply acts to worsen the overinclusiveness of schizophrenia as a diagnosis and to reduce research into paraphrenia [31].

In the previous edition of this book, Munro set out his proposal for the diagnostic criteria of paraphrenia, using a DSM-style format [5]. The criteria were then revised in a subsequent publication and are outlined below.

Diagnostic criteria for paraphrenia [31]

Diagnostic criteria for paraphrenia specify a delusional disorder of at least 6 months' duration characterized by the following:

1 Preoccupation with one or more semi-systematized delusions, often accompanied by auditory hallucinations. These delusions are not encapsulated from the rest of the personality as in delusional disorder.
2 Affect notably well preserved and appropriate. Even in acute phases, there is an ability to maintain rapport with the interviewer.
3 None of the following: intellectual deterioration, visual hallucinations, incoherence, flat or grossly inappropriate affect, or grossly disorganized behavior at times other than during the acute episode.
4 Disturbance of behavior is understandable in relation to the content of the delusions and hallucinations.
5 Only partially meets Criterion A for schizophrenia. No significant organic brain disorder.
Associated Features: The illness is associated with distress and agitation, and irrational behavior may appear as delusions become more vivid and judgment lessens. Patients may accuse others of persecution, complain to the authorities, or occasionally show aggression to imagined pursuers.
Age of Onset: Traditionally thought to be middle or old age, but this is unproven.
Course: A chronic illness, ameliorated but not cured by treatment.
Impairment: Intellectual functioning is unimpaired. Daily living, occupational activity, social functioning, and quality of marriage are likely to deteriorate during exacerbations.
Complications: Some paraphrenia cases appear to deteriorate to schizophrenia. In elderly patients, dementia may sometimes supervene.
Predisposing Factors: Deafness, social isolation, migrant status, and other severe stressors may play a part. It is possible, though evidence is uncertain, that premorbid paranoid and schizoid personality disorders occur more commonly with paraphrenia than by chance. Celibacy, lower-than-normal marital rates, and reduced fertility have been mentioned, possibly indicating abnormal personality traits.
Gender Ratio: Uncertain, but seems to become more common in females with advancing age.

Familial Pattern: There is a low frequency of schizophrenia in families of paraphrenia patients, suggesting that there is little or no genetic link between the two disorders.

Differential Diagnoses: Delusional disorder; schizophrenia, especially paranoid schizophrenia; major mood disorder with delusions; dementia; severe schizoid, schizotypal, or paranoid personality disorder; schizoaffective disorder; severe obsessive-compulsive disorder with near-bizarre features and rituals.

Treatment: It can be tentatively said that paraphrenia, like paranoid schizophrenia, responds to standard neuroleptic medications. Behavioral therapy may reduce the degree of delusional preoccupation, but psychotherapy is not of primary value.

Treatment Outcome: Clinical outcome is often satisfactory, with a surprisingly complete return to near-normal. However, treatment compliance is not always good, and relapse seems quite common. In older patients, age-related difficulties and adverse personality factors may make social rehabilitation more difficult than clinical improvement.

This description of paraphrenia was then applied to a case series of patients presenting to hospital with a psychotic illness. Over an 18-month period they identified 33 patients who met the criteria for paraphrenia. They concluded that their study provided evidence to support the theory that paraphrenia (as defined by Kraepelin but updated by Munro) is a recognizable diagnostic entity and that it is distinguishable from paranoia/delusional disorder and from paranoid schizophrenia [31]. There have been further attempts to identify cases of paraphrenia, using the criteria as proposed by Munro [32]. In order to provide greater validation of paraphrenia it seems that it might be helpful for others to conduct further studies using Munro's description of paraphrenia.

Discussion

The validity of paraphrenia as a diagnosis has been controversial for a century. Current psychiatric practice rarely affords the opportunity of observing the progression of untreated psychotic illnesses over many years, a profoundly positive change for people with psychosis and for the health professionals whose aim it is to alleviate suffering. In addition, antipsychotics do not have specific actions on different types of psychotic illnesses. Therefore, people are treated with "generic" antipsychotic medications, often before the full clinical picture is clear. This is likely to impair our ability to differentiate between subtle variations in psychosis and therefore it is easy to adopt the opinion that the diagnosis of schizophrenia is all encompassing. If psychiatric treatments were effective in 100 percent of cases and removed distressing symptoms for everyone, this position might be defensible. However, where heterogeneity exists it is important first to review the diagnosis. Thirty-six percent of Kraepelin's patients with paraphrenia still had a diagnosis consistent with paraphrenia after 10 years and more recent studies have shown that paraphrenia can be recognized as a distinct illness. It seems that research into paraphrenia has been limited, first by the findings of Mayer and the subsequent interpretation of his work, and then by the hijacking of the term *paraphrenia* for the description of late-life psychosis, and finally by the omission of paraphrenia from prominent classification systems. In the art of medicine, diagnosis allows us to advise about many things, particularly treatment and prognosis. The comparative lack of research into paraphrenia means that the opportunity for this is limited. If nothing else, then greater recognition of paraphrenia should lead to more interest, greater research, and thus greater understanding of the spectrum of paranoid disorders.

References

1 Kahlbaum K, 1863, Die Gruppirung der Psychischen Krankheiten. Kafemann, Danzig.
2 Casanova M, Stevens J, Brown R, Royston C, Bruton C, 2002, Disentangling the pathology of schizophrenia and paraphrenia. Acta Neuropathol, 1003: 313–320.
3 McKenna P, 2007, Schizophrenia and Related Syndromes. 2nd edition, Routledge, New York.
4 Kraepelin E, 1919, Dementia Praecox and Paraphrenia. Translated by Barclay M; edited by Robertson G. Robert Krieger, New York, 1971.
5 Munro A, 1997, Paraphrenia, in: Bhugra D, Munro A, editors. Troublesome disguises: Underdiagnosed psychiatric syndromes. Blackwell Science, Oxford, 91–111.
6 Mayer, 1921 in Sato A and Ihda S, 2002, Paraphrenia and Late Paraphrenia. Psychogeriatrics, 2: 20–25.
7 Mayer, 1921 in Casanova M, 2010, The pathology of paraphrenia. Curr Psychiatry Rep, 12: 196–201.
8 Mayer, 1921 in Fish F, 1960, Senile schizophrenia. J Men Sci, 106: 938–946.
9 Leonhard, 1936 in Fish F, 1958, Leonhard's classification of schizophrenia, J Men Sci, 104: 943–971.
10 Fish F, 1958, Leonhard's classification of schizophrenia. J Men Sci, 104: 943.
11 Petho B, Tolna J, Tusnády G, Farkas M, Vizkeleti G, Vargha A, Czobor P, 2008, The predictive validity of the Leonhardean classification of endogenous psychoses: A 21–33-year follow-up of a prospective study ("BUDAPEST 2000"). Eur Arch Psychiatry Clin Neurosci, 258: 324–334.
12 Fish F, 1964, The influence of the tranquilizers on the Leonhard schizophrenic syndromes. Encephale, 53(suppl): 245–249.
13 Ban T, 2004, Neuropsychopharmacology and the genetics of schizophrenia: A history of the diagnosis of schizophrenia. Prog Neuropsychopharmacol Biol Psychiatry, 28: 753–762.
14 Roth M, Morrissey J, 1952, Problems in the diagnosis and classification of mental disorder in old age; with a study of case material. J Ment Sci, 98: 66–80.

15 Roth M, 1955, The natural history of mental disorder in old age. J Ment Sci, 101: 281–301.

16 Kay D, Roth M, 1961, Environmental and hereditary factors in the schizophrenias of age ("late paraphrenia") and their bearing on the general problem of causation in schizophrenia. J Ment Sci, 107: 649–686.

17 Holden N, 1987, Late paraphrenia or the paraphrenias? A descriptive study with a 10-year follow-up. Brit J Psychiat, 150: 635–639.

18 Post F, 1966, Persistent Persecutory States of the Elderly. Pergamon Press, Oxford.

19 Howard R, Rabins P, Seeman M, Jeste D, the International Late-Onset Schizophrenia Group, 2000, Late-onset schizophrenia and very-late-onset schizophrenia-like psychosis: An international consensus. Am J Psychiatry, 157: 172–178.

20 Howard R, Almeida O, Levy R, 1994, Phenomenology, demography and diagnosis in late paraphrenia. Psychol Med, 24: 397–410.

21 Almeida O, Howard R, Levy R, David A, 1995 (a), Psychotic states arising in late life (late paraphrenia): Psychopathology and nosology. Brit J Psychiat, 166: 205–214.

22 Almeida O, Howard R, Levy R, David A, 1995 (b), Psychotic states arising in late life (late paraphrenia): The role of risk factors. Brit J Psychiat, 166: 215–228.

23 Herbert M, Jacobson S, 1967, Late paraphrenia. Brit J Psychiat, 113: 461–469.

24 Naguib M, Levy R, 1987, Late paraphrenia: Neuropsychological impairment and structural brain abnormalities on computed tomography. Int J Geriatr Psychiatry, 2: 83–90.

25 Burns A, Carrick J, Ames D, Naguib M, Levy R, 1989, The cerebral cortical appearance in late paraphrenia. Int J Geriatr Psychiatry, 4: 31–34.

26 Miller B, Lesser I, Boone K, Hill E, Mehringer M, Wong K, 1991, Brain lesions and cognitive function in late-life psychosis. Brit J Psychiat, 158: 76–82.

27 Howard R, Forstl H, Almeida O, Burns A, Levy R, 1992, Computer-assisted CT measurements in late paraphrenics with and without Schneiderian first-rank symptoms: A preliminary report. Int J Geriatr Psychiatry, 7: 35–38.

28 Flint A, Rifa S, Eastwood M, 1991, Late-onset paranoia: Distinct from paraphrenia. Int J Geriatr Psychiatry, 6: 103–109.

29 Lagodka A, Robert P, 2009, Is late-onset schizophrenia related to neurodegenerative processes? A review of literature. Encephale, 35: 386–393.

30 Almeida, O, Howard R, Forstl H, Levy R, 1992, Should the diagnosis of late paraphrenia be abandoned? Psychol Med, 22: 11–14.

31 Ravindran A, Yatham L, Munro A, 1999, Paraphrenia redefined. Can J Psychiatry, 44: 133–137.

32 Pelizza L, Bonazzi F, 2010, What's happened to paraphrenia? A case-report and review of the literature. Acta Biomed, 81: 130–140.

CHAPTER 3

Brief reactive psychoses

Jüergen Zielasek and Wolfgang Gaebel

Department of Psychiatry and Psychotherapy, Medical Faculty, Heinrich Heine University, LVR-Clinics Düsseldorf, Düsseldorf, Germany

Introduction

"Brief Reactive Psychoses" is a designation for a group of transient psychotic disorders occurring after stressful events [1, 2]. Some issues of terminology and conceptualization arise: Different designations have been used over time to describe a transient psychotic state following a stressful event. Jauch and Carpenter [1] provided a succinct summary by describing "reactive psychosis" by its relation to a precipitating stressor, by the briefness in duration of the episode, by the absence of chronicity, and by a return to the previous level of functioning. This summary was derived from previous concepts developed by Jaspers on the reactive psychoses, which were characterized by rapid onset, full return to normal once the stressor was removed, and psychotic thoughts comprehensibly related to the nature of the stressor [3]. Other examples are Magnan's "bouffée delirante," Leonhardt's "cycloid psychosis," and Wimmer's "psychogenic psychosis," the latter basically reflecting Jaspers's criteria [4] but also containing 33 percent schizophrenia cases [5]. The concept of a brief reactive psychosis had become increasingly used in Scandinavian countries in the second half of the last century and was also used to describe what are now considered culture-bound psychotic states precipitated by external events like "yak," "latah," "koro," and others. In the Scandinavian tradition, it was important that the psychotic reaction bore a relation to acute mental trauma, that the content of the delusion reflected the traumatic experience, that the course was benign and that termination of the psychosis was expected upon "liquidation of the traumatic experience" [6]. Thus, Jaspers's central features of reactive psychoses can be found in the Scandinavian conceptualization. Only the elements of the brief duration and of the immediate temporal relationship of the trauma and the psychotic reaction were retained in later international definitions. Faergeman's monograph published in 1963 was the first English publication on this topic [5] and McCabe's monograph [7] was the first

Troublesome Disguises: Managing Challenging Disorders in Psychiatry, Second Edition.
Edited by Dinesh Bhugra and Gin S. Malhi.
© 2015 John Wiley & Sons, Ltd. Published 2015 by John Wiley & Sons, Ltd.

detailed investigation of 40 cases, which—in 90 percent—fulfilled Jaspers's criteria. The latter study, for example, showed that Jaspers's criterion of a comprehensible relation of the psychotic contents to the traumatic event could be ascertained in 33 of the 40 cases. Only 12.5 percent of cases showed Schneiderian first-rank symptoms of schizophrenia. "Brief Reactive Psychoses" were first incorporated in the American Diagnostic and Statistical Manual in its second edition (DSM-II) in 1968, but no explicit diagnostic criteria were given. With DSM-III in 1980, a list of six criteria was introduced (described in detail in the section on "Diagnosis" in this chapter). This disorder was not included by this name in the various versions of the International Classification of Disorders (ICD) published by the World Health Organization (WHO). In ICD-10, the clinical picture of "brief reactive psychosis" can be classified under a different name (i.e., "acute and transient psychotic disorder," or ATPD), but ATPD is a group of disorders among which the reactive psychoses only are a part. Therefore, ATPD (ICD-10) is not identical with the "brief psychotic disorder" (DSM-5), and neither ATPD nor "brief psychotic disorder" are identical with "brief reactive psychosis." A brief overview of the history of the concept of "brief reactive psychoses" is given in Table 3.1 and a recent summary of the historic and conceptual issues can be found in a doctoral thesis by Krstev [8].

Table 3.1 History of the concept of brief reactive psychosis and classification of brief reactive psychoses.

Time	Feature
Late 19th-early 20th century	Concepts of acute and transient, in some concepts also reactive psychoses developed Examples: Magnan's "bouffée delirante" Wimmer's "psychogenic psychosis" Leonhardt's "cycloid psychosis"
1967	ICD-8 includes "reactive psychosis"
1968	DSM-II mentions "brief reactive psychosis"
1980	DSM-III lists explicit diagnostic criteria for "brief reactive psychoses" ICD-9 moves "reactive psychosis" into the chapter "other non-organic psychoses"
1990	DSM-IV puts reactive and non-reactive psychoses into one common category ("brief psychotic disorder") and adds a specifier for the presence of "marked stressor(s)"
1992	ICD-10 introduces "acute and transient psychotic disorders" including a specifier "with or without associated acute stress"
2013	DSM-5 retains the concept of "brief reactive psychosis" with or without marked stressor(s), and adds a catatonia and a severity specifier ICD-11: suggestion to retain the diagnostic principles of ATPD, but to move the ATPD subtypes into different chapters to better differentiate between prototypical ATPD, brief schizophrenia-like psychoses, and brief purely delusional disorders

Given the different conceptualizations of "brief reactive psychoses" over time and in the different classification systems, a central issue is which clinical characteristics should be used to characterize brief reactive psychoses, what is known about their prevalence, and whether there are treatment guidelines that may be followed. Finally, open questions for future research need to be identified. This review will therefore focus on the following questions: (1) classification; (2) epidemiology; (3) treatment; (4) open questions for future research.

Classification

DSM

DSM-III was the first and only classification system for mental disorders to explicitly operationalize "brief psychotic disorder" (diagnosis code 298.80 [9]). The definition included the sudden onset of a psychotic disorder of at least a few hours' duration, with a maximum duration of 2 weeks. The psychotic symptoms had to follow "immediately" a recognizable psychosocial stressor "that would evoke significant symptoms of stress in almost everyone." The loss of a loved one or the psychological trauma of combat were mentioned as examples of such stressors. According to DSM-III, invariably emotional turmoil ensues. Characteristic symptoms of psychosis were incoherence or loosening of associations, delusions, hallucinations, and behavior that was grossly disorganized or catatonic. Thus, "psychotic" was used in DSM-III not in Jaspers's wider sense, but in a more narrow sense. DSM-III adds other associated features, including perplexity, a feeling of confusion, bizarre behavior, suicidality, and aggressiveness. Disturbances of affect and speech are also listed. Hallucinations and delusions were described as transient. Disorientation and memory impairment were considered to occur often. A return to the premorbid level of functioning would "usually" occur within a day or two. A maximum disease duration of 2 weeks was the upper limit. Of note, one of Jaspers's original criteria, namely that the psychotic state must resolve quickly once the stressor was removed, was not included, but a maximum duration time criterion was introduced [2]. As exclusion criteria, DSM-III mentions that no period of increasing psychopathology may have preceded the psychosocial stressor and no organic mental disorder, manic episode, or factitious disorder with psychological symptoms may have been present. DSM-III-R introduced several changes, including that the maximum duration was prolonged to 1 month, the prodrome exclusion was specified as "the prodromal symptoms of schizophrenia," overwhelming perplexity or confusion could substitute for a lack of emotional turmoil, schizotypal personality disorder and a psychotic mood disorder had to be excluded [1].

DSM-IV/DSM-IV-TR [10] added those brief psychotic disorders occurring without stressors (i.e., non-reactive brief psychotic disorders) into the diagnosis code 298.80, which had been used for the "brief reactive psychosis" in DSM-III, so that this code in DSM-IV was renamed "brief psychotic disorder" and included all brief psychotic disorders, that is, those with or without marked stressor(s). DSM-IV-TR explicitly states that the brief psychotic disorder with marked stressor(s) had been called "brief reactive psychosis" in DSM-III. The precipitating event was defined in DSM-IV-TR as "one or more events that, singly or together, would be markedly stressful to almost anyone in similar circumstances in that person's culture." Disease duration was at least 1 day and not more than 1 month. Similarly to DSM-III, confusion and emotional turmoil are mentioned as associated features. Thus, compared to DSM-III, DSM-IV still included the "brief reactive psychotic disorders," but not anymore as a separate mental disorder, and confirmed the longer duration criterion introduced in DSM-III-TR (1 month instead of 2 weeks). This may reflect the tendency of DSM-IV to deemphasize the putative causality of stressors for mental disorders. The reasons for the increase of the duration of symptoms are unclear.

In DSM-5, a brief reactive psychosis was again not included as a unique mental disorder. However, DSM-5 retained the category of "Brief Psychotic Disorder" (298.8) [11], which still includes the specifier "with or without marked stressor(s)." Thus, a brief reactive psychosis would be classified as a "Brief Psychotic Disorder with marked stressor(s)." The key features are the sudden onset (i.e., within 2 weeks and usually without a phase of prodromal symptoms) of positive psychotic symptoms (i.e., delusions, hallucinations, disorganized speech, or grossly disorganized or catatonic behavior). In DSM-5, these symptoms must last at least 1 day, but not longer than 1 month. Eventually, there is a full return to the premorbid level of functioning within 1 month. Culturally sanctioned responses are excluded. The most striking difference compared to DSM-IV-TR is the introduction of a catatonia specifier and of a severity specifier, but this is a general new feature of the psychotic disorders in DSM-5 and does not particularly pertain to the brief psychotic disorders.

ICD

The World Health Organization International Classification of Disorders (ICD) has a section on mental disorders, but currently does not contain a "brief reactive psychotic disorder." Based upon requests from Scandinavia [12], the eighth edition (ICD-8) was the first to incorporate reactive psychosis as part of the nomenclature, and ICD-9 moved it into the category "other non-organic psychoses." ICD-10 moved this disorder into the chapter of "acute and transient psychotic disorders" (ATPD) together with the other (nonreactive) acute and transient psychotic disorders (F23 [13]). ATPD is characterized by an acute onset (within 2 weeks) of a "polymorphic" (i.e., rapidly changing and variable) acutely psychotic state. A psychotic state is defined as "the presence of hallucinations, delusions, or a limited number of severe abnormalities of behavior, such as gross excitement and overactivity, marked psychomotor retardation, and catatonic behavior" (ICD-10, p. 3–4 [13]). "Associated acute stress" may be specified, but ICD-10 states that this condition may arise without associated stress. A stress-association requires that first psychotic symptoms occur within 2 weeks of one or more events that would be regarded stressful to most people in similar circumstances. ICD-10 mentions bereavement, unexpected loss of partner or job, marriage, or the psychological trauma of combat, terrorism, or torture. In ICD-10, complete recovery is expected to be reached within 2–3 months, but ICD-10 acknowledges that there may be cases with persistent symptoms. Six separate psychotic disorders belong to this chapter:

F23.0 Acute polymorphic psychotic disorder without symptoms of schizophrenia
F23.1 Acute polymorphic psychotic disorder with symptoms of schizophrenia
F23.2 Acute schizophrenia-like psychotic disorder
F23.3 Other acute predominantly delusional psychotic disorders
F23.8 Other acute and transient psychotic disorders
F23.9 Acute and transient psychotic disorder, unspecified

Evaluating the index episode in ATPD patients, Marneros and coworkers [14] found delusions in 98 percent of all cases and hallucinations in 76 percent. Disturbances of drive and psychomotor disturbances were present in 86 percent, depressed mood in 74 percent, and maniform symptoms in 76 percent. Anxiety was found in 76 percent. Very characteristic was a fluctuating symptomatology, with rapidly changing delusions in 48 percent and rapidly changing mood in 69 percent. Of note, suicidality occurred in 36 percent during the acute episode [15] and is still the leading cause of excess mortality in acute and transient psychotic disorders besides cardiovascular diseases [16, 17]. In post-hoc analyses, only minor differences of the psychopathological features could be differentiated in the various ATPD disorders and as compared to other psychotic disorders, but the clinical characteristics best differentiating ATPD from schizophrenia were rapidly changing delusional topics, rapidly changing mood, and anxiety [14].

In ICD-10, a fifth character is used to indicate the presence or not of acute stress:

F23.x0 Without associated acute stress
F23.x1 With associated acute stress

Thus, ATPD is a group of disorders and the brief reactive psychotic disorders may be subsumed in this group. Category F23.x1 in ICD-10 would correspond to a "brief reactive psychotic disorder" of DSM-5, except for the different maximum duration criteria.

ICD-10 is currently under revision and for ATPD the essential clinical features of acute onset, polymorphic and temporally variable clinical presentation, and short duration, will be retained. However, in order to better reflect a distinction between schizophrenic and purely delusional clinical types of these disorders, the original ICD-10 F23 categories will probably be reorganized: ICD-10 F23.0 "Acute polymorphic psychotic disorder without symptoms of schizophrenia" was chosen as the basis of the clinical guideline for 05 B 02 ATPD with a duration of up to 3 months, as it best reflects the polymorphic and varying clinical presentation typical of ATPD. The delusional subtype (F23.3) will be moved into the revised category 05 B 04 Delusional Disorder and the schizophrenic subtypes (F23.1 and F23.2) into 05 B 05 Other primary psychotic disorders [18] (Figure 3.1).

In ICD-10, the subtypes F23.1 and F23.2 are mainly acute cases of schizophrenia without the necessary duration yet, because symptoms need to have an acute onset and to meet the diagnostic criteria of schizophrenia (F20.x) during the majority of the time since the establishment of an obviously psychotic clinical picture. These "schizophrenia ATPD" categories probably were the "unstable" ones among the ATPD subtypes due to their programmed reclassification as "schizophrenia" during follow-up once the duration criterion for schizophrenia of 4 weeks was met. This category may also explain why "schizophrenia" was the diagnostic category into which "unstable" ATPD cases most often fell upon long-term follow up. However, schizophrenia—in contrast to ATPD—is not typically characterized by rapid fluctuations of

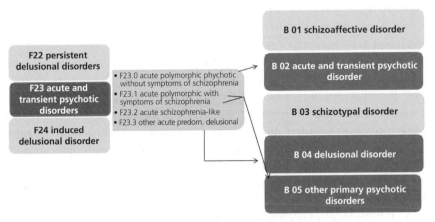

Figure 3.1 Proposal for the revision of the classification of acute and transient psychotic disorders in ICD-11 [18]. The proposal mainly suggests subdividing the ICD-10 group of "acute and transient psychotic disorders" into a group of polymorphic brief psychotic disorders with symptoms of schizophrenia (ICD-11 B05), with primary delusional symptoms (ICD-11 B04) and in those without symptoms of schizophrenia (ICD-11 B02).

psychotic or mood symptoms, and polymorphic clinical presentations are also not typical for schizophrenia. Thus, it seems warranted to place diagnostically unclear cases of "schizophrenia not yet having reached the necessary duration criterion" under "other primary psychotic disorders," and not under ATPD, until the necessary length of observation has been reached. This would also reflect the clinical observation that a psychopathological differentiation of ATPD from schizophrenia in the early course of the disease is feasible, especially regarding the rapid clinical fluctuations so characteristic of ATPD, which do not occur in schizophrenia. In ICD-10, classifying patients with schizophrenia symptoms as a subtype of ATPD falsely suggested that this was a temporally limited mental disorder and may have falsely contributed to the "diagnostic instability" of ATPD.

The advantage of this proposal is that transient predominantly delusional psychoses can be classified among their parent category, and that only the typical non-schizophrenic, non-purely delusional core ATPD phenotype characterizes the future diagnostic group of "acute and transient psychotic disorders." Essential diagnostic elements like acute onset, polymorphic clinical presentation and full remission within several months will be retained.

Taken together, "brief reactive psychosis" as a mental disorder can be found in both major international classification systems of mental disorders, but nowadays only as a subtype of broader categories of both reactive and non-reactive brief/transient psychotic disorders. Common features are an acute onset within 2 weeks, a polymorphic and temporally variable clinical picture [14], and full recovery within several weeks. Differences are the maximum duration criterion (1 month in DSM-5 vs. 2–3 months in ICD-10). Only few studies have addressed whether these similar clinical conceptualizations lead to a concordance of diagnoses in clinical practice. Comparing ICD-9, ICD-10, DSM-III-R and DSM-IV criteria, Pitta and Blay [19] found that the number of patients in the different categories was highly different, and that the results of the different classification systems in relationship to the original concept as laid down in ICD-9 was limited. The published tables show that there was apparently a good agreement between the classification systems for the brief reactive psychoses, but the interpretation of these results was limited by the fact that it was not shown whether these diagnostic agreements were in identical patients. A clearer result was presented in a study by Pillmann and coworkers [20] comparing ICD-10 ATPD with DSM-IV brief psychotic disorder. This study showed that 62 percent of those who fulfilled the ATPD criteria also fulfilled the DSM-IV criteria of brief psychotic disorder, but 31 percent of "brief reactive psychosis" patients had a schizophreniform disorder. Patients with DSM-IV "brief reactive psychosis" had a shorter duration of the illness episode and more acute onset compared to those ATPD patients who did not meet DSM-IV criteria of brief reactive psychosis. The ICD-8 diagnosis of a brief reactive psychosis was compared in Denmark with ICD-10 ATPD and showed little continuity. It conformed more to the acute delusional ATPD subtype and associated stress was recorded only in a minority of ATPD cases (5.3 percent) [21]. These studies indicate that although the basic concepts and criteria between the classification systems are quite similar, different patient groups may be subsumed longitudinally and transsectionally under the various designations, and that the DSM-IV time duration criterion may be too narrow. Patients with acute psychotic disorders and a good prognosis are not completely covered by the DSM-IV criteria for brief reactive psychosis. As the DSM-IV-criteria are basically the same as in DSM-5, this conclusion is probably also valid for DSM-5.

In order to achieve a reasonably certain diagnosis, the plan of action in cases of suspected brief reactive psychoses should be to evaluate the actual clinical picture and the history of the patient thoroughly regarding the following key aspects:

- Polymorphic, temporally variable clinical picture of hallucinations, delusions, disordered thinking and emotional upset
- Acute onset within a short time frame (i.e., at most several days), following the exposure to an extremely severe stressor, and rapid progression to a full psychotic clinical picture within a few days
- Exclusion of other mental disorders, somatic disorders or substance-related conditions

While this information may be readily available transsectionally after the psychotic picture has started, further observation may be necessary to clarify that the fourth essential criterion—rapid and full remission within 2–3 months—can be ascertained. More problematic is if a patient is first seen during the acute initial phase, when it is unclear whether complete remission will occur. Such equivocal cases should be coded as an unspecified psychotic disorder until further follow-up clarifies the course characteristics.

Epidemiology

A central problem for epidemiological studies is that persons with "brief reactive psychoses" may be classified in different mental disorders, especially in times when ICD-8, ICD-9 or DSM-III were used [4], but also still today given the differences between brief reactive psychosis in DSM-5 and ATPD in ICD-10. Modern studies using ATPD as the core diagnostic feature include a majority of patients without marked stressors or with schizophrenia and may therefore not be applicable to "brief reactive psychoses." However, comparing these populations may at least indicate the range of expected epidemiological findings.

Older epidemiological studies showed large variations in the prevalence of reactive psychosis: it was diagnosed in 1.6–11 percent of all psychiatric first admissions (reviewed by Jauch and Carpenter [1]). Reactive psychoses mainly occur in adulthood and the average age of onset was in the range of 30–39 years. Using the specific and restrictive diagnostic criteria of DSM-III, a field study of 11,589 mental disorder patients found "brief reactive psychosis" in only 0.3 percent of all cases [2]. Among the brief psychotic disorders, stressors could be identified in 39–72 percent of cases [2]. In a study on 15–60 years old first onset non-affective psychosis patients hospitalized in England, 20 (9 percent) of the 221 psychoses were brief psychoses (defined in the study as full remission within 6 months; i.e., not strictly following the restrictive duration criterion of DSM-III-R or ICD-10) and only seven (3 percent) were acute brief psychoses (i.e., onset within 2 weeks following the ICD-10 criteria [22]). In a critique of the duration criterion, Jauch and Carpenter [2] reviewed the available studies and found that only approximately 35 percent of all original "brief reactive psychosis" patients would fulfill this restrictive duration criterion.

Krstev [8] studied first-onset psychosis cases (age range 16–30 years) of whom 30 percent were considered "reactive psychosis." There was a quicker recovery in reactive psychosis, but stressors were mainly identified many months before the onset of symptoms and the onset of psychosis was rather slow (over weeks and months). Also, follow-up indicated that "reactive" cases had similar psychotic symptomatology after 9 months and 15 months, leaving open the question whether brief reactive psychosis in this young adult group was a distinct syndrome or a less severe initial stage of an incipient chronic psychosis.

For ATPD, hospital register studies showed that 5–20 percent of all patients from the ICD-10 group F2 (schizophrenia, schizotypal and delusional disorders) were classified as ATPD [23]. In an intake cohort sample from England investigating non-hospitalized patients with a first contact with the mental health system due to a psychotic disorder, the rate of persons with ATPD was higher in the outpatient setting as compared to the previous studies in inpatients (19 percent in out-patients (32 of 168 persons [24]) vs. 9 percent in inpatients [25]). This indicates that persons with ATPD may often not be in contact with inpatient services. The study showed that acute onset and early remission did not predict favorable outcome over 3 years of follow-up, and that the outcome was better than in schizophrenia. Another studied used data from patients in 13 countries with any first contact with the medical system due to a non-affective remitting psychotic disorder initially diagnosed as schizophrenia (World Health Determinants of Outcome Study [22]). The annual incidence rate was higher in women (0.140 per 10,000) than men (0.040 per 10,000) and about 10-fold higher in developing as compared to developed countries (0.878 per 10,000 women and 0.486 per 10,000 men). In a Danish case registry study of psychiatric inpatient admissions and outpatient contacts, the incidence of ATPD was 0.96 cases per 10,000 population, but the preponderance in women was low (0.98 cases per 10,000 women vs. 0.94 cases per 10,000 men [26]). The mean age was higher for women (46.2 years) than men (37.8 years). Interestingly, the readmission rate to hospital treatment was 83 percent and the stability rate of the initial ATPD diagnosis was low (39 percent), with schizophrenia as the most frequent new diagnosis upon readmission. This is in agreement with older studies (reviewed by Jauch and Carpenter [1]). Other studies in ATPD found that the relapse rate was 79 percent after a first episode, and this was as high as in schizophrenia [27]. The relapses occurred mostly within 1–2 years after the initial episode. About 30 percent of ATPD patients had long-lasting, stable remissions with good functioning over at least 2 years [27]. Similar results were obtained when DSM-IV criteria for "brief psychotic disorder" were applied [28]: about two-thirds of patients with schizophrenia or brief psychotic disorder had relapses approximately 1–2 years following the index episode, and psychosocial outcomes were more favorable in brief psychotic disorders than in schizophrenia. Long-term observations showed that while general functioning declined in patients with schizophrenia, this was not the case in patients with ATPD. "Diagnostic stability" of ATPD was high, in that among relapsing patients with ATPD, most had another episode of ATPD (approximately two-thirds of all patients with relapses), one-third had an affective episode, and only a minority had schizoaffective episodes (13.8 percent) or schizophrenia (6.9 percent) [29]. As a rule, diagnostic stability increased with repeated admissions, and lower relapse rates were reported from developing as compared to more developed countries (see note 26 for a discussion of this topic). Disease duration is similar in developed and developing countries (modal duration of 2–4 months, indicating that the longer ICD-10-criterion for duration may be more appropriate than the shorter DSM-5 criterion [30]). Considering regional or life-event-associated variations, in a literature review on Asian ATPD cases, a high degree of diagnostic instability over time was shown [31]. Migrant populations have a higher incidence compared to non-migrant populations, shown, for example, for ATPD for Asian foreign domestic workers [31], but there are only few studies and these are limited by methodological problems and a lumping together of ATPD and other brief psychotic disorders into unspecific categories like "other non-affective psychotic disorders," so that associations of course and outcome of specific psychotic disorders with ethnicity, urbanicity, or other factors are not well established [32]. Taken together, the epidemiological data show brief reactive psychosis to be a rare mental disorder following DSM-criteria, but a more frequent mental disorder following ICD-criteria probably due to a too restrictive duration criterion in

DSM. There is an age-related gender distribution, with women dominating at a higher age and men at a younger age. There are indications that the incidence is higher in developing countries and persons with a migration background.

Treatment

We could not find studies or recommendations explicitly addressing the treatment of ATPD or brief reactive psychoses. Reviewing the literature and searching treatment guidelines for non-schizophrenic psychotic disorders, Jäger and coworkers [23] found neither controlled clinical trials nor explicit guideline treatment recommendations for ATPD or brief reactive psychoses. Usually, symptomatic treatment with antipsychotic drugs in brief reactive psychoses and ATPD will be initiated, but no guidance can be derived from literature evidence regarding the best choice of drug, expected response rates or the necessary duration of treatment. Another unsolved question is how to predict and prevent relapses. There are no clinical, demographic or genetic studies which may help to identify those ATPD patients with increased rates of relapses, in whom—given the epidemiological disease course data—preventive administration of antipsychotic drugs would be warranted. Studies are lacking showing the efficacy of preventive administration of antipsychotic medication in persons following the remission of a brief reactive psychosis.

Open questions for future research

The main open questions are related to the pathophysiology of brief reactive psychoses, because understanding the pathophysiology may lead to novel diagnostic, preventive or therapeutic approaches. The main open questions are: (1) why do some individuals experience acute and brief psychotic reactions following acute and severe stress, while others do not show such reactions under identical circumstances? and (2) what is the role of trauma in the pathogenesis of psychotic disorder in general, and how would this be applicable to the brief reactive psychoses?

Individual factors related to the development of brief reactive psychoses

There are no known clinical, demographic, neuroimaging, or genetic markers that may aid in the prediction of the development of brief reactive psychoses in persons exposed to extreme stressors, or in the prediction and prevention of relapses. There are no known preventive measures against brief reactive psychoses except the avoidance of extremely stressful life events. A Danish register study indicates that the occurrence of ATPD is modestly associated with other mental disorders in family members of the person with ATPD [33]. Jauch and Carpenter [1] reviewed family studies in reactive psychosis probands and found increased rates of reactive psychosis in psychotic family members of these probands and a 14 percent concordance for reactive psychosis in monozygotic twins. However, case numbers were small and no individual prediction is possible on the basis of such findings. Studies are lacking regarding specific sociodemographic or neurobiological/genetic factors associated with increased rates of psychotic reactions following extreme stress.

The role of trauma in the pathogenesis of psychotic disorders

Figure 3.2 shows the principal associations between an acute psychotic disorder and precipitating stressful life events. A recent review on life events and psychosis came to the conclusion that there was some evidence that the exposure to adult adverse life events was associated with an increased risk of psychosis and "subclinical psychotic experiences." However, the methodological quality of studies was considered low, precluding firm conclusions [34]. For the purpose of this review, it seems appropriate to distinguish between the immediate

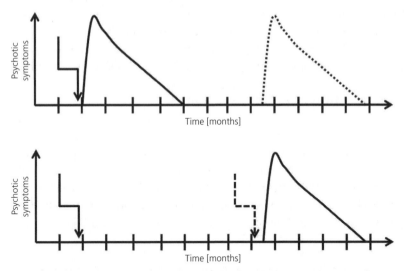

Figure 3.2 Temporal relationship between traumatic life events and psychotic disorders. Arrows indicate the occurrence of a catastrophic stressor. In the upper panel, psychotic symptoms occur immediately and with a rapid progression to a full psychotic clinical picture within a very short time (at most several days). Symptoms subside over weeks or months and full recovery is attained. Relapses (usually without a second stressor) may occur (indicated by the dotted line). In the lower panel, a traumatic event has no immediate temporal relationship with the psychotic symptoms, but may raise the susceptibility to subsequent stressors, which may not even reach the intensity of the first stressor (second stressor indicated by the dotted arrow).

consequences of trauma for the pathogenesis of psychotic disorders, and delayed effects. The *acute* reaction toward severe traumatic events mainly involves the sympathetic nervous systems and the hypothalamus-pituitary-adrenal gland system. While there is no known direct psychotogenic effect of sympathetic nervous system activation, excess production of cortisol may have immediate psychotogenic effects, probably mediated via the upregulation of dopamine production [35]. This may explain the time lag of several days or weeks between an exposure to acute stressors and the acute psychotic reaction. Termination of the acute stress exposure may lead to a down regulation of this neurohormonal psychotogenic response. A major methodological issue is that previous experimental clinical work in this area has been performed in patients with schizophrenia or at ultra-high risk for psychosis and has used rather mild "acute" stress like that associated with the Trier Social Stress Test [36–38].

Both the sympathetic and the neurohormonal systems play a role in the aftermath of all kinds of psychosocial stressors, and both systems were shown to be involved in the pathophysiology of psychotic symptoms (reviewed by Walker and Diforio [39] and Walker et al. [40]). While much discussion has centered on the chronic effects of such changes in neurotransmission and hormonal regulation (see below), some studies and case reports have shown that reducing cortisol production may have immediate beneficial effects on symptomatic psychoses in patients with Cushing syndrome [41]. This indicates that even if hormonal dysregulation may have become chronic, there are still immediate clinical effects on mental functions that may be amenable to treatment. More research is obviously needed to clarify how these alterations lead to psychotic symptoms. It is also still unclear whether there are genes involved in the pathophysiology of psychotic disorders, which may determine whether an individual will have a psychotic reaction immediately following a traumatic live event. Some evidence correlating minor stressful live events with affective reactions and more intense moment-to-moment variations of subtle psychotic experiences indicates that there may be a very close and immediate relationship [42]. Another aspect is whether there are acute effects of brief psychotic reactions on other health conditions, and some initial evidence suggests that there are adverse, but temporary, effects on glucose homeostasis of acute psychotic exacerbations in patients with schizophrenia [43, 44]. It is currently unclear whether there are predisposing genes or characteristic neuroendocrine responses which may be responsible for the inter-individual differences in the type and timing of psychotic reactions toward acute severe stressors. Studies in persons who have or have had a brief reactive psychosis are lacking, and there are no studies assessing neurohormonal functions in the different disease stages of brief reactive psychosis.

Among the *delayed* effects, it is noteworthy that epidemiological studies showed that early childhood and recent adversity were significantly associated with each other [45]. This suggests that early childhood adversity may somehow either increase the likelihood of later adversity or that there are individuals who by unknown mechanisms are more susceptible to experience traumatic events. This study also showed that exposure to early life adverse events enhanced the sensitivity to the psychotogenic effects of recent traumatic events, and that there was a threshold effect at the level of severe recent adversity in eliciting psychotic symptoms. However, "recent" in this study was defined as having occurred between interview dates, and this may have been a time period of several years. This would not be compatible with the "recency" criterion of a short interval of time between traumatic life events and the occurrence of psychotic symptoms as defined in DSM-IV-TR "brief reactive psychosis" chapter. Also, the study population was a non-clinical epidemiological sample of adolescents and young adults, which may not be representative for the typical higher age of "brief reactive psychosis" patients. Thus, while probably not suitable to proof the concept of "brief reactive psychosis," this study shows that there may be remote effects of early childhood traumatization, which manifest themselves clinically later in life, and this may be of importance for the pathophysiology of adult brief reactive psychoses. On a background of increased chronic stress, the cortisol response to acute moderate stress becomes attenuated in individuals at ultra-high risk of psychosis [38], but how this finding bears on the pathophysiology of acute psychotic reactions is unknown.

A final question is "When is a trauma traumatic?" In a clinical study, Modestin and Bachmann [46] showed that "life events" occurred in all psychotic disorders and even "uncontrollable life events" and "life events of major upset" were not specific to "reactive/psychogenic psychoses." This may lead to chance associations between "reactive" psychotic states and life events, and a central issue will be to conclusively show that a certain life event was responsible for a psychotic reaction. Given the knowledge about the long-term consequences of early life traumatization, in the sense of a sensitization toward future psychotic reactions, it seems difficult to clearly state whether a recent or past traumatic life event or stressor was *the* responsible factor. One promising research approach may be to search for structural or functional alterations of brain networks following stress exposure similar to research in post-traumatic stress disorder [47, 48], which may then correspond with immediate or delayed psychotic reactions.

In summary, while the acute psychotogenic effects of extreme traumatic events can be explained by acute neurohormonal effects mainly on the cortisol and dopamine systems, it is still unclear which pathophysiologic relation exists between early life or chronic stress and the later development of psychotic disorders, and which genetic or other factors determine whether a psychotic reaction in an individual person exposed to a certain marked stressor occurs.

Conclusion

The concept of "brief reactive psychoses" was subject to a number of changes of the clinical criteria over the last 100 years. Dropping one of Jaspers's criteria for the reactive psychoses, namely that the psychotic disorder would have to remit once the stressor was removed, in DSM-III seems to have been a paradigm shift leading to the lumping of reactive and non-reactive brief psychotic disorders in international classification systems of mental disorders ("brief psychotic disorders" in DSM and "acute and transient psychotic disorders" in ICD). There is a lack of representative, large-scale epidemiological and therapeutic studies in this area. Associations between stressors and psychotic disorders have been studied extensively, but do not seem to be a specific feature of the "brief reactive psychoses" as they may occur in any psychotic disorder. While there are reasonable assumptions about the pathophysiology of stress-associated psychotic disorders, the field is far from proving that the observed temporal associations between stress and psychotic states were causative. In order to develop a clearer picture, one research avenue would need to establish such causative relationships. While the functional outcome of brief psychotic disorders is generally more favorable than in schizophrenia, there is an excess mortality of patients with acute and transient psychotic disorders mainly due to suicidality and a high relapse rate leading to repeated hospitalizations. A second research avenue could therefore focus on the treatment of brief reactive psychosis (with or without stressor), in which controlled clinical trials addressing the efficacy of antipsychotic medication for limiting the acute psychotic episode and for reducing relapse rates would be necessary. Studies into the genetic or other neurobiological underpinnings of stress-induced psychotic states would be necessary with a view to develop novel preventive strategies based on insights into the pathophysiology of reactive psychotic disorders.

References

1 Jauch DA, Carpenter WT. (1988) Reactive psychoses I. Does the pre-DSM-III concept define a third psychosis? *J Nerv Ment Dis* 176, 72–81.
2 Jauch DA, Carpenter WT. (1988) Reactive psychoses II. Does DSM-II-R define a third psychosis? *J Nerv Ment Dis* 176, 82–86.
3 Jaspers K. (1913) *General Psychopathology*. Hoenig J and Hamilton MW (Translators). Manchester University Press (1963), Manchester, UK.
4 Strömgren E. (1986) The development of the concept of reactive psychoses. *Psychopathology* 20, 62–67.
5 Faergeman PM. (1963) *Psychogenic Psychoses*. Butterworth, London.
6 Retterstol N. (1983) Course of paranoid psychoses in relation to diagnostic grouping. *Psychiatr Clin* 16, 198–206.

7 McCabe MS. (1975) Reactive psychoses. A clinical and genetic investigation. *Acta Psychiatrica Scand Suppl* 259, 1–133.

8 Krstev H. (2011) Reactive psychosis in a first-episode psychosis population. Thesis. Victoria University, 2011. http://vuir.vu.edu.au/17943/1/Helen_Krstev.pdf.

9 American Psychiatric Association. (1980) *Diagnostic and Statistical Manual (DSM-III)*. 3rd ed. American Psychiatric Association, Washington.

10 American Psychiatric Association. (2000) *Diagnostic and Statistical Manual (DSM-IV-TR)*. 4th ed. American Psychiatric Association, Washington.

11 American Psychiatric Association. (2013) *Diagnostic and Statistical Manual of Mental Disorders*. 5th ed. American Psychiatric Publishing, Washington.

12 Dahl AA. (1994) The validity of the Scandinavian concept of reactive psychoses. *Seishin Shinkeigaku Zasshi* 96, 660–675.

13 World Health Organization. (1992) *The ICD-10 Classification of Mental and Behavioural Disorders: Clinical Descriptions and Diagnostic Guidelines*. World Health Organization, Geneva.

14 Marneros A, Pillmann F, Haring A, et al. (2005) Is the psychopathology of acute and transient psychotic disorder different from schizophrenic and schizoaffective disorders? *Eur Psychiatry* 20, 315–320.

15 Pillmann F, Balzuweit S, Haring A, et al. (2003) Suicidal behavior in acute and transient psychotic disorders. *Psychiatry Res* 117, 199–209.

16 Castagnini AC, Bertelsen A. (2011) Mortality and causes of death of acute and transient psychotic disorders. *Soc Psychiatry Psychiatr Epidemiol* 46, 1013–1017.

17 Castagnini A, Foldager L, Bertelsen A. (2013) Excess mortality of acute and transient psychotic disorders: Comparison with bipolar affective disorder and schizophrenia. *Acta Psychiatr Scand.* 2013. Doi: 10.1111/acps.12077.

18 Gaebel W, Zielasek J, Cleveland HR. (2013) Psychotic disorders in ICD-11. *As J Psychiatry* 6, 263–265.

19 Pitta JCN, Blay SL. (1997) Psychogenic (reactive) and hysterical psychoses: A cross-system reliability study. *Acta Psychiatr Scand* 95, 112–118.

20 Pillmann F, Haring A, Balzuweit S, et al. (2002) The concordance of ICD-10 acute and transient psychosis and DSM-IV brief psychotic disorder. *Psychol Med* 32, 525–533.

21 Castagnini A, Bertelsen A, Munk-Jørgensen P, et al. (2007) The relationship of reactive psychosis and ICD-10 acute and transient psychotic disorders: Evidence from a case register-based comparison. *Psychopathology* 40, 47–53.

22 Susser E, Wanderling J. (1994) Epidemiology of nonaffective acute remitting psychosis vs schizophrenia: Sex and sociocultural setting. *Arch Gen Psychiatry* 51, 294–301.

23 Jäger M, Frasch K, Weinmann S, Becker T. (2007) [Treatment guidelines for non-schizophrenic psychotic disorders?] *Psychiatr Prax* 34, 370–376 [Article in German].

24 Singh SP, Burns T, Amin S, et al. (2004) Acute and transient psychotic disorders: Precursors, epidemiology, course and outcome. *Br J Psychiatry* 185, 452–459.

25 Susser E, Fennig S, Jandorf L, et al. (1995) Epidemiology, diagnosis, and course of brief psychoses. *Am J Psychiatry* 152, 1743–1748.

26 Castagnini A, Bertelsen A, Berrios GE. (2008) Incidence and diagnostic stability of ICD-10 acute and transient psychotic disorders. *Compr Psychiatry* 49, 255–261.

27 Pillmann F, Marneros A. (2005) Longitudinal follow-up in acute and transient psychotic disorders and schizophrenia. *Br J Psychiatry* 187, 286–287.

28 Pillmann F, Haring A, Balzuweit S, et al. (2002) A comparison of DSM-IV brief psychotic disorder with "positive" schizophrenia and healthy controls. *Compr Psychiatr* 43, 385–392.

29 Marneros A, Pillmann F, Haring A, et al. (2003) What is schizophrenic in acute and transient psychotic disorder? *Schizophr Bull* 29, 311–323.

30 Mojtabai R, Varma VK, Susser E. (2000) Duration of remitting psychoses with acute onset. Implications for ICD-10. *Br J Psychiatry* 176, 576–580.

31 Udomratn P, Burns J, Farooq S. (2012) Acute and transient psychotic disorders: An overview of studies in Asia. *Int Rev Psychiatry* 24, 463–466.

32 Chorlton E, McKenzie K, Morgan C, et al. (2012) Course and outcome of psychosis in black Caribbean populations and other ethnic groups living in the UK: A systematic review. *Int J Soc Psychiatry* 58, 400–408.

33 Castagnini AC, Laursen TM, Mortensen PB, et al. (2013) Family psychiatric morbidity of acute and transient psychotic disorders and their relationship to schizophrenia and bipolar disorder. *Psychol Med* 43(11), 2369–2375.

34 Beards S, Gayer-Anderson C, Borges S, et al. (2013) Life events and psychosis: A review and meta-analysis. *Schizophr Bull* 39, 740–747.

35 Corcoran C, Walker E, Huot R, et al. (2003) The stress cascade and schizophrenia: Etiology and onset. *Schizophr Bull* 29, 671–692.

36 Brenner K, Liu A, Laplante DP, et al. (2009) Cortisol response to a psychosocial stressor in schizophrenia: Blunted, delayed, or normal? *Psychoneuroendocrinology* 34, 859–868.

37 Steen NE, Lorentzen S, Barrett EA, et al. (2011) Sex-specific cortisol levels in bipolar disorder and schizophrenia during mental challenge: Relationship to clinical characteristics and medication. *Prog Neuropsychopharmacol Biol Psychiatry* 35, 1100–1107.

38 Pruessner M, Béchard-Evans L, Boekestyn L, et al. (2013) Attenuated cortisol response to acute psychosocial stress in individuals at ultra-high risk for psychosis. *Schizophr Res* 146, 79–86.

39 Walker EF, Diforio D. (1997) Schizophrenia: A neural diathesis-stress model. *Psychol Rev* 104, 667–685.

40 Walker E, Mittal V, Tessner K. (2008) Stress and the hypothalamic pituitary adrenal axis in the developmental course of schizophrenia. *Annu Rev Clin Psychol* 4, 189–216.

41 Zielasek J, Bender G, Schlesinger S, et al. (2002) A woman who gained weight and became schizophrenic. *Lancet* 360, 1392.

42 Myin-Germeys I, van Os J. (2007) Stress-reactivity in psychosis: Evidence for an affective pathway to psychosis. *Clin Psychol Rev* 27, 409–424.

43 Shiloah E, Witz S, Abramovitch Y, et al. (2003) Effect of acute psychotic stress in nondiabetic subjects on beta-cell function and insulin sensitivity. *Diabetes Care* 26, 1462–1467.

44 Shiloah E, Kanety H, Cohen O, et al. (2007) Acute psychotic stress is associated with decreased adiponectin serum levels. *J Endocrinol Invest* 30, 382–387.

45 Lataster J, Myin-Germeys I, Lieb R, et al. (2012) Adversity and psychosis: A 10-year prospective study investigating synergism between early and recent adversity in psychosis. *Acta Psychiatr Scand* 125, 388–399.

46 Modestin J, Bachmann KM. (1992) Is the diagnosis of hysterical psychosis justified?: Clinical study of hysterical psychosis, reactive/psychogenic psychosis, and schizophrenia. *Compr Psychiatry* 33, 17–24.

47 Admon R, Milad MR, Hendler T. (2013) A causal model of post-traumatic stress disorder: Disentangling predisposed from acquired neural abnormalities. *Trends Cogn Sci* pii: S1364-6613(13)00104-6. Doi: 10.1016/j.tics.2013.05.005.

48 Li X, Zhu D, Jiang X, et al. (2013) Dynamic functional connectomics signatures for characterization and differentiation of PTSD patients. *Hum Brain Mapp.* Doi: 10.1002/hbm.22290 [Epub ahead of print].

CHAPTER 4
Cycloid psychoses

Andrea Schmitt, Berend Malchow, Peter Falkai, and Alkomiet Hasan
Department of Psychiatry and Psychotherapy, Ludwig-Maximilians-University, Munich, Germany

Historical aspects

From a historical viewpoint, the most important classificatory approach of severe psychotic diseases by Emil Kraepelin (1856–1926) strongly influenced modern concepts of psychiatry. He differentiated between "dementia praecox" with a deleterious outcome and "manic-depressive insanity" with good prognosis. According to his classification, acute psychoses with good prognosis are integrated into affective diseases. Meanwhile, the French psychiatrist Valentin Magnan (1835–1916) established the diagnosis *bouffée délirante*, including the sudden onset of delusions, intense symptoms with varying content, and complete remission [1]. In Germany, Carl Wernicke (1848–1905) was the first to describe "anxiety psychosis" and "motility psychosis," which describe anxious affects and paranoid psychosis as well as motor symptoms with hyperkinetic, akinetic, and mixed states and entail a good prognosis. His scholar, Karl Kleist (1879–1960), defined the term *cycloid psychoses,* including motility psychosis and confusional psychosis, not leading to mental deficits [2]. He suggested this group of psychoses to be caused by temporary dysfunctions of labile brain regions [1]. In his psychiatric school, cycloid psychoses belong to an atypical disorder representing a third form of psychosis apart from manic-depressive and schizophrenia psychoses. They may occur in patients predisposed to phasic illness with often spontaneous and full recovery and no residual symptoms.

Karl Leonhard (1904–1988) further developed Kleist's concept by adding anxiety-elation psychosis as third subform, thus extending it to a psychosis with rapid shift of mood and ecstatic feelings. Cycloid psychoses have been described as a group of acute psychoses with polymorph symptomatology and good prognosis due to complete remission. Leonhard considered three subforms entailing bipolar symptoms according to abnormalities in mood, thinking, and behavior. They consist of anxiety-elation, excited-inhibited

Troublesome Disguises: Managing Challenging Disorders in Psychiatry, Second Edition.
Edited by Dinesh Bhugra and Gin S. Malhi.

confusion, and hyperkinetic-akinetic motility psychosis [3]. To validate his innovative concept, he longitudinally observed about 700 patients at the University hospitals in Frankfurt and Berlin and separated the distinct cycloid psychoses from "unsystematic" schizophrenia with unstable symptoms and variable course and "systematic" schizophrenia with a chronic course and stable symptoms [4–6]. Unsystematic schizophrenia included "affective paraphrenia," "periodic catatonia," and "cataphasia" with unfavorable long-term outcome, while systematic schizophrenia consists of "hebephrenia," "paraphrenia," and "catatonia" and a non-episodic, progressive course of the disease. Contrastingly, cycloid psychoses exhibit a phasic and cyclic course with full recovery or only mild residual symptoms [7, 8]. As a prominent example, based on the classification of Leonhard, the psychiatric disease of Vincent van Gogh has been considered to be an anxiety-elation psychosis with fluctuating mood that influenced his biography [9].

In 1933, Jacob Kasanin [10] described the acute schizoaffective psychoses as an episodic psychotic disease with predominant affective symptoms, that was viewed to be a good-prognosis schizophrenia. In 1950, the Japanese psychiatrist Hilrstoehi Mitsuda [11] named periodical psychoses with favorable prognosis, rapid fluctuation, emotional disturbances, and positive psychotic symptoms "atypical psychoses" and considered them to be another genetic category than schizophrenia and manic-depressive psychosis. Based on clinical and family studies in Britain and Italy in the 1970s and 1980s, Carlo Perris and Ian Brockington developed operational diagnostic criteria for cycloid psychoses with polymorphous symptoms and confusion or distressed perplexity without distinguishing between specific subforms [12–14]. Meanwhile, several investigators supported the nosological validity of the concept of cycloid psychoses [15], among them the psychiatric school of Helmut Beckmann (1940–2006) and colleagues at the University of Würzburg, Germany, prominent for differentiating the psychopathology of psychoses in the classificatory tradition of Wernicke-Kleist-Leonhard.

Incidence

The group of cycloid psychoses is not rare; among psychotic patients hospitalized for the first time they may account for 13 percent of the cases [16]. Peralta and colleagues [17] estimated a total of 10–15 percent cases with cycloid psychoses. In another clinical sample, the 1-year incidence of cycloid psychoses has been assessed in 514 patients discharged in 1983 in Lund, Sweden. Out of 83 first hospitalization patients, 29 received the diagnosis functional psychosis. In this group, 4 females and 3 males fulfilled the diagnostic criteria for cycloid psychosis based on the definition of Leonhard and

Perris. Overall, the 1-year incidence for first admission in cycloid psychoses per 100,000 inhabitants of the age group 15–50 years was 5.0 in females and 3.6 in males [18]. The onset of disease occurs during the second or third decade of life with a mean age of 27.4 years [18]. While Leonhard calculated the proportion of females to be 57 percent (motility psychosis 74 percent) [19], later studies reported cycloid psychoses to be even more frequent in women, who represent 72–78 percent of the cycloid patients [17, 18, 20]. In contrast, no gender differences have been detected in schizophrenia [21].

Symptoms and course of the group of disorders

According to Leonhard's classification, symptoms of cycloid psychoses are expressed in a dichotomic manner. The anxiety-elation psychosis with rapid changes of anxiety and ecstatic mood consists of severe anxiety, accompanied by distrust and self-references, delusions of threat and persecution and affect-congruent sensory illusions or hallucinations. The other pole has been described as ecstatic mood with happiness and delusions of reference, calling, or salvation (often religious or political ideas) as well as affect-generated illusions or hallucinations such as divine messages or inspirations. The excited-inhibited confusion psychosis is composed of excitation on the one hand such as incoherence of thought and speech, fleeting misrecognition of persons, ideas of reference and hallucinations, and on the other hand of inhibition of thought with perplexedness and language impoverishment up to mutism. The hyperkinetic-akinetic motility psychosis entails a hyperkinetic pole with excess of movements, increase in expressive and reactive motions, severe distractibility by environment, and senseless motor activity. The akinetic pole is composed of reduction of expressive and reactive motions, reduction of voluntary movements, incoherence and lack of spontaneous speech, and akinetic stupor [22]. The symptoms may be confluent between the three subtypes, but all of them exhibit a phasic course with bipolarity and complete remission except for secondary effects of repeated illness, hospitalizations, and impaired functioning [15].

The Perris and Brockington criteria for cycloid psychoses comprise age between 15 and 50 years, acute psychosis, and sudden change from health to psychosis within hours to a few days plus symptoms across the spectrum of the three subforms primarily described by Leonhard. These demand at least four of the following symptoms: confusion from perplexity to severe disorientation with derealization or depersonalization, mood-incongruent delusions or paranoid symptoms inclusive ideas of reference, influence or persecution. Furthermore, hallucinations of any kind, deep feelings of happiness or ecstasy, deep anxiety and fear that something terrifying is about to happen, motility disturbances with increased or decreased activity, and particular concern about death or dying. They describe mood swings that are not sufficient to support the diagnosis of affective disorders. Symptoms are considered to be polymorph with opposite polar phases within a single episode [15].

Overall, after an acute onset the course of the disease has been described as cyclic with recurrent psychotic episodes lasting days to months and possible spontaneous remission. A mean onset of 32.1 years and 3.2 episodes during 7 years within the course of the disease has been observed in patients fulfilling the Perris and Brockington criteria [20]. Corresponding to the initial hypothesis of full remission, Beckmann and colleagues [23] verified lacking residual morbidity in reevaluating 31 of Leonhard's cycloid psychoses patients during a period of 4 years. The team thus could demonstrate stability and prognostic validity of the diagnosis. The investigation of another group of 108 female patients with psychotic disorders during a follow-up period of 30 years provided good evidence for stability and validity of diagnostic groups according to Leonhard's classifications of cycloid psychoses, bipolar disorder, and systematic schizophrenias [24]. In the subsequent prospective analysis of 276 psychosis patients, including 222 female patients for a period of 21–33 years, predictive validity of the diagnostic categories have been assessed. Leonhard's classifications of hebephrenias and schizophrenias were the most valid categories, followed by bipolar and cycloid psychoses [25]. Reevaluating 22 schizophrenia patients (ICD-10 and DSM-IIR diagnosis) by 4 independent raters using Leonhard's classification, a high interrater reliability was achieved in separating cycloid psychoses from systematic and unsystematic schizophrenias [26]. A prospective study reexamined 39 females with postpartum psychiatric disorders on average 12.5 years after the first episode of psychosis. Using Leonhard's classification, 54 percent of the patients suffered from cycloid psychosis with a motility psychosis predominating the clinical picture [27]. These results accord with previous reports of Wernicke [28], who considered puerperal psychoses predominantly to be motility psychosis. Schizophrenia, in contrast, is only rarely present in this group of disorders [29]. Outcome criteria such as Clinical Global Impression (CGI), Global Assessment of Functioning (GAF), symptoms as expressed by the Positive and Negative Syndrome Scale (PANSS), and quality of life as measured by the Lancashire Quality of Life Profile (QoL) have been assessed in 33 patients with cycloid psychoses compared to 44 schizophrenia patients after 13 years since first hospitalization [19]. According to the unfavorable course of the illness, schizophrenia patients developed symptoms earlier, revealed more frequent and longer periods of hospitalization, and received higher neuroleptic doses than patients with cycloid psychoses. Corresponding with the hypothesis of remission without residual symptoms, patients with cycloid psychoses displayed better scores in CGI, GAF, Strauss-Carpenter Outcome, and PANSS scales. Other than in schizophrenia, patients did not differ from healthy controls with respect to quality of life in three out of four domains. Furthermore, they specifically exhibit a favorable outcome in employment status and familial relations such as marriage and children [19]. In the entire group of psychotic disorders, symptoms of confusion, acute and late onset of the disease, and intact premorbid personality have been considered to be an important factor in remission quality [30]. Female patients with psychosis were shown to have an increased age at onset [21]. The good outcome in female patients may be related to their preponderance with respect to the diagnosis cycloid psychoses and may be due to positive effects of estrogen on outcome. Animal studies, for example, have shown that estradiol reduces catalepsy caused by the dopamine antagonist haloperidol and behavioral changes by the dopamine agonist apomorphine [31]. This led to the application of adjuvant estrogens as a therapeutic attempt in female patients with schizophrenia [32].

Classification in ICD-10, DSM-IV, and DSM-V

The group of schizophrenia and other psychotic diseases such as schizoaffective, schizotypal, and delusional disorders (in ICD-10 F20.x-F29.x, in DSM-IV 295.10–295.90, in DSM-V B00-B10) describes a range of psychotic syndromes sharing some common characteristics like reality distortion, disorganization, delusions, and hallucinations as well as affective symptoms, whereas length of the prodromal state, duration of the psychotic episode, and quality of remission differ significantly [33–35]. Therefore, the separation of good-prognosis disorders such as cycloid psychoses from diseases with an unfavorable outcome like schizophrenia is warranted. The number of publications dealing with cycloid psychoses, however, has declined during the last 25 years, due to its uncertain nosological status and unclear presentation in the modern, international classification systems. In examining the concordance of the diagnosis of cycloid psychoses according to Perris and Brockington's criteria with psychotic disorders across the ICD-10 and DSM-IV diagnostic systems, Peralta and Cuesta [36] assessed 660 psychotic inpatients. Of this sample, 68 patients met the criteria of cycloid psychoses and exhibited a wide range of ICD-10 and DSM-IV diagnoses for which reason they did not correspond closely to any of the international classification systems. The categorization under the diagnoses brief psychotic disorder (DSM-IV) or acute and transient psychotic disorder (ICD-10) was not successful because exceeding the "duration of disease" criterion is only up to one (DSM-IV) or three (or one when schizophrenia symptoms are present) (ICD-10) months. Moreover, the exclusion of a full affective syndrome speaks against proper classification of cycloid psychoses.

The ICD-10 category of acute and transient psychotic disorders (ATPD) defines a psychotic episode with acute onset within 2 weeks and a duration up to 3 months. The subgroup "acute polymorphic psychoses" without or with symptoms of schizophrenia (F.23.0 or F23.1) includes acute onset, rapidly changing symptoms, emotional turmoil, ecstasy, and alterations in psychomotor activity and shows significant concordance with the diagnosis of cycloid psychoses [37]. However, most of the studies investigating the nosological status of cycloid psychoses in the modern classification systems failed to show correspondence [17]. For example, only 55 percent of the cases diagnosed with ATPD according to ICD-10 met Perris and Brockington's criteria of cycloid psychoses. At follow-up after 5 years, patients with cycloid ATPD had more frequent recurrence and showed better remission and social functioning than those not diagnosed with cycloid psychoses [20]. Apart from the exclusion of major mood syndromes, ICD-10 based ATPD diagnoses are restricted to a limited duration of illness and cycloid episodes on average last 3 months or longer [17]. In a prospective study comparing patients with ATPD and persistent delusional disorders and persistence of delusions for at least 3 months, ATPD differed from the second group with respect to a larger female group, younger age at onset, higher richness and variety of symptoms, more re-hospitalizations, less chronicity of delusions, and higher global functioning during follow-up of 10–12 years [38]. The annual incidence of ATPD per 100,000 inhabitants amounted to 0.74 in men and 1.99 in women [39]. In Denmark again, the incidence of ATPD was 9.6 per 100,000 population, but in about half of the patients the diagnosis has been changed to schizophrenia or affective disorders during follow-up, reaching a diagnostic stability of only 39 percent [40]. The diagnostic heterogeneity of ATPD was also stressed by 1-year and 3-year follow-up studies, which later reclassified half of the patients to suffer from schizophrenia or affective disorders [39, 41]. The same has been explored in China, where diagnostic stability for ATPD over 5 years has been shown only for 35 percent and 29 percent of the patients developed schizophrenia [42].

The schizoaffective psychosis as described in ICD-10 and DSM-IV as an intermediate form between schizophrenia and affective disorders has been suggested to be a useful category for the cycloid patients with affective syndromes. However, all studies examining the relationship between schizoaffective and cycloid psychoses revealed only poor concordance due to the coexistence of schizophrenia symptoms and major affective disorder. Features of cycloid psychoses such as severe anxiety and ecstasy, brief changes in affectivity, and mood swing not meeting the criteria for a full affective disorder are not considered in the definition [17]. In a group of 70 patients diagnosed by first-episode schizoaffective disorder, schizophrenia, or schizophreniform disorder, patients with cycloid psychoses have been classified according to the

Perris and Brockington criteria. The cycloid patients presented less prodromal symptoms, shorter duration of episode, higher PANSS scores except for negative symptoms, and higher presence of depression or mania symptoms. Therefore they may represent a distinct clinical entity [43].

DSM-IV described features of cycloid psychoses in the less differentiated categories of brief psychotic disorder, schizophreniform disorder, and "psychotic disorder not otherwise specified," stressing the duration of the episode, but less considering the multifaceted psychopathology [44]. The brief psychotic disorder is characterized by an episode with at least one psychotic symptom, lasting less than 1 month, while schizophreniform disorder is defined as entailing two or more symptoms of schizophrenia lasting at least 1 month but less than 6 months. The psychotic disorder not otherwise specified includes psychotic symptoms with insufficient information for a specific diagnosis [45]. Lifetime prevalences for brief psychotic disorder have been calculated to be about 0.05 percent, for schizophreniform disorder 0.07 percent and 0.45 percent for psychotic disorder not otherwise specified [17]. Additionally, bipolar disorder with psychotic and catatonic features does not coincide with rapidly fluctuating affective, psychotic, and cognitive symptoms presented by cycloid psychoses [46]. Non-affective acute psychoses have been reported to have a higher incidence in developing compared to industrialized countries [47, 48]. However, it has to be noted that using different diagnostic systems across the studies aggravates comparisons. In a 15-year follow-up study of 197 patients comparing ICD-10 and DSM-IV diagnoses, the majority of patients initially diagnosed with ATPD, schizophreniform, and brief psychotic disorder later were classified as schizophrenia or affective disorder patients. Of the ATPD patients, 30 percent had a single episode, 50 percent an episodic-remitting, and 20 percent a chronic course of the disease [49].

The new ICD-11 classification is on the way to be revised by work groups under guidance of the WHO Advisory Group and scheduled for presentation to and adoption by the World Health Assembly, the WHO's governing body, in 2015 [50]. Major revisions are recommended for the ICD-10 ATPD category while retaining essential clinical features such as acute onset, brief duration, and the presence of polymorphic clinical symptoms. F23.0 (acute polymorph psychotic disorder without symptoms of schizophrenia) is classified as B 02 ATPD. In this group, the duration criterion has been extended up to 3 months. If symptoms last longer, schizophrenia (B 00) or delusional disorder (B 04) should be considered. The former F23.1 (acute polymorphic psychotic disorder with symptoms of schizophrenia) and F23.3 (acute schizophrenia-like psychotic disorder) diagnoses are proposed to be collapsed into B 05 (other primary psychotic disorders) if the episode lasts less than 4 weeks. In case of an episode lasting more than 4 weeks, schizophrenia B 00 should be diagnosed. In the recently published DSM-V a schizophreniform disorder for patients presenting symptoms for more than 1 month and less than 6 months and brief psychotic disorder with a duration of less than 1 month are included. Such patients with short duration would be classified in ICD-11 under ATPD or other primary psychotic disorder [51].

Etiology and neurobiology

Family studies revealed a threefold higher ATPD frequency in first-degree relatives of patients with ATPD compared to schizophrenia [52] and the same group subsequently showed that ATPD patients with a family history of mental disorders experienced fewer stress-related life [53]. Relatives of these patients seem to have an increased risk of cycloid psychoses [54]. However, relatives of patients with cycloid psychoses showed lower likelihood for psychoses and manic-depressive illness than patients with affective disorders, suggesting an etiological separation between cycloid psychoses and affective disorders [55]. The lack of heritability has been confirmed by a later study, which showed that the risk for functional psychoses in relatives of patients with cycloid psychoses does not differ from healthy controls [56]. It has to be noted that Beckmann and coworkers did not consider schizophrenia-like psychoses as diagnostic continuum, but rather as subgroups with distinct genetic, environmental, and psychosocial origin. In fact, psychosocial stress has been considered to play a role in the pathophysiology of the disease [57]. Twin studies [58] and Beckmann and Franzek [59] documented only low genetic loading for cycloid psychoses, which raises the question of the impact of environmental factors during neurodevelopment. The frequency and severity of birth complications for affected monozygotic twins was significantly higher than for unaffected subjects [59]. Furthermore, first-trimester respiratory infection induced by influenza or febrile cold has significantly been associated with cycloid psychoses and may predict earlier onset of the disease [60]. An inflammation process of the brain, predisposing occurrence of later psychoses, may not only be induced by prenatal infections, but also by preterm birth under 30 weeks of gestation [61].

Patients with non-specific abnormalities like frontal atrophy, ventricular enlargement, and asymmetry in cranial computer tomography (CCT) presented a higher prevalence of developing cycloid psychoses [62] Falkai and colleagues [63] described an increased ventricle-brain ratio in patients with cycloid psychoses compared to healthy controls and chronic schizophrenia patients. This finding could not be replicated in a magnetic resonance imaging study with a small sample, but the cycloid patients revealed decreased asymmetry of the planum temporale and larger corpus callosum [64]. In contrast to schizophrenia, a CCT study reported no differences in ventricular size compared to healthy controls in cycloid patients at first episode or after a follow-up period of 16 years [65]. A 99mTc-HMPAO-SPECT study did not find evidence for alterations of global perfusion in patients with cycloid psychoses [66, 67]. With respect to neurophysiology, cycloid patients featured normal P300 topographies and latencies, but higher amplitudes than controls, indicating a state of hyperarousal [68]. This increased arousal may be manifest as higher motor activity compared to patients with schizophrenia [69]. As a biochemical correlate, alterations of the noradrenergic system have been discussed [70], but post-mortem studies as well as modern neuroimaging approaches are missing.

Therapy

To date, no randomized, controlled treatment studies have been conducted. In a study of ATPD patients, 95 percent received an antipsychotic, 21 percent an antidepressant, and 7 percent lithium [71]. In acute psychotic disorders, atypical antipsychotics have been shown to exert beneficial effects on prefrontal cortex function [72]. Atypical antipsychotics at low doses are recommended for a period of at least 1 year [73, 74]. It has to be assumed that a portion of the patients have self-remitting episodes and therefore the attempt for discontinuation of medication is justified [17]. Electroconvulsive therapy may be beneficial in patients with motility psychosis [75, 76]. However, therapeutic strategies in cycloid psychoses are mainly based on clinical experience and expert-based recommendations.

Conclusion

Reliable diagnosis of cycloid psychoses is possible using the Leonhard and Perris and Brockington classifications. However, these classifications do not match well with modern, international diagnostic systems such as ICD or DSM. Apart from the variable course of psychotic disorders with the possibility of misdiagnosing prodromal symptoms as cycloid psychoses, rater-dependent inconsistencies based on experience with different psychopathological schools, and impaired compliance of patients with severe anxiety and psychosis have to be considered when classifying acute psychotic episodes like cycloid psychoses. Due to the lack of diagnostic consensus criteria and the dissemination of history-based classification rather in Central Europe than in the Anglo-American language area, research on cycloid psychoses declined during the last decades and neurobiological insights are scarce. However, it is worthwhile to draw further conclusions of the concept of cycloid psychosis in the interest of improving diagnostic criteria for good-outcome psychosis and developing valid treatment standards.

References

1 Pillmann F, Marneros A. Brief and acute psychoses: The development of concepts. *Hist Psychiatry*. 2003;14(2):161–77.

2 Neumarker KJ, Bartsch AJ. Karl Kleist (1879–1960): A pioneer of neuropsychiatry. *Hist Psychiatry*. 2003;14(56 Pt 4):411–58.

3 Leonhard K. Cycloid psychoses: Endogenous psychoses which are neither schizophrenic nor manic-depressive. *Ment Sci*. 1961;107:633–48.

4 Leonhard K. [The origin of cycloid psychoses]. *Psychiatrie, Neurologie, und medizinische Psychologie*. 1981;33(3):145–57.

5 Leonhard K. [Differential diagnosis and different etiologies of monopolar and bipolar phasic psychoses]. *Psychiatrie, Neurologie, und medizinische Psychologie*. 1987;39(9): 524–33.

6 Leonhard K. [Differential diagnosis of endogenous psychoses in relation to a symptom catalog]. *Psychiatrie, Neurologie, und medizinische Psychologie*. 1990;42(3):136–45.

7 Leonhard K. [The pre-psychotic temperament in monopolar and bipolar phasic psychoses]. *Psychiatria et neurologia*. 1963;146:105–15.

8 Leonhard K. [On monopolar and bipolar endogenous psychoses]. *Nervenarzt*. 1968; 39(3):104–6.

9 Strik WK. [The psychiatric illness of Vincent van Gogh]. *Nervenarzt*. 1997;68(5):401–9.

10 Kasanin J. The acute schizoaffective psychoses. *Am J Psychiatry*. 1933;90(1):97–126.

11 Hatotani N. The concept of 'atypical psychoses': Special reference to its development in Japan. *Psychiatry Clin Neurosci*. 1996;50(1):1–10.

12 Perris C, Brockington IF. Cycloid psychoses and their relation to the major psychoses. In: Perris C, Struwe G, Jansson B (eds.) *Biol Psychiatry*. Amsterdam: Elsevier; 1981. p. 447–50.

13 Brockington IF, Perris C, Kendell RE, Hillier VE, Wainwright S. The course and outcome of cycloid psychosis. *Psychol Med*. 1982;12(1):97–105.

14 Brockington IF, Perris C, Meltzer HY. Cycloid psychoses: Diagnosis and heuristic value. *J Nerv Ment Dis*. 1982;170(11):651–56.

15 Salvatore P, Bhuvaneswar C, Ebert D, Maggini C, Baldessarini RJ. Cycloid psychoses revisited: Case reports, literature review, and commentary. *Harv Rev Psychiatry*. 2008;16(3):167–80.

16 van der Heijden FM, Tuinier S, Kahn RS, Verhoeven WM. Nonschizophrenic psychotic disorders: The case of cycloid psychoses. *Psychopathology*. 2004;37(4):161–67.

17 Peralta V, Cuesta MJ, Zandio M. Cycloid psychosis: An examination of the validity of the concept. *Curr Psychiatry Rep*. 2007;9(3):184–92.

18 Lindvall M, Axelsson R, Ohman R. Incidence of cycloid psychosis. A clinical study of first-admission psychotic patients. *Eur Arch Psychiatry Clin Neurosci*. 1993;242(4):197–202.

19 Jabs BE, Krause U, Althaus G, Bartsch AJ, Stober G, Pfuhlmann B. Differences in quality of life and course of illness between cycloid and schizophrenic psychoses: A comparative study. *World J Biol Psychiatry*. 2004;5(3):136–42.

20 Pillmann F, Haring A, Balzuweit S, Bloink R, Marneros A. Concordance of acute and transient psychoses and cycloid psychoses. *Psychopathology*. 2001;34(6):305–11.

21 Hafner H, Behrens S, De Vry J, Gattaz WF. Oestradiol enhances the vulnerability threshold for schizophrenia in women by an early effect on dopaminergic neurotransmission. Evidence from an epidemiological study and from animal experiments. *Eur Arch Psychiatry Clin Neurosci*. 1991;241(1):65–8.

22 Leonhard K. *Classification of endogenous psychoses and their differential etiology.* 2nd ed. Wien, New York: Springer; 1999.

23 Beckmann H, Fritze J, Lanczik M. Prognostic validity of the cycloid psychoses. A prospective follow-up study. *Psychopathology*. 1990;23(4–6):205–11.

24 Tolna J, Peth B, Farkas M, Vizkeleti G, Tusnady G, Marosi J. Validity and reliability of leonhard's classification of endogenous psychoses: Preliminary report on a prospective 25- to 30-year follow-up study. *J Neural Transm*. 2001;108(6):629–36.

25 Petho B, Tolna J, Tusnady G, Farkas M, Vizkeleti G, Vargha A, et al. The predictive validity of the Leonhardean classification of endogenous psychoses: A 21–33-year follow-up of a prospective study ("BUDAPEST 2000"). *Eur Arch Psychiatry Clin Neurosci*. 2008;258(6):324–34.

26 Pfuhlmann B, Franzek E, Stober G, Cetkovich-Bakmas M, Beckmann H. On interrater reliability for Leonhard's classification of endogenous psychoses. *Psychopathology*. 1997;30(2):100–5.

27 Pfuhlmann B, Stober G, Franzek E, Beckmann H. Cycloid psychoses predominate in severe postpartum psychiatric disorders. *J Affect Disord*. 1998;50(2–3):125–34.

28 Wernicke C. *Grundriss der Psychiatrie.* 2nd ed. Leipzig: Thieme; 1906.

29 Pfuhlmann B, Stoeber G, Beckmann H. Postpartum psychoses: Prognosis, risk factors, and treatment. *Curr Psychiatry Rep*. 2002;4(3):185–90.

30 Bailer J, Brauer W, Rey ER. Premorbid adjustment as predictor of outcome in schizophrenia: Results of a prospective study. *Acta Psychiatr Scand*. 1996;93(5):368–77.

31 Hafner H, Behrens S, De Vry J, Gattaz WF. An animal model for the effects of estradiol on dopamine-mediated behavior: Implications for sex differences in schizophrenia. *Psychiatry Res*. 1991;38(2):125–34.

32 Louza MR, Marques AP, Elkis H, Bassitt D, Diegoli M, Gattaz WF. Conjugated estrogens as adjuvant therapy in the treatment of acute schizophrenia: A double-blind study. *Schizophr Res*. 2004;66(2–3):97–100.

33 World Health Organization. *ICD-10: international statistical classification of diseases and related health problems.* 2nd ed. Geneva: World Health Organization; 2004.

34 American Psychiatric Association. *Diagnostic and statistical manual of mental disorders.* Washington, DC: American Psychiatric Association; 1994.

35 American Psychiatric Association. *Diagnostic and statistical manual of mental disorders.* 5th ed. Arlington, VA: American Psychiatric Association; 2013.

36 Peralta V, Cuesta MJ. The nosology of psychotic disorders: A comparison among competing classification systems. *Schizophr Bull*. 2003;29(3):413–25.

37 Marneros A, Pillmann F, Haring A, Balzuweit S, Bloink R. Is the psychopathology of acute and transient psychotic disorder different from schizophrenic and schizoaffective disorders? *Eur Psychiatry*. 2005;20(4):315–20.

38 Pillmann F, Wustmann T, Marneros A. Acute and transient psychotic disorders versus persistent delusional disorders: A comparative longitudinal study. *Psychiatry Clin Neurosci*. 2012;66(1):44–52.

39 Singh SP, Burns T, Amin S, Jones PB, Harrison G. Acute and transient psychotic disorders: Precursors, epidemiology, course and outcome. *Br J Psychiatry*. 2004;185:452–59.

40 Castagnini A, Bertelsen A, Berrios GE. Incidence and diagnostic stability of ICD-10 acute and transient psychotic disorders. *Compr Psychiatry*. 2008;49(3):255–61.

41 Jorgensen P, Bennedsen B, Christensen J, Hyllested A. Acute and transient psychotic disorder: A 1-year follow-up study. *Acta Psychiatr Scand.* 1997;96(2):150–54.

42 Chang WC, Pang SL, Chung DW, Chan SS. Five-year stability of ICD-10 diagnoses among Chinese patients presented with first-episode psychosis in Hong Kong. *Schizophr Res.* 2009;115(2–3):351–57.

43 Garcia-Andrade RF, Diaz-Marsa M, Carrasco JL, Lopez-Mico C, Saiz-Gonzalez D, Aurecoechea JF, et al. Diagnostic features of the cycloid psychoses in a first psychotic episode sample. *J Affect Disord.* 2011;130(1–2):239–44.

44 Orlikov AB. Two case reports of confusion psychosis: Should we reevaluate the place of cycloid psychoses in modern psychiatry? *Prim Care Companion CNS Disord.* 2011;13(1): PCC.10l01024.

45 Nugent KL, Paksarian D, Mojtabai R. Nonaffective acute psychoses: Uncertainties on the way to DSM-V and ICD-11. *Curr Psychiatry Rep.* 2011;13(3):203–10.

46 Srihari VH, Lee TS, Rohrbaugh RM, D'Souza DC. Revisiting cycloid psychosis: A case of an acute, transient and recurring psychotic disorder. *Schizophr Res.* 2006;82(2–3):261–64.

47 Susser E, Wanderling J. Epidemiology of nonaffective acute remitting psychosis vs schizophrenia. Sex and sociocultural setting. *Arch Gen Psychiatry.* 1994;51(4):294–301.

48 Verma VK, Malhotra S, Jiloha RC. Acute non-organic psychotic state in India: Symptomatology. *Indian J Psychiatry.* 1992;34(2):89–101.

49 Moller HJ, Jager M, Riedel M, Obermeier M, Strauss A, Bottlender R. The Munich 15-year follow-up study (MUFUSSAD) on first-hospitalized patients with schizophrenic or affective disorders: Comparison of psychopathological and psychosocial course and outcome and prediction of chronicity. *Eur Arch Psychiatry Clin Neurosci.* 2010;260(5):367–84.

50 Gaebel W, Zielasek J, Cleveland HR. Classifying psychosis: Challenges and opportunities. *Int Rev Psychiatry.* 2012;24(6):538–48.

51 Gaebel W. Status of psychotic disorders in ICD-11. *Schizophr Bull.* 2012;38(5):895–98.

52 Das SK, Malhotra S, Basu D. Family study of acute and transient psychotic disorders: Comparison with schizophrenia. *Soc Psychiatry Psychiatr Epidemiol.* 1999;34(6):328–32.

53 Das SK, Malhotra S, Basu D, Malhotra R. Testing the stress-vulnerability hypothesis in ICD-10-diagnosed acute and transient psychotic disorders. *Acta Psychiatr Scand.* 2001;104(1):56–8.

54 Perris C. A study of cycloid psychoses. *Acta Psychiatr Scand Suppl.* 1974;253:1–77.

55 Pfuhlmann B, Jabs B, Althaus G, Schmidtke A, Bartsch A, Stober G, et al. Cycloid psychoses are not part of a bipolar affective spectrum: results of a controlled family study. *J Affect Disord.* 2004;83(1):11–19.

56 Jabs B, Althaus G, Bartsch A, Schmidtke A, Stober G, Beckmann H, et al. [Cycloid psychoses as atypical manic-depressive disorders. Results of a family study]. *Nervenarzt.* 2006;77(9):1096–100, 102–4.

57 Peralta V, Cuesta MJ. Cycloid psychosis. *Int Rev Psychiatry.* 2005;17(1):53–62.

58 Pfuhlmann B, Franzek E, Beckmann H. Absence of a subgroup of chronic schizophrenia in monozygotic twins. Consequences for considerations on the pathogenesis of schizophrenic psychoses. *Eur Arch Psychiatry Clin Neurosci.* 1999;249(1):50–4.

59 Beckmann H, Franzek E. The genetic heterogeneity of "schizophrenia." *World J Biol Psychiatry.* 2000;1(1):35–41.

60 Stober G, Kocher I, Franzek E, Beckmann H. First-trimester maternal gestational infection and cycloid psychosis. *Acta Psychiatr Scand.* 1997;96(5):319–24.

61 Hagberg H, Gressens P, Mallard C. Inflammation during fetal and neonatal life: Implications for neurologic and neuropsychiatric disease in children and adults. *Ann Neurol.* 2012;71(4):444–57.

62 Franzek E, Becker T, Hofmann E, Flohl W, Stober G, Beckmann H. Is computerized tomography ventricular abnormality related to cycloid psychosis? *Biol Psychiatry.* 1996;40(12):1255–66.

63 Falkai P, Bogerts B, Klieser E, Mooren I, Waters H, Schlüter U. Cranial computed tomography in schizophrenics, patients with cycloid psychosis and controls. In: Beckmann H, Neumärker K (eds.). *Endogenous Psychoses: Leonhard's Implication on Modern Psychiatry.* Berlin: Ullstein-Mosby; 1995. p. 213–15.

64 Falkai P, Franzek E, Schneider T. Neuroradiologische Befunde basierend auf der Nosologie von Leonhard. *Nervenarzt.* 1996;67(suppl. 1):89.

65 Hoffler J, Braunig P, Kruger S, Ludvik M. Morphology according to cranial computed tomography of first-episode cycloid psychosis and its long-term-course: Differences compared to schizophrenia. *Acta Psychiatr Scand.* 1997;96(3):184–87.

66 Bartsch A, Seybold S, Koeck P, Jabs B, Fallgatter A, Reiners C, et al. Cycloid psychoses in video-demonstrations and 99mTc-HMPAO-SPECT findings. *World J Biol Psychiatry.* 2001; 97(2):97.

67 Köck P, Bartsch A, Seybold S, Müller T, Jabs B, Stöber G, et al. Cerebrale Tc-99 m-HMPAO-SPECT bei zykloiden und chronisch schizophrenen Psychosen im Akutstadium und nach Teilremission. *J Funct Mol Imaging.* 2001;40(A81).

68 Strik WK, Fallgatter AJ, Stoeber G, Franzek E, Beckmann H. Specific P300 features in patients with cycloid psychosis. *Acta Psychiatr Scand.* 1996;94(6):471–76.

69 Walther S, Horn H, Koschorke P, Muller TJ, Strik W. Increased motor activity in cycloid psychosis compared to schizophrenia. *World J Biol Psychiatry.* 2009;10(4 Pt 3):746–51.

70 Strik WK. Anxiety as a primary symptom in cycloid psychosis. *CNS Spectr.* 2000; 5(9):47–51.

71 Marneros A, Pillmann F. *Acute and Transient Psychoses.* Cambridge: Cambridge University Press; 2004.

72 Ehlis AC, Zielasek J, Herrmann MJ, Ringel T, Jacob C, Fallgatter AJ. Beneficial effect of atypical antipsychotics on prefrontal brain function in acute psychotic disorders. *Eur Arch Psychiatry Clin Neurosci.* 2005;255(5):299–307.

73 Thomas P, Alptekin K, Gheorghe M, Mauri M, Olivares JM, Riedel M. Management of patients presenting with acute psychotic episodes of schizophrenia. *CNS Drugs.* 2009; 23(3):193–212.

74 Gaebel W, Weinmann S, Sartorius N, Rutz W, McIntyre JS. Schizophrenia practice guidelines: International survey and comparison. *Br J Psychiatry.* 2005;187:248–55.

75 Little JD, Ungvari GS, McFarlane J. Successful ECT in a case of Leonhard's cycloid psychosis. *J ECT.* 2000;16(1):62–7.

76 Montgomery JH, Vasu D. The use of electroconvulsive therapy in atypical psychotic presentations: A case review. *Psychiatry.* 2007;4(10):30–9.

CHAPTER 5

Borderline personality disorder

John M. Oldham

Senior Vice President and Chief of Staff, The Menninger Clinic, Barbara and Corbin Robertson Jr. Endowed Chair for Personality Disorders, Professor and Executive Vice Chair, Menninger Department of Psychiatry and Behavioral Sciences, Baylor College of Medicine, Houston, Texas, U.S.

Phenomenology

Borderline personality disorder (BPD) is a prevalent and disabling condition characterized by emotion dysregulation and interpersonal instability. In the early days when the term began to appear in the clinical literature, BPD was thought to be "on the border" between the psychoses and what were formerly called the neuroses [1]. In the United States, however, the criteria defining BPD that were included in the third edition of the Diagnostic and Statistical Manual of Mental Disorders (DSM-III) [2] of the American Psychiatric Association (APA), published in 1980, characterized BPD as a disorder of emotion dysregulation and impulse dyscontrol, and schizotypal PD was recognized as the PD aligning more closely with the psychoses. These distinctions have remained applicable in DSM-IV [3] and in DSM-5, [4] and BPD might more accurately be thought of as a condition close to the border of the mood disorders and the impulse control disorders.

To make a DSM-5 BPD diagnosis, at least five of nine criteria must be present; abbreviated versions of these nine criteria are shown on Table 5.1. Since DSM-5 utilizes a polythetic system and any five of the nine criteria suffice to establish a BPD diagnosis, considerable heterogeneity is inevitable; it has been estimated that there can be 256 different criteria combinations in the case of BPD [5]. In addition to extensive heterogeneity of the borderline diagnosis, co-morbid conditions are common in patients with BPD. In one representative study, about 84 percent of patients with BPD also met criteria for at least one "Axis I" disorder (a term reflecting the multi-axial diagnostic system of DSM-III and DSM-IV, which was abandoned in DSM-5), principally mood disorders, anxiety disorders, and substance use disorders [6].

Patients with BPD typically have severe impairment in functioning. In addition to emotion dysregulation and impulsivity, self-injurious behavior is

Troublesome Disguises: Managing Challenging Disorders in Psychiatry, Second Edition.
Edited by Dinesh Bhugra and Gin S. Malhi.
© 2015 John Wiley & Sons, Ltd. Published 2015 by John Wiley & Sons, Ltd.

Table 5.1 DSM-IV diagnosis of borderline personality
disorder (at least 5 must be present).

Fear of abandonment
Difficult interpersonal relationships
Uncertainty about self-image or identity
Impulsive behavior
Self-injurious behavior
Emotional changeability or hyperactivity
Feelings of emptiness
Difficulty controlling intense anger
Transient suspiciousness or "disconnectedness"

common, and suicide risk is significant. It has been estimated that in clinical populations, between 8 and 10 percent of BPD patients die by suicide; risk factors include co-morbid mood or substance use disorders, history of sexual abuse, and family history of suicide [7]. Among emerging findings about other characteristics of patients with BPD are the presence of significantly disturbed sleep profiles [8], and possible alterations in inflammatory mechanisms [9].

Neurobiology

Patterns of family transmission of BPD have been identified for some time [10], and there has been growing interest in the heritability of BPD [11–15]. The estimated heritability of personality disorders as a group is in the 20–40 percent range, comparable to anxiety disorders and depressive disorders, and the heritability of BPD itself is estimated to be between 30 and 40 percent [16].

New technologies have been increasingly utilized to explore patterns of neuropathology and pathophysiology in all patients with brain disorders, including those with BPD. Volumetric abnormalities in limbic structures have been reported in patients with BPD, particularly reduced volume in the hippocampus and the amygdala [17]; a question has been raised, however, about whether these changes are accounted for by BPD itself or by co-morbid conditions such as post-traumatic stress disorder [18], but recent work suggests that the volume reductions are "candidate endophenotypes" for BPD and not secondary to co-morbid pathology [19]. One important hypothesis arising from neuroimaging studies is that the normally robust connectivity between the amygdala and the prefrontal cortex, thought to facilitate inhibitory control over the amygdala, is compromised in patients with BPD, hence their frequent failure to down-regulate amygdala-generated emotionality in response to aversive stimuli [20]. This pattern of emotion dysregulation has been observed and described clinically, and it has been documented using "ecological momentary assessment" technology, involving "real-time" computer-based assessment of affective states [21]. Earlier work had revealed that borderline patients show greater activation than controls particularly in the left amygdala when viewing facial expressions [22].

There has been recent interest in the role of neuropeptides in borderline pathology. Oxytocin has been shown to enhance the accuracy of recognition of facial expressions [23], and oxytocin levels have been reported to be low in BPD patients [24]. In one study of women with BPD, low oxytocin levels were suggested to have resulted from traumatic childhood experiences, particularly emotional neglect and abuse [25], and indeed a striking difference has been shown between borderline patients and controls with respect to interpersonal trust after the administration of intranasal oxytocin (enhancing trust in control subjects but not in borderlines) [26]. Similarly, a profound incapacity for borderline patients to maintain cooperation with a partner in an experimental paradigm has been demonstrated, correlated with altered activity of the anterior insular cortex in BPD patients, suggesting that the norms used in perception of social gestures are pathologically perturbed or missing altogether in patients with BPD [27]. These findings are particularly compelling in light of the growing recognition of disruptions in the attachment process early in the lives of many children and adolescents who later develop borderline pathology [28]. Gunderson has emphasized the importance of interpersonal hypersensitivity in borderline patients [29], and Koenigsberg has summarized work describing disturbed attachment styles in borderline patients as either "preoccupied" or "unresolved" [30].

Theoretical models of borderline pathogenesis and symptom formation

Figure 5.1 portrays a sequential theoretical model of the pathogenesis of borderline personality disorder [7], reflecting the bidirectional nature of heritable risk and disruptions in attachment, leading to instability of interpersonal relationships as the "signature" disturbance characteristic of borderline patients.

Figure 5.2 portrays a theoretical model of symptom expression in borderline patients, reflecting the vulnerability conferred by heritable risk factors in these patients. This vulnerability is activated by stressful stimuli, generally in the social and interpersonal realm, leading to highly symptomatic states of extreme distress. Behavior during these periods of stress, though listed as symptomatic criteria for borderline personality disorder, can actually be thought of as compensatory efforts to achieve relief, such as dissociative states, self-injurious behavior, or suicidality.

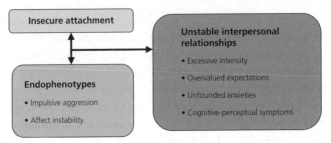

Figure 5.1 Sequential theoretical model of BPD pathogenesis.

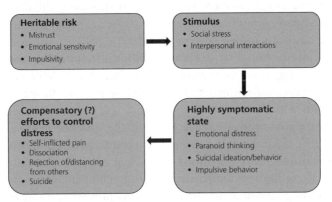

Figure 5.2 Theoretical model of BPD symptom expression.

Longitudinal studies

There have been a number of longitudinal studies focusing on clinical populations that included borderline patients, but these historical studies were based primarily on non-standardized clinical observations [31–34]. Two methodologically rigorous, independent longitudinal studies have more recently yielded important data about the course of borderline patients over time: the Collaborative Longitudinal Personality Disorders Study (CLPS) [35] and the McLean Study of Adult Development (MSAD) [36]. Both multi-year programs are naturalistic follow-along studies utilizing standardized assessment instruments at regular intervals, similar to highly informative studies of schizophrenia and also of depression. In order to evaluate whether personality disorders are "stable and enduring over time" as stated in DSM-IV (and in DSM-5), a definition of remission was needed. A rigorous threshold was established to define remission in the CLPS protocol. In order to enroll in the study, for example, patients with borderline personality disorder had to endorse at least 5 out of 9 DSM-IV criteria. In order to be classified as in remission, patients had to endorse no more than 2 criteria for at least one continuous year. Surprisingly, at the end of 10 years, about 85 percent of the patients with borderline personality disorder were in remission utilizing this definition. However, analysis of the Global

Assessment of Functioning revealed that functional remission was much slower to appear [35]. Similar findings were shown in the MSAD study. At the 16-year point, a range of 78–99 percent of borderline patients achieved remission (in this case defined as no longer meeting the study criteria for a period of at least 2 years), although only 40–60 percent showed restoration of good social and vocational functioning [36]. Generally, these findings have been interpreted to suggest that over time, borderline patients "shed" some of the reactive, stress-related symptoms but that trait-based defining criteria are much slower to resolve; such conclusions support the view that the DSM-IV defining criteria represent hybrid groupings of symptoms and traits. Another report from the CLPS data reinforces that view, in which the 10-year rank-order corrected stability of personality traits was 0.60–0.90, compared to 0.25–0.65 for DSM-IV-defined personality disorders themselves [37].

Treatment

An evidence-based practice guideline for the treatment of patients with borderline personality disorder was developed by the American Psychiatric Association and published in 2001, which recommended psychotherapy as the primary, or core, treatment for the disorder, augmented by adjunctive symptom-targeted pharmacotherapy [38]. At that time, randomized controlled trials had been published, demonstrating the effectiveness of dialectical behavior therapy (DBT) [39] and mentalization-based therapy (MBT) [40] for borderline patients. Subsequently, evidence-based guidelines have been developed in The Netherlands [41], the United Kingdom [42], and most recently in Australia [43]. There is remarkable consistency in the recommendations of all of these guidelines, sustaining the emphasis on psychotherapy as the primary treatment for borderline personality disorder. In addition to DBT and MBT, randomized controlled trials have been published demonstrating the effectiveness of other forms of psychotherapy, including cognitive behavior therapy [44], schema-focused therapy [45], transference-focused therapy [46], and systems training for emotional predictability and problem solving [47]. Adjunctive pharmacotherapy remains useful, though new studies suggest that time-limited use of mood stabilizers or second generation antipsychotics may be helpful, perhaps more so than selective serotonin reuptake inhibitors, which were tentatively prioritized in the early APA report.

DSM-5 alternative model

Since the publication of DSM-IV, a consensus has emerged that personality disorders are best conceptualized dimensionally, since there are many problems with the more traditional categorical disease model [48, 49]. It has been argued that many psychiatric conditions are characterized by symptoms that are also normally distributed in the population, such as major depression, autism, and especially the personality disorders, and that the DSM-IV personality disorders may need a "big re-design" [50, 51]. Among the problems that have been identified with the DSM-IV categorical system are excessive co-occurrence of disorders; extensive heterogeneity within categories; and arbitrary distinctions between normal personality, abnormal traits, and clear disorders. A goal of the DSM-5 Personality and Personality Disorders Work Group of the APA was to explore the possibility of a dimensional approach to the personality disorders.

A new model for the personality disorders was eventually developed by the Work Group that might best be described as a hybrid dimensional and categorical diagnostic system. This new approach is included in Section III (the section on "Emerging Measures and Models") of DSM-5, as an Alternative Model for Personality Disorders. (See Skodol et al. [52] for a review of the data supporting the Alternative Model.) The generic defining features of a personality disorder were simplified into two criteria, to reflect impairment in personality functioning (at the moderate or greater level, with moderate as level 2 on a 4-point scale [a threshold arrived at empirically]), and the presence of pathological personality traits. The first criterion, impairment in personality functioning, is specified as impairment in self-functioning (in terms of identity and self-direction) and impairment in interpersonal functioning (in terms of empathy and intimacy). The second criterion, the presence of pathological personality traits, is specified as pathology in any of five trait domains: negative affectivity, detachment, antagonism, disinhibition, and psychoticism. The Alternative Model includes detailed descriptions of the nature of the impairment in functioning and of the pathological personality traits for six personality disorders: antisocial, avoidant, borderline, narcissistic, obsessive-compulsive, and schizotypal. Reviews of the literature led the Work Group to conclude that the remaining four DSM-IV personality disorders (dependent, histrionic, paranoid, and schizoid) were best understood as types of pathological personality traits, and they can be diagnosed (along with many other variations) as "Personality Disorder, Trait-Specified."

Using the DSM-5 Alternative Model, borderline personality disorder is diagnosed by the presence of moderate or greater impairment in personality functioning, identified by the presence of difficulties in at least two of the following areas: (1) identity, (2) self-direction, (3) empathy, and (4) intimacy (Criterion A), and narrative text specifies the nature of typical impairment in each area, in borderline patients. In addition, the presence of four or more pathological personality traits must be identified in the trait domains of negative affectivity, disinhibition, and antagonism (one of the four must be either in the domain of disinhibition or the domain of antagonism). Narrative text is also provided in the Level of Personality Functioning Scale to guide clinicians in assessing whether the impairment in functioning is at the moderate or greater level.

Some concerns were raised during the DSM-5 development process by experienced clinicians that the draft model being considered for the personality disorders would be too complex for clinical use. In fact, however, the number of items required for DSM-5 personality disorder diagnoses was reduced by 43 percent, compared to DSM-IV, and in the DSM-5 Field Trials, high percentages of clinicians found the new model moderately, very, or extremely useful compared to DSM-IV. In fact, the percentages of clinicians reporting these rankings were higher for the personality disorders than for schizophrenia spectrum and other psychotic disorders, bipolar and related disorders, any depressive disorders, and any anxiety disorders. Additionally, in a study involving 334 clinicians, in 14 out of 18 comparisons the clinicians found the DSM-5 model to be more clinically useful than DSM-IV [53]. Finally, it interesting to note that the pooled test-retest reliability for BPD using the Alternative Model showed an intraclass Kappa of 0.54, in the "good" range, and better than schizophrenia, mild neurocognitive disorder, and major depressive disorder [54].

Conclusion

A great deal of progress has been made in our understanding of patients who suffer from borderline personality disorder. Early unfortunate notions that these patients were willfully "difficult" were based on lack of recognition of the heritable, developmental, and neurobiological underpinnings of the condition. Substantial advances in our knowledge have led to evidence-based practice guidelines that demonstrate many forms of effective treatment for BPD, and longitudinal studies have shown that over time, borderline patients become far less symptomatic. Functional impairment and disability, however, are less likely to resolve at the same pace, and these areas need to be primary priorities for treatment.

References

1 Gunderson JG. (2009) Borderline personality disorder: ontogeny of a diagnosis. *American Journal of Psychiatry* 166, 530–539.
2 American Psychiatric Association. (1980) *Diagnostic and Statistical Manual of Mental Disorders, 3rd Edition.* American Psychiatric Association, Washington, DC.
3 American Psychiatric Association. (1994) *Diagnostic and Statistical Manual of Mental Disorders, 4th Edition.* American Psychiatric Association, Washington, DC.

4 American Psychiatric Association. (2013) *Diagnostic and Statistical Manual of Mental Disorders*, 5th *Edition*. American Psychiatric Association, Arlington, VA.

5 Johansen M, Karterud S, Pedersen G, et al. (2004) An investigation of the prototypic validity of the borderline DSM-IV construct. *Acta Psychiatrica Scandinavica* 109, 289–298.

6 Lenzenweger MF, Lane MC, Loranger AW, Kessler RC. (2007) DSM-IV personality disorders in the national comorbidity survey replication. *Biological Psychiatry* 62(6), 553–564.

7 Oldham JM. (2006) Borderline personality disorder and suicidality. *American Journal of Psychiatry* 163(1), 20–26.

8 Fleischer M, Schäfer M, Coogan A, Häßler F, Thome J. (2012) Sleep disturbances and circadian CLOCK genes in borderline personality disorder. *Journal of Neural Transmission* 199(10), 1105–1110.

9 Diaz-Marsa M, MacDowell KS, Guemes I, et al. (2012) Activation of the cholinergic anti-inflammatory system in peripheral blood mononuclear cells from patients with borderline personality disorder. *Journal of Psychiatric Research* 46(12), 1610–1617.

10 Loranger AW, Oldham JM, Tulis EH. (1982) Familial transmission of DSM III borderline personality disorder. *Archives of General Psychiatry* 39, 795–799.

11 Joyce PR, McHugh PC, McKenzie JM, et al. (2006) A dopamine transporter polymorphism is a risk factor for borderline personality disorder in depressed patients. *Psychological Medicine* 36, 807–813.

12 Kendler KS, Myers J, Reichborn-Kjennerud T. (2011) Borderline personality disorder traits and their relationship with dimensions of normative personality: a web-based cohort and twin study. *Acta Psychiatrica Scandinavica* 123, 349–359.

13 Ni X, Sicard T, Bulgin N, et al. (2007) Monoamine oxidase A gene is associated with borderline personality disorder. *Psychiatric Genetics* 17, 153–157.

14 Ni X, Chan D, Chan K, et al. (2009) Serotonin genes and gene-gene interactions in borderline personality disorder in a matched case-control study. *Progress in Neuro-Psychopharmacology & Biological Psychiatry* 33, 128–133.

15 Wagner S, Baskaya Ö, Dahmen N, et al. (2010) Modulatory role of the brain-derived neurotrophic factor Val66Met polymorphism on the effects of serious life events on impulsive aggression in borderline personality disorder. *Genes, Brain and Behavior* 9, 97–102.

16 Kendler KS. (2011) *The genetic epidemiology of personality disorders: Results from the Norwegian Institute of Public Health Twin Registry. Presented at the Annual Meeting of the American College of Psychiatrists*, San Francisco, California.

17 O'Neill A, Frodl T (2012) Brain structure and function in borderline personality disorder. *Brain Structure and Function* 217, 767–782.

18 Schmahl C, Berne K, Krause A, et al. (2009) Hippocampus and amygdala volumes in patients with borderline personality disorder with or without posttraumatic stress disorder. *Journal of Psychiatry and Neuroscience* 34, 289–295.

19 Ruocco A, Amirthavasagam S, Zakzanis KK. (2012) Amygdala and hippocampal volume reductions as candidate endophenotypes for borderline personality disorder: a meta-analysis of magnetic resonance imaging studies. *Psychiatry Research: Neuroimaging* 201, 245–252.

20 New A, Hazlett EA, Buchsbaum MS, et al. (2007) Amygdala-prefrontal disconnection in borderline personality disorder. *Neuropsychopharmacology* 32, 1629–1640.

21 Santangelo P, Bohus M, Ubner-Priemer UW. (2012) Ecological momentary assessment in borderline personality disorder: a review of recent findings and methodological challenges. *Journal of Personality Disorders* published ahead of print. Doi: 10.1521/pedi_2012_26_067.

22 Donegan NH, Sanislow CA, Blumberg HP, et al. (2003) Amygdala hyperreactivity in borderline personality disorder: implications for emotional dysregulation. *Biological Psychiatry* 54(11), 1284–1293.

23 Domes G, Heinrichs M, Gläscher J, et al. (2007) Oxytocin attenuates amygdala responses to emotional faces regardless of valence. *Biological Psychiatry* 62(10), 1187–1190.

24 Stanley B, Siever LJ. (2010) The interpersonal dimension of borderline personality disorder: toward a neuropeptide model. *American Journal of Psychiatry* 167, 24–39.

25 Bertsch K, Schmidinger I, Neumann I, Herpertz SC. (2013) Reduced plasma oxytocin levels in female patients with borderline personality disorder. *Hormones and Behavior* 63(3), 424–429.

26 Bartz J, Simeon D, Hamilton H, et al. (2010) Oxytocin can hinder trust and cooperation in borderline personality disorder. *Social Cognitive and Affective Neuroscience* 6(5), 556–563.

27 King-Casas B, Sharp C, Lomax-Bream L, et al. (2008) The rupture and repair of cooperation in borderline personality disorder. *Science* 321, 806–810.

28 Fonagy P, Bateman A, Lorenzini N, Campbell C. (2014) Development, attachment and childhood experiences. In: Oldham JM, Skodol AE, Bender DS (eds.) *American Psychiatric Press Textbook of Personality Disorders*, 2nd Edition. American Psychiatric Press, Arlington, VA.

29 Gunderson JG, Lyons-Ruth K. (2008) BPD's interpersonal hypersensitivity phenotype: a gene-environment-developmental model. *Journal of Personality Disorders* 22(1), 22–41.

30 Koenigsberg HW. (2011) *Update on the Neurobiology of Borderline Personality Disorder. Presented at the Annual Meeting of the American College of Psychiatrists*, San Francisco, California.

31 McGlashan TH. (1986) The Chestnut Lodge follow-up study: long-term outcome of borderline personalities. *Archives of General Psychiatry* 43, 20–30.

32 Stone M (1990). *The Fate of Borderline Patients: Successful Outcome and Psychiatric Practice*. Guilford Press, New York, NY.

33 Paris J, Zweig-Frank H. (2001) A 27-year follow-up of patients with borderline personality disorder. *Comprehensive Psychiatry* 42(6), 482–487.

34 Wallerstein RS. (1989) The psychotherapy research project of the Menninger Foundation: an overview. *Journal of Consulting and Clinical Psychology* 57(2), 195–205.

35 Gunderson JG, Stout RL, McGlashan TH, et al. (2011) Ten-year course of borderline personality disorder: psychopathology and function from the Collaborative Longitudinal Personality Study. *Archives of General Psychiatry* 68, 827–837.

36 Zanarini MC, Frankenburg FR, Reich DB, Fitzmaurice G. (2012) Attainment and stability of sustained symptomatic remission and recovery among patients with borderline personality disorder and axis II comparison subjects: a 16-year prospective follow-up study. *American Journal of Psychiatry* 169, 476–483.

37 Hopwood CJ, Morey LC, Donnellan MB, et al. (2013) Ten-year rank-order stability of personality traits and disorders in a clinical sample. *Journal of Personality* 81, 335–344.

38 American Psychiatric Association. (2001) *Practice Guideline for the Treatment of Patients with Borderline Personality Disorder*. American Psychiatric Association, Washington, DC.

39 Linehan MM. (1993) *Cognitive-Behavioral Treatment of Borderline Personality Disorder*. Guilford Press, New York, NY.

40 Bateman A, Fonagy P. (2001) Treatment of borderline personality disorder with psycho-analytically oriented partial hospitalization: an 18-month follow-up. *American Journal of Psychiatry* 158, 36–42.

41 Trimbos Instituut. (2008) *Practice Guideline on Diagnosis and Treatment of Adult Patients with a Personality Disorder* [in Dutch]. Trimbos Instituut, Utrecht, The Netherlands.

42 National Collaborating Centre for Mental Health. (2009) *Borderline Personality Disorder: The NICE Guideline on Treatment and Management.* British Psychological Society and Royal College of Psychiatrists, London, United Kingdom.

43 National Health and Medical Research Council. (2013) *Clinical Practice Guideline for the Management of Borderline Personality Disorder.* National Health and Medical Research Council, Melbourne, Australia.

44 Davidson K, Tyrer P, Gumpley A, Tata P, et al. (2006) A randomized controlled trial of cognitive behavior therapy for borderline personality disorder: rationale for trial, method, and description of sample. *Journal of Personality Disorders* 20(5), 431–449.

45 Young J, Klosko J. (2005) Schema therapy. In Oldham JM, Skodol AE, Bender DS (eds.) *American Psychiatric Publishing Textbook of Personality Disorders.* American Psychiatric Publishing, Washington, DC, pp. 289–306.

46 Clark JF, Levy KN, Lenzenweger MF, Kernberg OF. (2007) Evaluating three treatments for borderline personality disorder: a multiwave study. *American Journal of Psychiatry* 164, 922–928.

47 Blum N, St. John D, Pfohl B, et al. (2008) Systems Training for Emotional Predictability and Problem Solving (STEPPS) for outpatients with borderline personality disorder: a randomized controlled trial and 1-year follow-up. *American Journal of Psychiatry* 165, 468–478.

48 Rounsaville BJ, Alarcon RD, Andrews G, et al. (2002) Basic nomenclature issues for DSM-V. In Kupfer DJ, First MB, Regier DE (eds.) *A Research Agenda for DSM-V.* American Psychiatric Association, Washington, DC, pp. 1–29.

49 Widiger TA, Simonsen E (2006) Alternative dimensional models of personality disorder: finding a common ground. In Widiger TA, Simonsen E, Sirovatka PJ, Regier DA (eds.) *Dimensional Models of Personality Disorders: Refining the Research Agenda for DSM-V.* American Psychiatric Press, Arlington, VA, pp. 1–22.

50 Hyman SH. (2010) The diagnosis of mental disorders: the problem of reification. *Annual Review of Clinical Psychology* 6, 155–179.

51 Kendler KS, Parnas J (eds.). (2012) *Philosophical Issues in Psychiatry II.* Oxford University Press, New York, NY.

52 Skodol AE, Bender DS, Oldham JM. (in press) An alternative model for personality disorders: DSM-5 Section III and beyond. In Oldham JM, Skodol AE, Bender DS (eds.) *American Psychiatric Press Textbook of Personality Disorders,* 2nd Edition. American Psychiatric Press, Arlington, VA.

53 Morey LC, Skodol AE, Oldham JM. (2014) Clinician Judgments of Clinical Utility: A Comparison of DSM-IV-TR Personality Disorders and the Alternative Model for DSM-5 Personality Disorders. *Journal of Abnormal Psychology* 123(2), 398–405.

54 Regier DA, Narrow WE, Clarke DE, et al. (2013) DSM-5 field trials in the United States and Canada, Part II: test-retest reliability of selected categorical diagnoses. *American Journal of Psychiatry* 170(1), 59–70.

CHAPTER 6

Recurrent self-harm

Rohan Borschmann[1] and Paul Moran[2]

[1]Clinical Psychologist, Institute of Psychiatry, King's College London, London, UK
[2]Reader/Honorary Consultant Psychiatrist, Institute of Psychiatry, King's College London, London, UK

What is self-harm?

Self-harm is an act with a non-fatal outcome in which an individual deliberately initiates behaviour (such as self-cutting), or ingests a substance, an illicit drug or non-ingestible substance or object, with the intention of causing harm to themselves [1]. Considerable variation is observed within this range of behaviours, and self-harm often includes self-cutting, overdosing, burning, scalding, swallowing dangerous objects or substances, picking/scratching, biting, hair pulling, head-banging, bruising, or any combination of these [2, 3].

While any act of self-harm may or may not be associated with the intent to die, non-suicidal self-injury (NSSI) is defined as an act of self-harm that is deliberate, contains no desire to die, and is for purposes not socially sanctioned such as tattooing or piercing the body for adornment [4, 5]. While NSSI can provide short-term relief from distress, it can have negative emotional, physical, and social consequences [4]. Emotionally, it can evoke more complex feelings of guilt and shame toward oneself [6]. Physically, it can lead to infection, scarring, or reduced functioning. Socially, it can be associated with stigma and exclusion from peer groups, which may contribute to the cycle starting again [4]. Despite being extensively researched (mostly in North America), NSSI does not appear as a disorder in either the *Diagnostic and Statistical Manual of Mental Disorders* (4th edition; DSM-IV) or the *International Statistical Classification of Diseases and Related Health Problems* (10th ed.; ICD-10) and is not a diagnostic criterion of any current depressive or anxious disorder. This lack of nosological recognition is to be acknowledged in the forthcoming DSM-V, with NSSI being classified as a syndrome in its own right [4], a move that has received a mixed reception [7, 8]. Critics of the NSSI construct have highlighted the fact that, despite the apparent lack of suicidal intent in people

Troublesome Disguises: Managing Challenging Disorders in Psychiatry, Second Edition.
Edited by Dinesh Bhugra and Gin S. Malhi.
© 2015 John Wiley & Sons, Ltd. Published 2015 by John Wiley & Sons, Ltd.

engaging in NSSI, it is strongly correlated with subsequent suicide [8]. For example, self-cutting (the most common method of NSSI) is a behavior that is often regarded as being of limited seriousness by clinical services [8]; however, research suggests that self-cutting resulting in hospital treatment is actually associated with a greater risk of eventual suicide than self-poisoning in both adults [9] and adolescents [10].

Many acts of body modification or destruction of one's bodily tissue have cultural or social meaning and are not linked to a desire to die or to relieve distress (or even to experience any pain). In the Western world, such behaviours may include tattooing, piercing on the head or body, and practices such as stretching one's earlobes as a display of bodily art. At the more extreme end, it has been documented that native tribesmen of the Ivory Coast plunge knives several inches into their abdomens during New Year celebrations in the belief that bad spirits will be driven away as a result of this act [5]. In some Pacific Island tribes, it is not uncommon for relatives of the newly deceased to engage in acts of self-mutilation (including cutting off their fingertips, extracting teeth, tattooing their tongues, and/or cutting off their ears) as a mark of respect for the deceased [5]. Despite the severity (and potential risk of accidental death) of these behaviours, it would be inappropriate to give them a psychiatric label as they are in keeping with local cultural norms. The remainder of this chapter will be focusing on self-harm that is not socially sanctioned and does not have cultural significance for the individual.

Prevalence and correlates of self-harm in the general population

Self-harm occurs in all cultures and is especially prevalent in young people, a group in whom rates of self-harm have risen in recent years [11, 12]. Approximately 4 percent of general adult populations report engaging in self-harm [6], and it is common among adolescents [13–15]. and college students [16–18]. Peak onset of self-harm coincides with the onset of puberty [19]. and about 10 percent of teenagers report having engaged in some form of self-harm [20], although longitudinal research indicates that 90 percent of teenagers who self-harm stop the behaviour as they enter into adulthood [21]. In the general population, self-harm is generally more common among women than men; among lesbian, gay, and bisexual people [22, 23]; among those living in areas of socio-economic deprivation [24]; and in those identifying with "Gothic" subculture [12, 25]. In the UK, Asian women are at higher risk of self-harm compared to their white counterparts, but there have been few studies comparing rates of self-harm among people of Caribbean, African, and other minority ethnic groups. The World Health Organization (WHO) reported that self-inflicted injuries accounted for approximately 800,000 deaths worldwide in 2001 [26]. Prevention of self-harm (along with suicide) is now included in health policy initiatives in several countries and is part of the Health-For-All targets of the WHO [27]. Self-harm is associated with substantial costs to health services, as it often results in admissions to emergency departments and subsequent psychiatric or general admissions, in addition to loss of productivity [28, 29]. In the UK, self-harm is one of the most common reasons for acute admission to hospital [30, 31], accounting for up to 200,000 hospital attendances each year in the UK [29], 40–50 percent of which are repeat episodes [32]. The vast majority of hospital admissions for self-harm relate to overdoses [33].

Why do people engage in recurrent self-harm?

Self-harm is not an illness; rather, it is a behavioural disorder that should alert clinicians to one or more underlying emotional problems. The functions of self-harm are extremely varied and include both internal and external factors [5, 34–36], including (but not limited to):
• Emotional regulation (i.e., to alleviate acute negative feelings)
• Self-punishment
• Sensation-seeking
• Distraction
• Expressing anger
• Attempting to "feel something"
• Attempting to escape from an intolerable situation
• Attempting to communicate with, or to influence, others
• To assert one's autonomy or establish a boundary between self and other
• To generate excitement

   A person who self-harms repeatedly might not always do so for the same reason each time, nor by the same method. Thus, assumptions about intent should not be made on the basis of a previous pattern of self-harm; each act must be assessed separately to determine the motivation behind it [37]. Paradoxically, the purpose of some acts of self-harm is to preserve life; a concept many health professionals may find difficult to understand [37]. The precipitants of self-harm are extremely varied [38–40], although common problems preceding acts of self-harm typically include social problems, difficulties with a partner or family member, finances, physical health, employment or studies, housing, or alcohol or drug misuse [25, 41, 42]. For many people, self-harm is a habitual coping mechanism and there is some evidence that these behaviours often continue even after personal problems have been resolved [43, 44]. It can provide immediate short-term relief, but often at considerable cost (such as permanent scars or damage to internal organs).

Furthermore, individuals often report more than one motivation for self-harming and different forms of self-harm can serve different functions [22]. For example, while taking an overdose may provide escape from a difficult situation, cutting oneself may serve to regulate dysphoric affect [36]. Rodham and colleagues [45] reported that self-cutters think about self-harming for a shorter period than self-poisoners before initiating the behaviour. They suggested that taking an overdose requires more time and planning than cutting oneself and, as such, may indicate a more serious intent and be more likely to require medical attention [45]. Recent research by Hawton and colleagues [46] has suggested that different forms of self-harm place people at different levels of risk for subsequent completed suicide, with cutting paradoxically posing a greater risk than self-poisoning.

Clinicians' attitudes toward self-harm

Individuals who self-harm are often viewed in a negative light by healthcare staff, particularly in emergency settings [47–52]. In turn, people who self-harm frequently describe their contact with health services as being difficult and characterised by ignorance, negative attitudes, and even punitive behaviour by health professionals [53]. One of the main reasons cited for such attitudes is that emergency practitioners do not always have sufficient time or resources to provide appropriate care for individuals presenting with self-inflicted injuries, leading to frustration toward these individuals [54]. and an extreme, punishing care (e.g., suturing without sufficient local anesthetic) [55]. Previous NICE guidelines regarding the treatment and management of self-harm [53] acknowledged that the experience of care for people who self-harm is often unacceptable and included recommendations about how members staff should relate to these individuals.

How often is there a "formal" underlying psychiatric disorder?

Most people who attend an emergency department following an act of self-harm will meet criteria for one or more psychiatric diagnoses at the time they are assessed [56]. The ICD-10 includes a diagnostic criterion for emotionally unstable personality disorder (EUPD) of "recurrent threats or acts of self-harm" [57]. Due to the very nature of the disorder, individuals with EUPD (otherwise classified as borderline personality disorder [BPD] in DSM-IV) are at an increased and ongoing risk of crises and self-harming behaviours [58–60]. Notwithstanding, the majority of individuals who engage in self-harming behaviour do not meet diagnostic criteria for EUDP. In addition, as many as a third of individuals with BPD do not self-harm [61]. On the other hand, depression and anxiety are very common correlates of self-harm [62, 63]. as are drug and alcohol misuse [64, 65].

What is the prognosis for people who repeatedly self-harm?

Self-harm is strongly associated with subsequent suicide [66]. In the UK, research has shown that approximately 1 percent of individuals presenting at emergency departments following an episode of self-harm go on to commit suicide within a year, with this figure rising to 3–5 percent within 10 years, 8.5 percent within 22 years and 10 percent across the lifespan [67, 68]. A prospective study of nearly 8,000 casualty attenders presenting following an episode of self-harm found that at 4-year follow-up, there was a 30-fold increase in suicide risk in the attenders compared with the general population [9]. Suicide rates were highest within the first 6 months after the index self-harm episode. For every completed suicide in the UK, it is estimated that 30 acts of self-harm take place [69] and, following an act of self-harm, the rate of suicide increases to between 50 and 100 times the rate of suicide in the general population [66, 70]. Approximately half of all people who commit suicide have a history of self-harm, with approximately 20–25 percent having had an episode within the preceding year [68]. As well having an increased risk of suicide, people who present to emergency departments after self-harm are at subsequent increased risk of both accidental death and also death from natural causes [71]. They are more likely to have compromised physical health and they experience a reduced life expectancy with disease of the circulatory and digestive systems being major contributors to years of life lost [72].

Economic costs

Self-harm is associated with significant economic costs to health services and society in general. Extrapolating from data gathered from three clinical centres in the UK, Hawton and colleagues [29] estimated that there were 220,000 episodes of self-harm dealt with by hospitals in England each year, with 40–50 percent of self-harm hospital episodes being related to repeat episodes [32]. Approximately 15 percent of individuals presenting at an emergency department following self-harm will present again within 12 months and even more will self-harm again without presenting [73]. As one might expect, recurrent self-harm has a cumulative effect on service costs, with the number of self-harm episodes being correlated with increased healthcare and social services costs [74]. The indirect costs of self-harm have not been quantified; however, they include absenteeism from work [53] and considerable strain on families and careers [75].

Treatments

While there are no proven effective treatments for recurrent self-harm, many interventions and guidelines for managing and preventing repetition of self-harm have been proposed [37, 67, 68]. The common goals of such interventions typically include reducing the repetition of self-harm and the desire to self-harm, preventing suicide, and improving social functioning and quality of life, while exerting minimal adverse effects [76]. In routine clinical practice, service users will receive a wide range of psychological interventions that may or may not focus primarily on their self-harm; addressing self-harm may occur in series or in parallel with other interventions the service user is receiving. The 2011 NICE guidelines on the management and prevention of self-harm [37] state that the key aims and objectives in the treatment of an individual who has self-harmed should include the following:

- Prompt assessment of physical and psychological need
- Effective engagement of the individual
- Prompt measures to minimise pain and discomfort
- Implementation of harm reduction strategies
- Prompt and supportive psychosocial assessment (including a risk assessment)
- Provision of information about the long-term treatment, management and risks associated with self-harm
- Provision of 3–12 sessions of a psychological intervention specifically structured for people who self-harm with the specific aim of reducing self-harm; this intervention may include cognitive-behavioural, psychodynamic or problem-solving elements
- Psychological, pharmacological and psychosocial interventions for any associated conditions (including BPD, depression, bipolar disorder, or schizophrenia)
- Prompt referral for further psychological, social, and psychiatric assessment and treatment when necessary

The guideline also recommends producing an integrated and planned approach to the problems precipitating the self-harming behaviour. These include the development of a care plan and a risk management plan in conjunction with the individual, their family, carers, or significant others, with printed copies provided for the individual and other key healthcare professionals.

As far as the acute management of self-harm is concerned, any attendance to an emergency department following an episode of self-harm should result in a psychosocial assessment of needs, regardless of the method of self-harm used [77]. Despite the publication of national guidelines, there continues to be considerable variation in the level of support offered to individuals presenting at emergency departments after an episode of self-harm. For example, hospital services tend to offer less help to individuals who have cut themselves even though they are far more likely to repeat than those who have self-poisoned [77]. Effective interventions for managing self-harm must also take into account the subjective goals of the individual engaging in self-harm, as these may vary considerably [77]. For example, while one individual's goal might be to permanently stop self-harming, recover from any underlying psychiatric disorder, and have a better quality of life, another individual's goal might be simply to reduce the frequency of self-harm or even to reduce the harm associated with each act of self-harm [37]. For others, the goal might be to improve their level of social or occupational functioning. As such, interventions aimed at reducing the repetition of self-harm may focus on the actual behaviours themselves, or they may take a more holistic approach by examining an individual's close relationships, cognitions, and social factors [37]. Qualitative research indicates that service users may have a preference for specialist community-based interventions that acknowledge that the management of self-harm may not necessarily involve its prevention [78].

There is little convincing evidence for the efficacy of interventions for self-harm [68]. However, several promising candidate interventions exist and these can be divided into three main categories: psychological interventions, psychosocial service-level interventions, and pharmacological interventions. A brief summary of each follows.

Psychological interventions

The rationale for most psychological interventions is that most self-harm is precipitated by emotional difficulties and interventions. Most psychological interventions are aimed at improving social functioning as well as reducing self-harming behaviour [53, 79]. Self-harm is associated with a wide variety of psychological problems and, as such, psychological interventions need to take account of this complexity. One key aim of many psychological interventions is to reduce self-harm through understanding the specific contributing factors in each individual [37].

Problem-solving therapy

There is some evidence to suggest that problem-solving skills may serve as a protective factor for further repetition of self-harm [37]. In addition, people who self-harm are more like to have detectable deficits in problem-solving skills [80]. Therefore, psychological treatments that attempt to enhance problem-solving skills may positively impact on recurrent self-harm [37, 79]. For example, one randomised controlled trial (RCT) comparing the effectiveness of interpersonal problem-solving skills Training (IPSST) with brief problem-solving therapy [79]. found that although there was no significant difference in the proportion of participants self-harming at 1-year follow-up, IPSST was significantly more effective in interpersonal cognitive problem-solving, self-rated personal problem-solving ability, perceived ability to cope with ongoing problems and self-perception. Although the available evidence suggests that problem-solving therapies may offer promise, clear evidence of efficacy is required.

Cognitive behaviour therapy (CBT)

Cognitive behaviour therapy (CBT) is a structured, time-limited, individual talking therapy that is focused on problems concerning dysfunctional emotions, behaviours, and cognitions. It is one of the most extensively researched forms of psychotherapy and, although originally developed as a treatment for depression, it has been successfully adapted for an increasingly wide range of disorders and problematic behaviours, including recurrent self-harm [31, 81, 82]. A 2008 systematic review and meta-analysis examining the effectiveness of cognitive-behavioural interventions to reduce self-harm and suicide behaviour [83] indicated that there was some evidence to indicate that CBT can reduce such behaviour in the short-term, although high-quality trials are needed to replicate this finding.

Psychosocial service-level interventions

The management of recurrent self-harm can involve stand-alone psychological therapies such as those listed above, or adjunctive treatments that operate alongside standard care, such as contact by letter, postcard, telephone, or provision of crisis cards [84]. One goal of many psychosocial interventions—in addition to reducing the frequency of self-harm—is to improve contact and engagement with health services following presentation to an emergency department. This is important because adherence to outpatient treatment programmes after an episode of self-harm is typically poor [53].

Emergency card interventions

Some studies have examined the impact of providing people who have self-harmed with an "emergency card" (which allowed easy access to on-call professionals in the event of difficulties at all times of the day and night) on the repetition of self-harm [85, 86]. These emergency cards also permitted participants to be admitted to a psychiatric ward for a brief period if they so desired. In one RCT, Morgan and colleagues [86] conducted a study using a sample of 212 first-time self-harmers. The experimental group received a "green card" indicating that a trainee psychiatrist was available at all times of the day and night via telephone if the participant experienced any further problems over the following 12-month period. The green card also encouraged participants to seek help at an early stage, so long as no self-harm had already occurred on that occasion. Data obtained after 1 year showed a significant reduction of actual or seriously threatened DSH in the experimental group, who also made considerably fewer demands on medical and psychiatric services, when compared with controls. Participants in the control group also used more health services than those in the experimental group, although this difference did not reach statistical significance [86].

Telephone supportive contact

Other studies have examined the effects of telephone contact with a therapist compared with treatment as usual on the treatment of recurrent self-harm [87, 88] In these studies, participants all had a past history of self-harm and had made a recent suicide attempt requiring medical intervention. The goal of the intervention was to increase participants' motivation and engagement with treatment and also to reduce the frequency of self-harm. There was insufficient evidence to determine the clinical effectiveness between telephone contact plus routine care and treatment as usual in relation to the frequency of self-harm and no conclusions could be drawn due to the small evidence base.

Postcard interventions

Carter and colleagues [89] conducted an RCT designed to reduce the rate of repetition of hospital-treated deliberate self-poisoning. A total of 772 individuals referred from a hospital emergency department in Australia were included in the study, 378 in the experimental group and 394 in the control group. Individuals in the experimental group were sent eight postcards over a 1-year period following their attendance, while the control group received standard care only. At 1-year follow-up, there were no significant differences in the number of participants who had one or more repeat episodes of deliberate self-poisoning in the experimental group compared to those in the control group [89]. However, the number of repeat episodes per individual was significantly lower in the experimental group than the control group, as was the total number of days spent in hospital. This low-cost intervention (approximately $15 per participant for stationary and postage) was also associated with evidence of cost effectiveness, resulting from the associated reductions in service use. A recently published 5-year follow-up of the trial participants found that the postcard intervention was associated with a 50 percent reduction in self-poisoning events and a one-third reduction in psychiatric admissions over the 5-year period [90]. The authors noted that this translated into substantial savings in general hospital and psychiatric hospital bed days. The results of trials of other brief contact interventions are mixed with one trial confirming the positive findings from the Cater and colleagues study [91], one study showing no effect [92] and one study reporting an increase in self-harm following a brief contact intervention consisting of an information sheet and two telephone calls following a hospital presentation for self-harm [93].

Many other psychosocial interventions, such as admission to hospital or discharge to GP, nurse-led case management and intensive intervention plus outreach work have been examined in various trials [37, 68, 84, 94]. However, the majority of these trials have yielded insufficient evidence to determine clinically meaningful effects between interventions and standard care in the reduction of the proportion of participants who repeated self-harm [37] and considerable uncertainty therefore remains about which psychosocial interventions are the most effective for this population [37, 68].

Pharmacological interventions

At the time of writing, no pharmacological interventions have been clearly demonstrated to be of significant benefit in reducing rates of recurrent self-harm [76] and no drugs are currently licensed in the UK for the treatment of recurrent self-harm. The frequent use of pharmacological interventions for people who self-harm stems from the link between mental illness and self-harming behaviour; that is, although medications do not play a direct role in the management of self-harm, they play a considerable role in the management of associated conditions. However, strong evidence for the efficacy of any pharmacological intervention to reduce self-harm is lacking [37]. Antidepressants and antipsychotics are commonly prescribed to people who self-harm. The evidence on whether some antidepressants are associated with self-harm is mixed. A retrospective study by Donovan and colleagues [95] compared the risk of self-harm by any method in 2776 individuals who had been prescribed either tricyclic antidepressants (TCAs) or selective serotonin reuptake inhibitors (SSRIs). Their results showed that significantly more self-harm events occurred following the prescription of SSRIs than TCAs, though the authors acknowledged that it is difficult to attribute the cause of such acts to any antidepressant medication in light of the complex clinical picture surrounding self-harm. More recently, studies have shown that selective serotonin reuptake inhibitors (SSRIs), such as Paroxetine, and serotonin–norepinephrine reuptake inhibitors (SNRIs), such as Venlafaxine, may be associated with higher rates of both suicidal behaviour [96] and suicide [97]. Findings from recent meta-analyses and systematic reviews [98, 99]. investigating the association between SSRIs and self-harm and suicide have raised doubt about the safety of SSRIs, suggesting that they are associated with an increase in self-harm and completed suicide in adolescents. A meta-analysis of safety data derived from trials of SSRIs [100] found weak evidence of an increased risk of self-harm after SSRI use and concluded that, although increased risks of suicide and self-harm caused by SSRIs cannot be ruled out, larger trials with longer follow-up periods are needed to assess the balance of risks and benefits more fully. The main limitation of trials in this area is that the majority have too few participants to detect clinically meaningful differences in rates of repetition of self-harm between the experimental and control treatments [11]. Larger trials, adequately powered to detect such differences, are therefore needed as a matter of urgency.

Treatment in people with borderline personality disorder

In clinical practice, people with borderline personality disorder (BPD) constitute an important subgroup of individuals who recurrently self-harm. The evidence base for the treatment of self-harm in this subgroup is better developed compared to the generic evidence on the treatment of self-harm.

Dialectical behaviour therapy (DBT)

Dialectical behaviour therapy (DBT) is a multi-modal, psychological treatment programme, combining weekly individual therapy and weekly psychoeducational and skills group training for a period of about 12 months. It combines cognitive-behavioural techniques for emotion regulation with concepts of distress tolerance, acceptance, and mindfulness [101, 102]. DBT emphasises clear and precise definition of treatment targets, ongoing assessment of current behaviours, and a collaborative working relationship between client and therapist [103]. The treatment goals of individual DBT therapy are organised hierarchically by importance in the following order: (1) reduction of self-harm and life-threatening behaviours; (2) reduction of any behaviours that interfere with the process of therapy; and (3) reduction of any behaviours that significantly interfere with the individual's quality of life [101]. The treatment was originally developed for women who self-harm and, at the time of writing, DBT remains the psychological intervention with the strongest evidence base for its effectiveness in reducing repetition of recurrent self-harm among women with BPD.

Mentalization-based treatment (MBT)

Mentalization-based treatment (MBT) is a complex psychological intervention (consisting of both group and individual therapy) for people with BPD and most research into MBT has therefore used samples of people with BPD. MBT is based on the premise that BPD is a developmental disorder of attachment, where the fundamental disturbance is a failure to mentalize (i.e., the ability to understand one's own and others' mental states) [104, 105]. The intervention is designed to increase the patient's capacity to self-reflect. The focus in MBT is on stabilizing the sense of self [105] and the overall aims are threefold: (1) to promote mentalizing about oneself; (2) to promote mentalizing about others; and (3) to promote mentalizing of important interpersonal relationships [106]. Findings from a recent trial comparing MBT with structured clinical management [107] in 134 outpatients showed that participants randomised to the MBT treatment arm displayed a steeper decline of suicide attempts than participants in the structured clinical management arm. However, it is noteworthy that participants in both groups showed substantial improvement over the course of the trial.

Conclusion

Self-harm is a significant problem across the lifespan and is the leading predictor of suicide, as well as contributing to substantial public health costs. Many psychological, psychosocial, and pharmacological interventions have been investigated in clinical trials in an attempt to manage and reduce self-harming behaviour. However, due in part to the small numbers of participants included in many of the trials investigating treatment interventions for self-harming behaviour, there remains considerable doubt about which interventions are effective with this population in reducing subsequent self-harming behaviour and/or suicide attempts [11, 68]. At present, DBT appears to be the most effective psychological intervention for reducing self-harm behaviour among women with BPD who self-harm. It has been previously recommended that future trials of the treatment of self-harm should be large enough to determine whether the intervention being tested reduces repetition of self-harm whilst simultaneously examining other relevant outcomes such as levels of service use, quality of life, mood, social functioning, and interpersonal difficulties [47]. Such trials are required to highlight effective interventions for recurrent self-harm.

References

1 Madge N, Hewitt A, Hawton K, De Wilde EJ, Corcoran P, Fekete S, et al. Deliberate self-harm within an international community sample of young people: Comparative findings from the Child & Adolescent Self-harm in Europe (CASE) Study. *Journal of Child Psychology and Psychiatry*. 2008;49(6):667–77.
2 Brooke S, Horn N. The meaning of self-injury and overdosing amongst women fulfilling the diagnostic criteria for 'borderline personality disorder.' *Psychology and Psychotherapy: Theory, Research and Practice*. 2010;83:113–28.

3 Gunderson J, Ridolfi ME. Borderline personality disorder: Suicidality and self-mutilation. *Annals of the New York Academy of Sciences.* 2001;932:61–77.

4 Wilksonson P. Non-suicidal self-injury. *European Child and Adolescent Psychiatry.* 2013;22 (Suppl 1):S75–S9.

5 Favazza AR. *Bodies under siege: Self-mutilation, nonsuicidal self-injury, and body modification in culture and psychiatry.* 3rd ed. Baltimore, USA: Johns Hopkins University Press; 2011.

6 Briere J, Gil E. Self-mutilation in clinical and general population samples: Prevalence, correlates, and functions. *American Journal of Orthopsychiatry.* 1998;68:609–20.

7 Plener PL, Fegert JM. Non-suicidal self-injury: State of the art perspective of a proposed new syndrome for DSM V. *Child and Adolescent Psychiatry and Mental Health.* 2012;6:9–10.

8 Kapur N, Cooper J, O'Connor RC, Hawton K. Non-suicidal self-injury v. attempted suicide: New diagnosis or false dichotomy? *British Journal of Psychiatry.* 2013;202:326–8.

9 Cooper J, Kapur N, Webb R, Lawlor M, Guthrie E, Mackway-Jones K, et al. Suicide after deliberate self-harm: A 4-year cohort study. *American Journal of Psychiatry.* 2005;162:297–303.

10 Hawton K, Bergen H, Kapur N, Cooper J, Steeg S, Ness J, et al. Repetition of self-harm and suicide following self-harm in children and adolescents: Findings from the Multicentre Study of Self-Harm in England. *Journal of Child Psychology and Psychiatry.* 2012;53: 1212–9.

11 Hawton K, Townsend E, Arensman E, Gunnell DJ, Hazell P, House A, et al. Psychosocial and pharmacological treatments for deliberate self harm. *Cochrane Database of Systematic Reviews.* 1999;(4):Art. No.: CD001764.

12 Young R, Sweeting H, West P. Prevalence of deliberate self harm and attempted suicide within contemporary Goth youth subculture: Longitudinal cohort study. *British Medical Journal.* 2006;332:1058–61.

13 Lloyd-Richardson EE, Perrine N, Dierker L, Kelley ML. Characteristics and functions of nonsuicidal self-injury in a community sample of adolescents. *Psychological Medicine.* 2007;37:1183–92.

14 Plener PL, Libal G, Keller F, Fegert JM, Muehlenkamp JJ. An international comparison of adolescent nonsuicidal self-injury (NSSI) and suicide attempts: Germany and the USA. *Psychological Medicine.* 2009;39:1549–58.

15 Ross S, Heath N. A study of the frequency of self-mutilation in a community sample of adolescents. *Journal of Youth and Adolescence.* 2002;31:67–77.

16 Favazza AR, DeRosear L, Conterio K. Self-mutilation and eating disorders. *Suicide and Life-Threatening Behavior.* 1989;19:352–61.

17 Gratz KL. Measurement of deliberate self-harm: Preliminary data on the Deliberate Self-Harm Inventory. *Journal of Psychopathology and Behavioral Assessment.* 2001;23(4): 253–63.

18 Whitlock J, Eckenrode J, Silverman D. Self-injurious behaviors in a college population. *Pediatrics.* 2006;117(6):1939–48.

19 Patton G, Hemphill SA, Beyers JM, Bond L, Toumbourou JW, McMorris BJ, et al. Pubertal stage and deliberate self-harm in adolescents. *Journal of the American Academy of Child and Adolescent Psychiatry.* 2007;46(4):508–14.

20 Hawton K, Saunders KEA, O'Connor RC. Self-harm and suicide in adolescents. *Lancet.* 2012;379:2373–82.

21 Moran P, Coffey C, Romaniuk H, Olsson C, Borschmann R, Carlin JB, et al. The natural history of self-harm during adolescence and young adulthood: Population-based cohort study. *Lancet.* 2011;379:236–243.

22 Skegg K. Self-harm. *Lancet.* 2005;366:1471–83.

23 Deliberto TL, Nock MK. An exploratory study of correlates, onset, and offset of non-suicidal self-injury. *Archives of Suicide Research.* 2008;12(3):219–31.

24 Hawton K, Harriss L, Hodder K, Simkin S, Gunnell D. The influence of the economic and social environment on deliberate self-harm and suicide: An ecological and person-based study. *Psychological Medicine.* 2001;31:827–36.

25 Moorey S. Managing the unmanageable: Cognitive behaviour therapy for deliberate self-harm. *Psychoanalytic Psychotherapy.* 2010;24(2):135–49.

26 WHO. Suicide huge but preventable public health problem, says WHO. 2005. World Health Organization. Downloaded from http://www.who.int/mediacentre/news/releases/2004/pr61/en/ (accessed September 19, 2013).

27 World Health O. *Health-for-all targets. The health policy for Europe. Summary of the updated edition (EUR ICP HSC 013).* Copenhagen: World Health Organisation; 1992.

28 Barbe RP, Rubovszky G, Venturini-Andreoli A, Andreoli A. The treatment of borderline personality disorder patients with current suicidal behaviour. *Clinical Neuropsychiatry.* 2005;2(5):283–91.

29 Hawton K, Bergen H, Casey P, Simkin S, Palmer B, Cooper J, et al. Self-harm in England: A tale of three cities. Multicentre study of self-harm. *Social Psychiatry and Psychiatric Epidemiology.* 2007;42(7):513–21.

30 Evans MO, Morgan HG, Hayward A, Gunnell DJ. Crisis telephone consultation for deliberate self-harm patients: Effects on repetition. *British Journal of Psychiatry.* 1999;175:23–7.

31 NICE. *Borderline personality disorder: Treatment and management.* NICE Clinical Guideline 78. National Institute for Health and Clinical Excellence. London: British Psychological Society; 2009.

32 Platt S, Hawton K, Kreitman N, Fagg J, Foster J. Recent clinical and epidemiological trends in parasuicide in Edinburgh and Oxford: A tale of two cities. *Psychological Medicine.* 1988;18:405–18.

33 O'Connor RC, Sheehy NP, O'Connor DB. Fifty cases of general hospital suicide. *British Journal of Health Psychology.* 2000;5:83–95.

34 APA. *Diagnostic and statistical manual of mental disorders.* 4th ed., text revision (DSM-IV-TR). Arlington, VA: American Psychiatric Association; 2000.

35 Klonsky ED. The functions of deliberate self-injury: A review of the evidence. *Clinical Psychology Review.* 2006;27:226–39.

36 Paris J. An evidence-based approach to managing suicidal behavior in patients with BPD. *Social Work in Mental Health.* 2008;6(1–2):99–108.

37 NICE. *Self-harm: Longer-term management.* National Clinical Guideline 133. London: National Institute for Health and Clinical Excellence; 2011.

38 Favazza AR. Why patients mutilate themselves. *Hospital and Community Psychiatry.* 1989;40(2):137–45.

39 Gratz KL. Risk factors for and functions of deliberate self-harm: An empirical and conceptual review. *Clinical Psychology: Science and Practice.* 2003;10(2):192–205.

40 Scoliers G, Portzky G, Madge N, Hewitt A, Hawton K, de Wilde EJ, et al. Reasons for adolescent deliberate self-harm: A cry of pain and/or a cry for help? Findings from the child and adolescent self-harm in Europe (CASE) study. *Social Psychiatry and Psychiatric Epidemiology.* 2009;44(8):601–7.

41 Hawton K, Fagg J, Simkin S, Bale E, Bond A. Trends in deliberate self-harm in Oxford, 1985-1995. *British Journal of Psychiatry.* 1997;171:556–60.

42 Nock MK. Why do people hurt themselves? New insights into the nature and functions of self-injury. *Current Directions in Psychological Science.* 2009;18(2):78–83.

43 Sakinofsky I, Roberts R. Why parasuicides repeat despite problem resolution. *British Journal of Psychiatry.* 1990;156:399–405.

44 Sakinofsky I, Roberts R, Brown Y, Cumming C, James P. Problem resolution and repetition of parasuicide: A prospective study. *British Journal of Psychiatry.* 1990; 156(395):399.

45 Rodham K, Hawton K, Evans E. Reasons for deliberate self-harm: Comparison of self-poisoners and self-cutters in a community sample of adolescents. *Journal of the American Academy of Child and Adolescent Psychiatry.* 2004;43:80–7.

46 Bergen H, Hawton K, Waters K, Ness J, Cooper J, Steeg S, et al. How do methods of non-fatal self-harm relate to eventual suicide? *Journal of Affective Disorders.* 2012;136:526–33.

47 House A, Owens D, Patchett L. Deliberate self harm. 1999. *Quality in Health Care.* 8: 137–43.

48 Creed FH, Pfeffer JM. Attitudes of house-physicians towards self-poisoning patients. *Medical Education.* 1981;15(5):340–5.

49 Ramon S, Bancroft JHJ, Skrimshire AM. Attitudes towards self-poisoning among physicians and nurses in a general hospital. *British Journal of Psychiatry.* 1975;127:257–62.

50 Cleaver K. Characteristics and trends of self-harming behaviour in young people. *British Journal of Nursing.* 2007;16(3):148–52.

51 Perego M. Why A&E nurses feel inadequate in managing patients who deliberately self-harm. *Emergency Nurse.* 1999;6(9):24–7.

52 Greenwood S, Bradley P. Managing deliberate self harm: The A&E perspective. *Accident and Emergency Nursing.* 1997;5:134–6.

53 NICE. *Self-harm: The short-term physical and psychological management and secondary prevention of self-harm in primary and secondary care.* Clinical guidelines. London: National Institute for Health and Clinical Excellence; 2004.

54 Anderson M, Standen P, Nazir S, Noon JP. Nurses and doctors attitudes towards suicidal behaviour in young people. *International Journal of Nursing Studies.* 2000;37:1–11.

55 Taylor TL, Hawton K, Fortune S, Kapur N. Attitudes towards clinical services among people who self-harm: Systematic review. *British Journal of Psychiatry.* 2009;194(2):104–10.

56 Haw C, Hawton K, Houston K, Townsend E. Psychiatric and personality disorders in deliberate self-harm patients. *British Journal of Psychiatry.* 2001;178:48–54.

57 World Health Organization (WHO). *International statistical classification of diseases and related health problems (ICD-10).* 1992.

58 Links PS. Developing effective services for patients with personality disorders. *Canadian Journal of Psychiatry.* 1998;43:251–9.

59 McMain SF, Links PS, Gnam WH, Guimond T, Cardish RJ, Korman L, et al. A randomized trial of dialectical behavior therapy versus general psychiatric management for borderline personality disorder. *American Journal of Psychiatry.* 2009;166(12):1365–74.

60 Skodol AE, Gunderson JG, Pfohl B, Widiger TA, Livesley WJ, Siever LJ. The borderline diagnosis I: Psychopathology, comorbidity, and personality structure. *Biological Psychiatry.* 2002;51:936–50.

61 Lieb K, Zanarini MC, Schmahl C, Linehan MM, Bohus M. Borderline personality disorder. *Lancet.* 2004;364(9432):453–61.

62 Klonsky ED, Oltmanns TF, Turkheimer E. Deliberate self-harm in a nonclinical population: Prevalence and psychological correlates. *American Journal of Psychiatry.* 2003;160:1501–8.

63 Brunner R, Parzer P, Haffner J, Steen R, Roos J, Klett M, et al. Prevalence and psychological correlates of occasional and repetitive deliberate self-harm in adolescents. *Archives of Pediatrics and Adolescent Medicine.* 2007;2007(161):7.

64 Kapur N, Cooper J, King-Hele S, Webb R, Lawlor M, Rodway C, et al. The repetition of suicidal behavior: A multicenter cohort study. *Journal of Clinical Psychiatry*. 2006;67(10): 1599–609.

65 Sinclair JM, Hawton K, Gray A. Six year follow-up of a clinical sample of self-harm patients. *Journal of Affective Disorders*. 2010;121(3):247–52.

66 Owens D, Horrocks J, House A. Fatal and non-fatal repetition of self-harm. Systematic review. *British Journal of Psychiatry*. 2002;181:193–9.

67 Crawford M, Thomas O, Kham N, Kulinskaya E. Psychosocial interventions following self-harm: Systematic review of their efficacy in preventing suicide. *British Journal of Psychiatry*. 2007;190:11–7.

68 Hawton K, Arensman E, Townsend E, Bremner S, Feldman E, Goldney R, et al. Deliberate self harm: Systematic review of efficacy of psychosocial and pharmacological treatments in preventing repetition. *British Medical Journal*. 1998;317:441–7.

69 Gelder M, Mayou R, Cowen P. Suicide and deliberate self-harm. In: Gelder M, Mayou R, Cowen P (eds.) *Shorter Oxford textbook of psychiatry*, 4th ed. Oxford, UK: Oxford University Press; 2001. p. 507–32.

70 Hawton K, Harriss L, Hall S, Simkin S, Bale E, Bond A. Deliberate self-harm in Oxford, 1990-2000: A time of change in patient characteristics. *Psychological Medicine*. 2003; 33(6):987–95.

71 Hawton K, Harriss L, Zahl D. Deaths from all causes in a long-term follow-up study of 11583 deliberate self-harm patients. *Psychological Medicine*. 2006;36(3):397–405.

72 Bergen H, Hawton K, Waters K, Ness J, Cooper J, Steeg S, et al. Premature death after self-harm: A multicentre cohort study. *Lancet*. 2012;380:1568–74.

73 Guthrie E, Kapur N, Mackway-Jones K, Chew-Graham C, Moorey J, Mendel E, et al. Randomised controlled trial of a brief psychological intervention after deliberate self poisoning. *British Medical Journal*. 2001;323:165–69.

74 Sinclair JM, Gray A, Rivero-Arias O, Saunders KE, Hawton K. Healthcare and social services resource use and costs of self-harm patients. *Social Psychiatry and Psychiatric Epidemiology*. 2011;46:263–71.

75 Oldershaw A, Richards C, Simic M, Schmidt U. Parents' perspectives on adolescent self-harm: Qualitative study. *British Journal of Psychiatry*. 2008;193:140–4.

76 Mustafa Soomro G. Deliberate self-harm (and attempted suicide). *Clinical Evidence (BMJ)*. 2008;12:1012–26.

77 Lilley R, Owens D, Horrocks J, House A, Noble R, Bergen H, et al. Hospital are and repetition follow self-harm: Multicentre comparison of self-poisoning and self-injury. *British Journal of Psychiatry*. 2008;192:440–5.

78 Hume M, Platt S. Appropriate interventions for the prevention and management of self-harm: A qualitative exploration of service-users' views. *BMC Public Health*. 2007;7:9–17.

79 McLeavey BC, Daly RJ, Ludgate JW, Murray CM. Interpersonal problem-solving skills training in the treatment of self-poisoning patients. *Suicide and Life-Threatening Behavior*. 1994;24(4):382–94.

80 McAuliffe C, Corcoran P, Keeley HS, Arensman E, Bille Brahe U, De Leo D, et al. Problem solving ability and repetition of deliberate self-harm: A multicentre study. *Psychol Med*. 2006;36(1):45–55.

81 Butler AC, Chapman JE, Forman EM, Beck AT. The empirical status of cognitive-behavioral therapy: A review of meta-analyses. *Clinical Psychology Review*. 2006;26(1):17–31.

82 Arntz A. Treatment of borderline personality disorder: A challenge for cognitive-behavioural therapy. *Behaviour Research and Therapy*. 1994;32(4):419–30.

83 Tarrier N, Taylor K, Gooding P. Cognitive-behavioral interventions to reduce suicide behavior: A systematic review and meta-analysis. *Behavior Modification.* 2008;32:77.

84 Kapur N, Cooper J, Bennewith O, Gunnell DJ, Hawton K. Postcards, green cards and telephone calls: Therapeutic contact with individuals following self-harm. *British Journal of Psychiatry.* 2010;197:5–7.

85 Evans J, Evans M, Morgan HG, Hayward A, Gunnell DJ. Crisis card following self-harm: 12-month follow-up of a randomized controlled trial. *British Journal of Psychiatry.* 1999;187:186–7.

86 Morgan HG, Jones EM, Owen JH. Secondary prevention of non-fatal deliberate self-harm: The green card study. *British Journal of Psychiatry.* 1993;163:111–2.

87 Cedereke M, Monti K, Ojehagen A. Telephone contact with patients in the year after a suicide attempt: Does it affect treatment attendance and outcome? A randomised controlled study. *European Psychiatry.* 2002;17:82–91.

88 Vaiva G, Ducrocq F, Meyer P, Mathieu D, Philippe A, et al. Effect of telephone contact on further suicide attempts in patients discharged from an emergency department: Randomised controlled study. *British Medical Journal.* 2006;332(7552):1241–5.

89 Carter GL, Clover K, Whyte IM, Dawson AH, D'Este C. Postcards from the EDge project: Randomized controlled trial of an intervention using postcards to reduce repetition of hospital treated deliberate self-poisoning. *British Medical Journal.* 2005;331:805.

90 Carter GL, Clover K, Whyte IM, Dawson AH, D'Este C. Postcards from the EDge: 5-year outcomes of a randomised controlled trial for hospital-treated self-poisoning. *British Journal of Psychiatry.* 2013;202:372–80.

91 Hassanian-Moghaddam H, Sarjami S, Kolahi A-A, Carter GL. Postcards in Persia: Randomised controlled trial to reduce suicidal behaviours 12 months after hospital-treated self-poisoning. *British Journal of Psychiatry.* 2011;198:309–16.

92 Robinson J, Yuen HP, Gook S, Hughes A, Cosgrave E, Killackey E, et al. Can receipt of a regular postcard reduce suicide-related behaviour in young help seekers? A randomized controlled trial. *Early Intervention in Psychiatry.* 2012;6:145–52.

93 Kapur N, Gunnell D, Hawton K, Nadeem S, Khalil S, Longson D, et al. Messages from Manchester: Pilot randomised controlled trial following self-harm. *British Journal of Psychiatry.* 2013;203:73–4.

94 Beautrais AL, Gibb SJ, Faulkner A, Fergusson DM, Mulder RT. Postcard intervention for repeat self-harm: Randomised controlled trial. *British Journal of Psychiatry.* 2010;197:55–60.

95 Donovan S, Clayton A, Beeharry M, Jones S, Kirk C, Waters K, et al. Deliberate self-harm and antidepressant drugs: Investigation of a possible link. *British Journal of Psychiatry.* 2000;177:551–6.

96 Kraus JE, Horrigan JP, Carpenter DJ, Fong R, Barrett PS, Davies JT. Clinical features of patients with treatment-emergent suicidal behavior following initiation of paroxetine therapy. *Journal of Affective Disorders.* 2010;120(1):40–7.

97 Rubino A, Roskell N, Tennis P, Mines D, Weich S, Andrews E. Risk of suicide during treatment with venlafaxine, citalopram, fluoxetine, and dothiepin: retrospective cohort study. *BMJ.* 2007;334(7587):242.

98 Barbui C, Esposito E, Cipriani A. Selective serotonin reuptake inhibitors and risk of suicide: A systematic review of observational studies. *Canadian Medical Association Journal.* 2009;180(3):291–7.

99 Dubicka B, Hadley S, Roberts C. Suicidal behaviour in youths with depression treated with new-generation antidepressants Meta-analysis. *British Journal of Psychiatry.* 2006;189(5):393–8.

100 Gunnell D, Saperia J, Ashby D. Selective serotonin reuptake inhibitors (SSRIs) and suicide in adults: Meta-analysis of drug company data from placebo controlled, randomised controlled trials submitted to the MHRA's safety review. *BMJ.* 2005; 330(7488):385.

101 Linehan MM, Armstrong HE, Suarez A, Allmon D, Heard HL. Cognitive-behavioral treatment of chronically parasuicidal borderline patients. *Archives of General Psychiatry.* 1991;48:1060–4.

102 Linehan MM, Dimeff LA, Reynolds SK, Comtois KA, Welch SS, Heagerty P, et al. Dialectical behavior therapy versus comprehensive validation therapy plus 12-step for the treatment of opioid dependent women meeting criteria for borderline personality disorder. *Drug and Alcohol Dependence.* 2002;67:13–26.

103 Linehan MM. *Skills training manual for treating borderline personality disorder.* New York, NY: Guilford Press; 1993.

104 Bateman A, Fonagy P. Effectiveness of partial hospitalization in the treatment of borderline personality disorder: A randomized controlled trial. *American Journal of Psychiatry.* 1999;156(10):1563–9.

105 Bateman A, Fonagy P. Mentalization-based treatment of BPD. *Journal of Personality Disorders.* 2004;18(1):36–51.

106 Bateman A, Ryle A, Fonagy P, Kerr IB. Psychotherapy for borderline personality disorder: Mentalization based therapy and cognitive analytic therapy compared. *International Review of Psychiatry.* 2007;19(1):51–62.

107 Bateman A, Fonagy P. Randomized controlled trial of outpatient mentalization-based treatment versus structured clinical management for borderline personality disorder. *American Journal of Psychiatry.* 2009;166:1355–64.

CHAPTER 7

Finding the truth in the lies: A practical guide to the assessment of malingering

Holly Tabernik and Michael J. Vitacco

Department of Psychiatry and Health Behavior, Georgia Regents University, Augusta, Georgia, U.S.

Introduction

Mental health professionals rely primarily on a patient's self-report to diagnosis and develop treatment interventions. The reliance on self-report is often effective when a therapeutic alliance exists between the patient and the professional, with the shared goal revolving around the alleviation of mental health suffering and achievement of optimal functioning. However, there are other clinical evaluations in which the evaluee's self-interests are not necessarily parallel with the professional's task. As an illustrative example, let us consider the most commonly requested forensic evaluation referral: competency to stand trial. In this instance, the hypothetical case involves the court ordering an evaluation of Mr. Jones, who is charged with the murder of his wife. Like many defendants, Mr. Jones has a goal of receiving the least serious consequences possible or avoiding prosecution all together. In an effort to achieve his goal, the defendant may attempt to feign or exaggerate mental health symptoms in order to avoid criminal prosecution. In contrast, the clinician's goal is to provide an accurate diagnostic impression and professional opinion regarding the defendant's capacity to proceed to trial, both of which may be detrimental to the defendant.

Likewise, consider a situation in which Ms. Smith is charged with murdering her husband, after which she is referred to a mental health professional to undergo an evaluation of her mental state at the time of the crime. The defendant is claiming she was acutely psychotic at the time of the alleged offense. After interviewing the defendant and conducting extensive psychological testing, the clinician opined Ms. Smith is malingering in order to avoid criminal prosecution. Ms. Smith is subsequently

Troublesome Disguises: Managing Challenging Disorders in Psychiatry, Second Edition.
Edited by Dinesh Bhugra and Gin S. Malhi.

tried and found both guilty and criminally responsible for killing her husband, at which point she is sent to prison and not provided mental health services. As both of these scenarios illustrate, a clinician's ability to successful differentiate between people with a bona fide mental illness versus people who are exaggerating symptoms of mental illness is extremely important and has a variety of long-term consequences.

The goals of this chapter are relatively straightforward:

- Discuss and critically evaluate current conceptualizations of malingering.
- Provide general information on malingering models and note how models can and should inform clinical practice.
- Introduce the idea of an additive approach to the assessment of malingering, during which a clinician uses a number of clinical tools to evaluate malingering.
- Select appropriate methodologies to detect malingering, with an emphasis on forensic populations.

Current conceptualization of malingering

According to the *Diagnostic and Statistical Manual of Mental Disorders*, 5th ed. (DSM-5) [1], malingering involves intentionally fabricating or grossly exaggerating symptoms in an effort to obtain external incentives or some type of secondary gain. The DSM-5 provides examples of external incentives, including: financial compensation, avoiding work, avoiding criminal prosecution, and obtaining drugs. The DSM-5 and its earlier counterparts suggest that malingering should be suspected if two or more of the following are present: medicolegal situations, a large discrepancy between the person's claimed symptoms and objective data, a lack of cooperation with evaluation and treatment, and the presence of antisocial personality disorder.

Although the DSM-5 and its earlier editions are the most commonly used resource for making mental health diagnoses, a large number of conceptual weaknesses and practical concerns have been cited related to using this resource to diagnosis malingering [2]. First, scholars have argued the DSM criteria for malingering have an implicit judgment of "badness" relying on characterological traits (i.e., antisocial personality disorder), which provide little explanatory power concerning the accurate diagnosis of malingering. The DSM relies on contextual variables (medicolegal evaluations) and interpersonal variables (uncooperativeness during the evaluation), all of which are highly subjective, and none having significant empirical support [3]. Take the proposed connection between antisocial personality disorder (APD) and malingering. In a recent study conducted by Pierson, Rosenfeld, Green, and Belfi [4], forensic patients with APD were no more likely to be suspected of malingering by clinicians or to exceed acceptable cutoff scores on the Structured Interview of Reported Symptoms [5] (SIRS) than patients not diagnosed with APD. Additionally, research has consistently failed to support the connection between a medicolegal evaluation and malingering, which is especially evident when considering the relatively large discrepancy in base rates of malingering across studies of forensic evaluations [6, 7].

Moreover, another DSM index suggests that mental health professionals consider malingering when an individual is uncooperative with treatment. Using this criterion, almost all patients involuntarily committed to a mental health facility would fall under the rubric of suspicion, regardless of the underlying reason for their admission. This would include any patient admitted due to a severe suicide attempt as well as the patient with a documented long-standing mental health history who is experiencing complications from medicine interactions. Lastly, the DSM directs professionals to consider malingering whenever a large discrepancy exists between clinical distress and objective findings. Despite this proposition the DSM falls short on several key aspects including providing counsel on the directionality of this discrepancy, leaving professionals to rely on clinical judgment, and test results that by their very nature are often contradictory.

DSM criteria treat malingering as taxonic, leaving little room for clinicians to rely on empirically validated approaches. In contrast to the DSM, researchers, backed by data, have argued that malingering is a dimensional (exaggeration of symptoms on a continuum) rather than categorical (malingerer or honest dichotomy) variable [8]. Resnik [9] suggested the individuals may present with three types of malingering: (1) "pure malingering" (i.e., a complete fabrication of symptoms), (2) "partial malingering" (i.e., exaggeration of actual symptoms or reporting past symptoms as present currently), and (3) "false imputation" (i.e., deliberately linking symptoms to compensable events). Another fallacy unaddressed by DSM criteria is the assumption that many will feign indiscriminately and in every situation. Such an approach is not supported by the literature [2]. Instead, extant research points to general independence among types of malingering (i.e., cognitive, psychiatric, and physical [10]). In other words, most individuals who malinger do so with a specific set of symptoms they perceive will provide them the greatest benefit given the current situation. As such, clinicians should not assume "once a malingerer, always a malingerer," because each situation warrants its own investigation into the validity of the symptom presentation.

In addition to conceptual concerns about the use of the DSM in diagnosing malingering, there are a number of practical concerns as well. One practical difficultly clinicians face in assessing and ultimately diagnosing malingering is the absence of any instrument, psychological or other, that can accurately identify a person's motivation for fabricating mental health symptoms, making it nearly impossible to differentiate those who are malingering (externally motivated to exaggerate) from those with factious disorder or somatoform disorder (internally motivated to exaggerate in order to assume the sick role). Rogers and Vitacco [11] argued that since no test can measure motivation, mental health professionals are forced to speculate about whether a patient's motivation to feign is intrinsic or extrinsic based on self-report and clinical judgment and to render a diagnosis accordingly. Another practical issue identified by Berry and Nelson [2] is that the DSM description of malingering has barely changed in over three decades, although research in this area has continued to advance at a rapid pace. Lastly, the practical utility of the conditions identified in the DSM as potentially indicative of malingering (i.e., medicolegal situations, lack of cooperation) has also been called into question. Rogers [3, 11] used these criteria to differentiate malingerers from non-malingerers and reported correct classification rates of only 20 percent.

What can be gleamed from the previous paragraphs is a need for refinement in the diagnostic criteria for malingering. All told, findings suggest that criteria outlined by the DSM for malingering are more inaccurate than accurate with minimal validity.

Alternative models of malingering

The utility of the DSM-5 diagnostic criteria for malingering is of questionable; however, even though it lacks empirical backing many clinicians continue to exclusively rely on these criteria when rendering a diagnosis of malingering. This reliance on unvalidated diagnostic criteria may at least partially explain why prevalence estimates of malingering vary widely across and within similar settings. For example, malingering prevalence rates in forensic cases range from 15 to 18 percent [7, 12], while studies conducted in forensic-psychiatric hospital settings have varied rates from less than 10 percent [13] to more than 25 percent [14–16].

In an effort to rectify some of the aforementioned criticisms of the DSM's conceptualization of malingering, Rogers proposed the adaptational model of malingering [3]. The model includes three ideas: (1) a person perceives the evaluation/treatment as involuntary or adversarial, (2) the person perceives that he or she has either something to lose from being honest or something to gain from malingering, and (3) the person does not perceive a more effective means to achieve the desired goal [17]. This model provides testable constructs without imposing morality or judgment, and accounts for situational aspects of malingering. From that aspect, the model is consistent with decision theory, in which choices made under conditions of uncertainty are based on expected utility and likelihood of several courses of action [18].

Similarly, Slick, Sherman, and Iverson proposed a set of criteria for malingered neurocognitive dysfunction: (1) presence of substantial external incentive, (2) evidence from neuropsychological testing (i.e., performance below chance or what would be expected of the examinee), (3) evidence from self-report (i.e., self-reported symptoms are not consistent with behavioral observations), and (4) criteria 2 and 3 are not fully accounted for by psychiatric, neurological, or developmental factors [19]. The model proposed by Slick and colleagues provides testable hypotheses, which again is in contrast to the largely subjective criteria offered by the DSM.

The additive model for assessing malingering

Given the inherent difficulties associated with diagnosing malingering and the negative consequences of misdiagnosis, the authors propose an additive approach to the assessment and diagnosis of malingering. The goal of an additive model is to rely only on empirically validated strategies when making a formal diagnosis. This approach integrates information from multiple sources and carefully considers information suggesting feigning, but also information suggestive of a bona fide mental disorder. The authors specifically encourage the use of information obtained during a clinical interview, information from collateral sources (i.e., interviews with family and friends), and a review of available medical and mental health records. In addition to the clinical approach, it is essential to carefully consider data gathered from measures specifically designed to assess response style (e.g., the SIRS-2 [20]).

Of note, the authors are not proposing that each of the above pieces of evidence must be reviewed in every case; instead, information gathered during one step should help professionals determine if the next step is necessary. By taking an additive approach to identifying malingering, the rate of false positives (i.e., diagnosing a person as malingering who is not) and false negatives (i.e., failing to diagnosis a person as malingering who is in fact malingering) can be minimized and the accuracy of diagnosis can be improved. Yet, when finalizing a diagnosis of malingering, the authors firmly recommend using empirically based methods and instruments. By using these instruments clinicians go beyond the problematic approach presented by the DSM and are on firmer footing if the clinician is going to be part of an adversarial process. A comprehensive review of the many different types of malingering is beyond the scope of this chapter, so the authors have chosen to focus on two of the most common types of malingering faced by mental health professionals working in forensic settings: malingering of psychopathology and cognitive deficits. The following paragraphs are designed to provide a practical outline of how to apply each of the afore-mentioned steps to arrive at a well-reasoned and defensible diagnosis of malingering.

Symptom presentation and record review: Feigning of psychiatric symptoms

The first and perhaps most familiar step is to conduct a clinical interview and record review of the examinee. One of the inherent challenges of this process is separating feigned symptoms from actual psychopathology. Toward this end there have been several investigations into empirically based cues of malingering. When reviewing the available records, clinicians would be wise to look for discrepancies between a person's self-reported symptoms and their ability to function on a day-to-day basis [21]. Clinicians need to consider history of malingering or evidence of external gain (such as seeking shelter or avoiding criminal responsibility), with an eye toward acknowledging that previous history of malingering is not indicative the individual is currently feigning. It should be noted that people who have experienced mental health symptoms in the past are better at feigning these symptoms in an effort to achieve some external incentive in the present than people who have never experienced mental health symptoms [22].

Additionally, suspicions of malingering often occur during the clinical interview. For example, individuals who are malingering are generally more willing to discuss their symptoms, may attempt to control the interview, and sometimes give vague answers to direct questions when compared to genuine patients [23]. Clinicians should conduct a detailed inquiry into the nature of self-reported symptoms using open-ended questions whenever possible. For example, clinicians should use open-ended questions in order to obtain information about the onset, frequency, severity, and nature of mental health symptoms. One of the most commonly exaggerated mental health symptoms is hallucinations. Some common examples of suspicious hallucinations include continuous rather than intermittent, stilted language describing the alleged phenomenon, and the hallucinations are described in terms indicating they are unpredictable, unbearably distressing, and vague or inaudible [22]. Cornell and Hawk identified 14 clinical presentation variables often consistent with a malingered presentation: exaggerated behavior, endorsing bogus symptoms (i.e., symptoms suggested by the evaluator), symptoms that do not "cluster" (i.e., symptoms that cross a number of diagnostic categories), suicidal ideation, and visual hallucinations [6]. Individuals who are malingering may also take longer to complete testing and repeat questions before providing an answer [24]. Another way to differentiate malingerers from genuine patients is to look at the symptoms that the person is not endorsing. Specifically, individuals who are feigning tend to present with the following symptoms less often than genuine patients: incoherent speech, poor hygiene, flat affect, concrete thinking, ideas of reference, and grandiose delusions [24]. Consistent with the additive model, these characteristics should not be used to diagnose malingering. Instead, the characteristics should serve to signal the need for a more thorough evaluation with a structured approach that incorporates empirically validated strategies to detect malingering.

In line with the above suggestions, Rogers identified four empirically based detection strategies that can be used to differentiate genuine psychopathology from malingering, all of which can be addressed by a skilled clinician during a clinical interview: (1) rare symptoms (i.e., symptoms that occur infrequently in genuinely impaired populations), (2) symptom severity (i.e., considers the number of potentially disabling symptoms endorsed by genuine patients versus malingerers), (3) obvious versus subtle symptoms (i.e., symptoms of mental illness that are readily recognized by the nonprofessional as related to mental illness versus symptoms that are typically recognized by nonprofessionals), and (4) symptom selectivity (i.e., endorsement of a wide range of symptoms that cross diagnostic categories) [25]. These detection strategies have been useful for developing new response style measures as well as for clinicians who may rely more heavily on clinical interviewing techniques to detect malingering.

Feigning cognitive impairments

Clinical interview data and information gathered from records can also be instrumental in differentiating a person with a genuine cognitive impairment from a person who is feigning a cognitive impairment. As part of the evaluation of feigning cognitive impairments, a clinician should gather information about prior as well as present cognitive functioning in addition to information about significant life events that could impact current cognitive functioning (i.e., serious head injuries). For example, school, mental health, and employment records are all useful in providing information about an individual's level of cognitive and adaptive functioning. Reported memory impairments should also be explored, preferably in a manner not easily identified by the examinee. For example, memory impairments may be assessed during the process of an interview using questions that are out of order or by asking the same question more than once in a different way. For example, if an examinee reports an inability to remember anything about his childhood at the beginning of the interview, the clinician should look for opportunities during the rest of the interview to get the examinee to discuss childhood memories perhaps by relating them to present functioning.

Rogers and Correa identified six empirically based strategies that can be used to detect feigning cognitive impairment, each of which have been utilized by tests designed to detect the feigning of cognitive impairment [26]: (1) performance curve (i.e., failing easy questions but responding correctly to difficult questions), (2) magnitude of error (i.e., responses that are either too close or too far from the correct answer), (3) violation of basic learning principles (i.e., scoring worse on something after being educated about it), (4) floor effect (i.e., responding incorrectly to a very easy question such as what is two plus two), (5) symptom validity testing (i.e., scores below chance on a multiple choice test), (6) forced choice tests (i.e., compares a person's responses on a true/false test to a control group). These strategies will be discussed in greater detail in the next section describing instruments used to detect malingering.

Objective personality measures

There is now extensive research demonstrating that objective personality tests such as the Minnesota Multiphasic Personality Inventory 2nd ed., MMPI-2 [27] and the Personality Assessment Inventory (PAI [28]) are reasonably accurate measures of response style or test-taking attitudes. Although these scales are not measures of malingering per se, they are thought to be useful in identifying patterns of overreporting and underreporting of mental health symptoms.

The MMPI-2 is the most extensively researched multiscale personality inventory, with validity indices that have shown the ability to successfully differentiate individuals who are feigning psychopathology from individuals with a genuine presentation [29]. The MMPI-2 is a 567-item self-report instrument that was designed to measure psychopathology, and also includes several validity scales commonly used in research as a measure of response style. In the most comprehensive meta-analysis of the MMPI-2 and feigning composed of data from 65 MMPI-2 feigning studies plus 11 MMPI-2 diagnostic studies, Rogers and colleagues found the largest effect sizes for Fp (Infrequency-Psychopathology), F (Infrequency), and Ds (Gough's dissimulation scale) for detecting feigning [30]. Rogers and colleagues identified F (mean *Cohen's d* = 2.21) and Fp (mean *Cohen's d* = 1.90) as particularly useful in detecting individuals who endorse rare symptoms. The Ds scale produced a large effect size (mean *Cohen's d* = 1.62) and relied on a strategy employing erroneous stereotypes (i.e., symptoms that are commonly misperceived as related to mental illness) [30]. Overall, Rogers and colleagues found that the Fp scale showed promise as a measure of feigning psychopathology, because it yielded the strongest effect sizes and consistent cut scores across settings and diagnostic categories. Other validity scales that have garnered varying levels of empirical support are the Fb (Back Infrequency) and F - K (Infrequency minus Correction) scales. Although these numbers seem promising, even the most accurate MMPI-2 scales fail to detect 5–15 percent of malingers [31], a statistic that lends direct support to an additive approach to the detection of malingering. Even the most researched measure of feigning mental illness does not accurately classify all malingerers, demonstrating that clinicians must employ additional testing in cases where malingering is suspected.

The PAI is a 344-item self-report multiscale measure of personality patterns and psychopathology that, like the MMPI-2, includes validity indices useful in examining response styles. The PAI has three indices developed for the detection of malingering: Negative Impression Scale (NIM), the Rogers Discriminant Function Scale (RDF), and the Malingering Index (Mal). The NIM is composed of items rarely endorsed in community and normative samples. The Mal is based on eight profile characteristics often associated with attempts to feign mental illness [32]. For example, patients with high levels of depression often report a strong desire to seek treatment, so if a test-taker reports high levels of depression but low levels of treatment motivation then malingering may be suspected. Finally, the RDF is based on a weighted combination of 20 PAI scale scores and a constant value [33]. While preliminary research showed that each of the above indices held promise in the detection of malingering, recent research has demonstrated variable levels of support, especially for the RDF and the Mal as screening measures in the detection of malingering [34]. However, Hawes and Boccaccini conducted a meta-analysis using 19 published articles, 6 unpublished theses or dissertations, and an unpublished conference presentation. Results of this meta-analysis indicated all three of the indices were relatively strong predictors of uncoached malingering (NIM *Cohen's* $d=1.48$, Mal *Cohen's* $d=1.15$, RDF *Cohen's* $d=1.13$) and coached malingering (NIM *Cohen's* $d=1.59$, Mal *Cohen's* $d=1.00$, RDF *Cohen's* $d=1.65$) [35]. In using the PAI to detect malingering, clinicians are on the strongest empirical ground if relying on the NIM scale.

Although both the MMPI-2 and the PAI have achieved some level of empirical support for their use as measures of response style and feigning, clinicians should use caution not to put too much emphasis on their utility. A number of potential problems exist when relying too heavily on validity indices from multiscale inventories to differentiate people with genuine mental health symptoms from malingers. One primary concern rests with a lack of discriminant validity for these scales; often, individuals with bona fide psychopathology have elevated validity scales. This is especially evident on the MMPI-2. This is not to say that the MMPI-2 and PAI do not offer important information that can be used to detect and ultimately diagnosis malingering, but it does indicate other information should also be considered, including information gathered from tests designed specifically to detect feigning.

Feigning measures

Although an extensive review of the measures designed to identify feigned psychiatric symptoms and cognitive impairments is beyond the scope of this chapter, the following paragraphs will provide a description of the most commonly used measures. The Structured Interview of Reported Symptoms (SIRS) [5] is the most commonly cited measure specifically designed to detect feigned psychiatric symptoms. The SIRS was recently revised and a second edition of the measure was published (SIRS-2) [20] in 2010. The SIRS-2 is a 172-item structured interview that takes approximately 45 minutes to administer. The SIRS and SIRS-2 are not measures of psychopathology, and are designed to detect malingering and related response styles. The SIRS-2 is composed of eight primary scales: Rare Symptoms (RS), Symptom Combinations (SC), Improbable or Absurd Symptoms (IA), Blatant Symptoms (BL), Subtle Symptoms (SU), Selectivity of Symptoms (SEL), Severity of Symptoms (SEV), and Reported versus Observed Symptoms (RO). Both the SIRS and the SIRS-2 have been extensively validated using a variety of research designs, including simulation studies and known-group designs [36–38]. However, the SIRS and SIRS-2 have been criticized because they require substantial clinician resources (e.g., a lengthy structured interview in addition to a file review). Additionally, other critics argue that while the SIRS is commonly described as an objective test, it also relies on clinical judgment to score answers, which means that it is not free of the error inherent in human subjectivity [39]. Of note, according to the SIRS-2 professional manual, interrater reliability estimates for the primary scales range from 0.91 to 1.00 [20], indicating high rater agreement and minimal effects of clinical judgment on SIRS/SIRS-2 scoring.

A number of shorter measures have been designed to screen for malingering of psychiatric symptoms. The Miller Forensic Assessment of Symptoms (M-FAST) [40] and the Structured Inventory of Malingered Symptomatology (SIMS) [41] are among the most commonly used screens. The M-FAST is a 25-item structured interview designed to screen for feigning mental health symptoms in approximately 5 minutes. The M-FAST is composed of seven rationally derived scales: reported versus observed (RO), extreme symptomatology (ES), rare combinations (RC), unusual hallucinations (UH), unusual symptom course (USC), negative image (NI), and suggestibility (S). The M-FAST has shown excellent psychometric properties in forensic populations [42, 43]. The SIMS was developed to identify feigning of specific conditions using a self-report, true-false format [44]. The 75 items are scored on five nonoverlapping scales: low intelligence, affective disorder, neurological impairment, psychosis, and amnesia. Vitacco and colleagues [16] evaluated the effectiveness of the SIMS, M-FAST, and the Evaluation of Competency to Stand Trial-Revised Atypical Presentation Scale (ECST-R ATP) [45] with a sample of 100 patients involved in competency to stand trial evaluations. The researchers used the SIRS to categorize people into one of two groups (malinger or nonmalinger). In comparing the groups, the M-FAST, SIMS, and ATP scales produced very large effect sizes overall with few exceptions. The results supported the strength of using these relatively brief scales and demonstrated their utility in differentiating individuals malingering from those classified as honest responders. Given their design, these measures can be used to quickly identify people whose effort/response style needs further evaluation.

Several measures have been designed to assess malingering related to cognitive deficits and memory, including the Test of Memory Malingering (TOMM) [46] and the Validity Indicator Profile (VIP) [47]. The TOMM is a forced-choice test that employs a visual recognition procedure during which examinees are presented with a set of 50 black-and-white pictures and then asked to identify which of two pictures they were shown previously after no delay and after an approximately 15-minute delay [46]. Clinicians then compare the percentage of correct answers to norms of individuals who are cognitively intact and individuals who are cognitively impaired. The TOMM is among the most commonly used instruments to detect feigned memory impairment. It has been validated for use in a variety of different populations, including defendants referred for pretrial evaluations [48] and people who have been diagnosed with mental retardation [49]. According to the TOMM professional manual, a score below 45 on the second learning trial is indicative of "probable" malingering.

The VIP is a two-alternative forced choice test designed to identify when results of cognitive and neuropsychological tests may be invalid because of malingering or other problematic response styles [47]. The VIP consists of a 100 item nonverbal subtest during which examinees must complete picture-matrix problems, of variable complexity, and a 75-item verbal subtest during which examinees are presented with a stimulus word and asked to choose which of two other words has a similar meaning. Based on an examinee's response to questions, they are categorized as either "compliant" (high effort to respond correctly), "careless" (low effort to respond correctly), "irrelevant" (low effort to respond incorrectly), or "malingering" (high effort to respond incorrectly). The developmental sample of the VIP, which was composed of over 1,000 people, demonstrated an overall classification rate of 79.8 percent for the nonverbal subtest and a 75.5 percent classification rate for the verbal subtest [50].

Although measures like the SIRS-2, TOMM, and M-FAST were specifically designed to assess response style, research cautions clinicians against relying too heavily on these measures without also considering the methodological limitations associated with them [13, 51]. For example, failure to recognize and consider the base rate of malingering in a given population may lead to higher false-positive rates. In minimizing errors, we continue to emphasize the need to use an additive approach to diagnosing malingering. We concur with the advice offered by Melton and colleagues, who stated, "Thus the forensic examiner's low threshold for suspecting dissimulation should be accompanied by a conservative stance with respect to reaching conclusions on that issue" (p. 57) [52].

Conclusion

Malingering has been a hot topic in psychology for several decades. As research into the conceptualization and detection of malingering expands, it has become increasingly important for clinicians to have a practical step-by-step process to identify and/or rule-out malingers in an efficient manner. Similar to the approach identified by Lewis, Simcox, and Berry [15], the current authors propose an additive model for the detection of malingering, during which a clinician begins with a clinical interview, behavioral observations, and file review. If the examinee endorses symptoms that are not consistent with records and/or are not consistent with those commonly identified by genuine mental health patients, then the clinician is strongly advised to administer a test designed to measure overall psychopathology and a specialized test of malingering. This step will help to identify true psychopathology as well as potentially confirming or disconfirming feigning. The clinician is again advised to evaluate all available evidence before coming to a conclusion about the validity of the examinee's symptom presentation.

There are several potential strengths of the proposed additive model for the detection of malingering. A strength of the additive model is that clinicians conserve time and resources. In order to assist with evaluations, we encourage clinicians to become familiar with the research literature in an effort to keep up with relevant malingering assessment instruments. Clinicians who follow the aforementioned steps and are familiar with recent research will find it easier to defend their opinion in an adversarial setting. The labeling of someone as malingering has a variety of potentially devastating consequences and as such should not be arrived at lightly. It is also important to consider that the presence of feigned symptoms does not automatically rule out genuine psychopathology. Instead, it is possible for a person who suffers from a mental illness to exaggerate symptoms at times, while attempting to downplay them at other times. Finally, a diagnosis of malingering should not be arrived at using a single test or piece of information; instead, a diagnosis of malingering should be based on the convergence of all the available evidence, and include formal testing of response styles.

References

1 American Psychiatric Association. *Diagnostic and Statistical Manual of Mental Disorders*, 5th ed. American Psychiatric Publishing: Washington, DC, 2013.

2 Berry DTR, Nelson NW. DSM-5 and malingering: A modest proposal. *Psychological Injury & Law* 2010; 3: 295–303.

3 Rogers R. Models of feigning mental illness. *Professional Psychology* 1990; 21, 182–88.

4 Pierson AM, Rosenfeld B, Green D, Belfi B. Investigating the relationship between antisocial personality disorder and malingering. *Criminal Justice & Behavior* 2011; 38: 146–56.

5 Rogers R, Bagby RM, Dickens SE. *Structured Interview of Reported Symptoms and Professional Manual*. Psychological Assessment Resources: Odessa, FL, 1992.

6 Cornell DG, Hawk GL. Clinical presentation of malingerers diagnosed by experienced forensic psychologists. *Law and Human Behavior* 1989; 13: 375–83.

7 Rogers R, Sewell KW, Goldstein A. Explanatory models of malingering: A prototypical analysis. *Law and Human Behavior* 1994; 18: 543–52.

8 Walters GD, Rogers R, Berry DTR, et al. Malingering as a categorical or dimensional construct: The latent structure of feigning psychopathology as measured by the SIRS and MMPI-2. *Psychological Assessment* 2008; 20: 238–47.

9 Resnik PJ. Malingering of posttraumatic disorder. In: Rogers R (ed.) *Clinical Assessment of Malingering and Deception*, 2nd ed. Guilford: New York, 1997: 130–52.

10 Alwes YR, Clark JA, Berry DTR, Granacher RP. Screening for feigning in a civil forensic setting. *Journal of Clinical & Experimental Neuropsychology* 2008; 30: 1–8.

11 Rogers R, Vitacco MJ. Forensic assessment of malingering and related response styles. In: Van Dorsten B. (ed.) *Forensic Psychology: From Classroom to Courtroom*. Kluwer-Plenum: Boston, 2002: 83–104.

12 Rogers R, Salekin RT, Sewell, KW, Goldstein A, Leonard KA. Comparison of forensic and nonforensic malingerers: A prototypical analysis of explanatory models. *Law and Human Behavior* 1998; 22: 353–67.

13 Heinze MC. Developing sensitivity to distortion: Utility of psychological tests in differentiating malingering and psychopathology in criminal defendants. *Journal of Forensic Psychiatry and Psychology* 2003; 14: 151–77.

14 Boccaccini MT, Murrie DC, Duncan SA. Screening for malingering in a criminal-forensic sample with the Personality Assessment Inventory. *Psychological Assessment* 2006; 18: 415–23.

15 Lewis JL, Simcox AM, Berry DTR. Screening for feigned psychiatric symptoms in a forensic sample by using the MMPI-2 and the Structured Inventory of Malingered Symptomology. *Psychological Assessment* 2002; 14: 170–76.

16 Vitacco MJ, Rogers R, Gabel J, Munizza J. An evaluation of malingering screens with competency to stand trial patients: A known-groups comparison. *Law and Human Behavior* 2007; 31: 249–60.

17 Rogers R, Cavanaugh JL. "Nothing but the truth": A reexamination of malingering. *Journal of Law and Psychiatry* 1983; 11: 443–60.

18 Von Neumann J, Morgenstern O. *Theory of Games and Economic Behavior*. Princeton University Press: Princeton, 1944.

19 Slick DJ, Sherman EMS, Iverson GL. Diagnostic criteria for malingered neurocognitive dysfunction: Proposed standards for clinical practice and research. *Clinical Neuropsychologist* 1999; 13: 545–61.

20 Rogers R, Sewell KW, Gillard ND. *Structured Interview of Reported Symptoms Professional Manual*, 2nd ed. Psychological Assessment Resources: Odessa, FL, 2010.

21 Kucharski LT, Ryan W, Vogt J, Goodloe E. Clinical symptom presentation in suspected malingerers: An empirical investigation. *Journal of the American Academy Psychiatry & the Law* 1998; 26: 579–85.

22 Resnick PJ, Knoll JL. Malingering psychosis. In: Rogers R (ed.) *Clinical Assessment of Malingering and Deception*, 3rd ed. Guilford Press: New York, 2008: 51–68.

23 Soliman S, Resnick PJ. Feigning in adjudicative competency evaluations. *Behavioral Science and the Law* 2010; 28: 614–29.

24 Meyer RG, Deitsch SM. The assessment of malingering in psychodiagnostic evaluations: Research-based concepts and methods for consultants. *Consulting Psychology Journal: Practice and Research* 1995; 47: 234–45.

25 Rogers R (ed.). *Clinical Assessment of Malingering and Deception*, 2nd ed. Guilford Press: New York, 1997.

26 Rogers R, Correa AA. Determinations of malingering: Evolution from case-based methods to detection strategies. *Psychiatry, Psychology, & Law* 2008; 15: 213–23.

27 Butcher JN, Dahlstrom WG, Graham JR, Tellegen A, Kaemmer B. *MMPI-2 Minnesota Multiphasic Personality Inventory 2 Professional Manual*. University of Minnesota Press: Minneapolis, MN, 1989.

28 Morey LC. *Personality Assessment Inventory: Professional Manual*. Psychological Assessment Resources: Odessa, FL, 1991.

29 Kucharski LT, Johnsen D. A comparison of simulation and known groups designs in the detection of malingering on the MMPI-2. *Journal of Forensic Science* 2002; 47: 1078–82.

30 Rogers R, Sewell KW, Martin MA, Vitacco MJ. Detection of feigned mental disorders: A meta-analysis of the MMMPI-2 and malingering. *Assessment* 2003; 10: 160–77.

31 Pelfrey WV. The relationship between malingerer's intelligence and MMPI-2 knowledge and their ability to avoid detection. *International Journal of Offender Therapy and Comparative Criminology* 2004; 48: 649–63.

32 Morey LC. *An Interpretive Guide to the Personality Assessment Inventory (PAI)*. Psychological Assessment Resources: Odessa, FL, 1996.

33 Rogers R, Sewell KW, Morey LC, Ustad KL. Detection of feigning mental disorders on the Personality Assessment Inventory: A discriminant analysis. *Journal of Personality Assessment* 1996; 67: 629–40.

34 Rogers R, Sewell KW, Cruise KR, Wang EW, Ustad K. The PAI and feigning: A cautionary note on its use in forensic-correctional settings. *Assessment* 1998; 5: 399–405.

35 Hawes SW, Boccaccini MT. Detection of overreporting of psychopathology on the Personality Assessment Inventory: A meta-analytic review. *Psychological Assessment* 2009; 21: 112–24.

36 McDermott BE, Sokolov G. Malingering in a correctional setting: The use of the Structured Interview of Reported Symptoms in a jail sample. *Behavioral Science & the Law* 2009; 27: 753–65.

37 Rogers R, Kropp PR, Bagby RM, Dickens, SE. Faking specific disorders: A study of the Structured Interview of Reported Symptoms (SIRS). *Journal of Clinical Psychology* 1992: 48: 643–48.

38 Rogers R, Vitacco MJ, Kurus SJ. Assessment of malingering with repeat forensic evaluations: Patient variability and possible misclassification on the SIRS and other feigning measures. *Journal of the American Academy of Psychiatry and the Law* 2010; 38: 109–14.

39 McCusker PJ, Moran MJ, Serfass L, Peterson KH. Comparability of the MMPI-2 F(p) and F scales and the SIRS in clinical use with suspected malingers. *International Journal of Offender Therapy and Comparative Criminology* 2003; 47: 585–96.

40 Miller HA. *M-FAST: Miller-Forensic Assessment of Symptoms Test Professional Manual.* Psychological Assessment Resources: Odessa, FL, 2001.

41 Windows MR, Smith GP. *SIMS: Structured Interview of Malingered Symptomatology Professional Manual.* Psychological Assessment Resources: Odessa, FL, 2004.

42 Guy LS, Kwartner PP, Miller HA. Investigating the M-FAST: Psychometric properties and utility to detect diagnosis specific malingering. *Behavioral Sciences & the Law* 2006; 24: 687–702.

43 Smith G. Brief screening measures for the detection of feigned psychopathology. In Rogers R (ed.) *Clinical Assessment of Malingering and Deception,* 3rd ed. Guilford: New York, 2008: 51–68.

44 Smith GP, Burger GK. Detection of malingering: Validation of the structured inventory of malingered symptomatology (SIMS). *Journal of the American Academy of Psychiatry and the Law* 1997; 25: 183–89.

45 Rogers R, Tillbrook CE, Sewell KW. *Evaluation of Competency to Stand Trial-Revised (ECST-R) Professional Manual.* Psychological Assessment Resources: Odessa, FL, 2004.

46 Tombaugh TN. *Test of Memory Malingering Professional Manual.* Multi-Health Systems: Toronto, Ontario, 1996.

47 Frederick RI. *Validity Indicator Profile Manual.* NCS Assessments: Minnetonka, MA, 1997.

48 Gierok SD, Dickson AL, Cole JA. Performance of forensic and non-forensic adult psychiatric inpatients on the test of memory malingering. *Archives of Clinical Neuropsychology* 2005; 20: 755–60.

49 Tombaugh TN. The test of memory malingering (TOMM): Normative data from cognitively intact and cognitively impaired individuals. *Psychological Assessment* 1997; 9: 260–8.

50 Frederick RI, Crosby RD. Development and validation of the validity indicator profile. *Law and Human Behavior,* 2000; 24: 59–82.

51 Franklin K. Malingering as a dichotomous variable: Case report on an insanity defendant. *Journal of Forensic Psychology Practice* 2008; 8: 95–107.

52 Melton GB, Petrila J, Poythress NG, Slobogin C. *Psychological Evaluations for the Court: A Handbook for Mental Health Professionals and Lawyers,* 3rd ed. Guilford: New York, 2007.

CHAPTER 8

Recurrent brief depression: "This too shall pass"?

David S. Baldwin[1] and Julia M. Sinclair[2]
[1] *Professor of Psychiatry and Head of Mental Health Group, Clinical and Experimental Sciences Academic Unit, Faculty of Medicine, University of Southampton, UK*
[2] *Senior Lecturer in Psychiatry, Clinical and Experimental Sciences Academic Unit, Faculty of Medicine, University of Southampton, UK*

Introduction

Psychiatrists and general practitioners should be aware of the need to distinguish between depressive symptoms, syndromes, and disorders. This awareness arises largely from observations in clinical practice, but also comes from the development of operationalized criteria for diagnosing depression, from early initiatives such as the Feighner criteria [1] and the research diagnostic criteria [2], to current schemes including the clinical descriptions included within the ICD-10 system [3] and the DSM-5 classification [4]. The various diagnostic systems have employed differing definitions for depressive disorders; for example, the criteria for "major" depression have varied with respect to the number and severity of symptoms, the duration of illness, the degree of personal distress, and the functional consequences of the condition (Table 8.1).

Psychiatrists see a poorly representative sample of the wider population of depressed patients, largely those who are most severely ill, with treatment-resistant symptoms, and with co-morbid disorders [5]. As a result, the definitions of depression derived from samples of psychiatric inpatients and outpatients may have limited relevance in primary care settings, where many depressed patients do not fulfill "accepted" criteria for major depressive episodes, because their illness is too mild, or too short, or not especially impairing. To address this problem, the more recent classifications have described a number of parallel depressive conditions, to include these important groups of depressed patients who could not otherwise be allocated a diagnosis. For example, the ICD-10 includes dysthymia to describe a persistent (at least 2

Troublesome Disguises: Managing Challenging Disorders in Psychiatry, Second Edition.
Edited by Dinesh Bhugra and Gin S. Malhi.
© 2015 John Wiley & Sons, Ltd. Published 2015 by John Wiley & Sons, Ltd.

Table 8.1 Diagnostic criteria for "major" depressive disorders.

	Feighner et al. [1]	RDC Spitzer et al. [2]		DSM-III APA 1980	DSM-III-R APA 1987	ICD-10 WHO [3]	DSM-IV APA 1994	DSM-5 APA [4]
		Major	Minor					
Low or dysphoric mood	+	+	+	+	+	−*	−†	−†
Duration (weeks)	4	2	1	2	2	2‡	2	2
Symptoms§	5/8	5/8	2/16	4/8	5/9	5/9	5/9	5/9
Impairment	No	Yes	No	No	No	Yes	Yes	Yes
Recurrence¶	No	No	No	No	No	No	No	No

*ICD-IO depressive episode (F32) requires presence of at least two of three "typical" symptoms (depressed mood, loss of interest and enjoyment, and reduced energy).
†DSM-IV and DSM-5 major depressive episode requires presence of at least one of two symptoms (depressed mood, loss of interest or pleasure).
‡ICD-IO depressive episode can be diagnosed earlier than 2 weeks, if symptoms are unusually severe and of rapid onset.
§Refers to minimum number of symptoms required for diagnosis.
¶Recurrence required to make diagnosis.

years) but mild depressive state; by contrast the DSM-5 uses "persistent depressive disorder" to describe long-lasting depressive illnesses previously recognised as either chronic but severe (chronic major depression), or chronic but mild (dysthymic disorder). Both ICD-10 and DSM-5 include a description of recurrent brief depression (RBD) within the broad group of depressive disorders.

Development of the concept of recurrent brief depression

Recurrent brief depression is not a new disorder, created to medicalize unhappiness or to satisfy a pressure for financial reimbursement. Short and mild depressive and hypomanic states were included within the broad category of manic-depressive illness by Kraepelin in 1889 [6], and transient states of severe affective disturbance were described 100 years ago [7, 8]. A condition similar to current conceptions of RBD was outlined shortly afterward [9] and was regarded as being particularly important in primary medical care. Patients were described as experiencing depressive episodes that were short-lived (lasting from a few hours to a few days), but that tended to recur frequently over the course of many years. Further accounts emphasized both the personality characteristics of affected individuals and the increased risk of suicide [10, 11].

However, despite its early recognition and readily apparent clinical importance, the syndrome of RBD was not subject to detailed investigation over the next 40 years. The research diagnostic criteria [2] included a category for diagnosing depressions that were short-lived and intermittent, but classified them as a form of minor depression, indicating that it was a mild disorder, of lesser clinical importance. Many studies of the prevalence of mild and short-lived affective disturbances in the general population have been performed, but there have been relatively few longitudinal studies of their incidence and longer-term course. The Zurich study [12], a prospective epidemiological investigation of depressive, neurotic, and psychosomatic syndromes, was the first modern investigation to lead to a renewed and heightened awareness of the clinical importance of short-lived (brief) but highly recurring and often markedly severe episodes of depression within the general population.

Arrival of modern diagnostic criteria: The Zurich study

In this influential investigation, a representative sample of (initially) young people from the Swiss Canton of Zurich has been interviewed repeatedly over the course of 35 years. Details of the study design and characteristics of the sample have been described elsewhere [12]. Participants within the cohort have been examined on many separate time points, using a specially designed interview schedule known as the SPIKE [13]. This interview covers a range of psychological and somatic syndromes, each of which is assessed according to the presence and number of symptoms; their duration, frequency, and recurrences; any treatment that has been received; and the presence of any family history.

Using SPIKE-derived data, the early interview phases showed that approximately one-half of the interviewees who had received treatment for depression did not fulfil the then-current DSM-III [14] criteria for major depression. These patients tended to experience depressive episodes that were short-lived but otherwise indistinguishable from major depressive episodes. In addition, around half of this group of patients experienced brief depressions that recurred at least monthly, and were associated with substantial social and occupational impairment. The early phases of the study revealed that approximately 5.0–10.0 percent of the general population experience intermittent brief depressions within any 1 year [15], and the period prevalence over the first 10 years (when the sample was aged between 20 and 30 years) was approximately 11 percent. The findings from this study subsequently led to the development of proposed diagnostic criteria for RBD.

The Zurich criteria, first delineated by Angst and colleagues [16, 17], stipulated that RBD is akin to DSM-III major depression with respect to symptoms, and similar to research diagnostic criteria [2] with respect to occupational impairment. However, RBD was distinguished from those two conditions, in requiring that depressive episodes last less than 2 weeks, but recur at least monthly over 1 year (Table 8.2). Broadly similar criteria for RBD are included within the ICD-10 and DSM-5: depressive episodes must last less than 14 days and should recur approximately monthly for at least 1 year. ICD-10 lists RBD within the group of "other recurrent mood [affective] disorders" [F38.1]. The DSM-5 places RBD within the group of "other specified depressive disorder" (311) (Table 8.3).

Table 8.2 Recurrent brief depression: the Zurich study criteria (from Angst and Dobler-Mikola [16]).

1 Dysphoric mood or loss of interest or pleasure
2 Four out of eight symptoms as listed for DSM-III major depression
  • Poor appetite or significant weight loss (when not dieting) or increased appetite or significant weight gain
  • Insomnia or hypersomnia
  • Psychomotor agitation or retardation
  • Loss of interest or pleasure in usual activities, or decrease in sexual drive
  • Loss or energy, fatigue
  • Feelings of worthlessness, self-reproach, or excessive or inappropriate guilt
  • Diminished ability to think or concentrate, slowed thinking or indecisiveness
  • Recurrent thoughts of death, suicidal ideation, wishes to be dead, or suicide attempts
3 Present less than 2 weeks but recurring at least monthly over 1 year
4 Reduced subjective capacity at work

Table 8.3 Recurrent brief depression in ICD-10 and DSM-5.

ICD-IO F38.I0 Recurrent brief depressive disorder
Recurrent brief depressive episodes, occurring approximately once a month over the past year. The individual depressive episodes all last less than 2 weeks (typically 2–3 days, with complete recovery) but fulfill the symptomatic criteria for mild, moderate, or severe depressive episode (F32.0, F32.1, F32.2).
Differential diagnosis
In contrast to those with dysthymia (F34.1), patients are not depressed for the majority of the time. If the depressive episodes occur only in relation to the menstrual cycle, F38.8 should be used with second code for the underlying cause (N94.8, other specified conditions associated with female genital organs and menstrual cycle).
DSM-5 311 Other specified depressive disorder
Recurrent brief depression: The concurrent presence of depressed mood and at least four other symptoms of depression for 2–13 days at least once per month (not associated with a menstrual cycle) for at least 12 consecutive months in an individual whose presentation has never met criteria for any other depressive disorder or bipolar disorder and does not currently meet active or residual criteria for any psychotic disorder.

Further epidemiological observations

Further support for the concept of RBD came from the findings of the World Health Organization study of psychological disorders in primary care [18]. From a group of 9697 consecutive general practice attenders, a sample of 1911 underwent a structured psychiatric interview. RBD was found to have a point prevalence of 3.7 percent, women being more commonly affected, and was seen to be a highly co-morbid condition, especially with major depression and generalized anxiety disorder, with a high (14 percent) lifetime rate of suicidal behaviour. Subsequent studies provided further support. For example, a sample of 300 primary care patients in Germany was assessed with respect to the number and duration of depressive symptoms: brief depression was diagnosed according to Zurich criteria, and found to have a point prevalence of 30 percent, more strictly-defined RBD having a point prevalence of 5.4 percent, the validity of brief depression appearing greater than that of "minor" depression (characterised by the presence of 3 or 4 depressive symptoms) [19]. Another study, performed in rural and urban Sardinia, and using a structured clinical interview, found that RBD had a lifetime prevalence of 6.9 percent, was frequently co-morbid with other mental disorders (particularly major depression), and associated with an increased risk of suicidal behaviour (9.1 percent), this being most marked in those with both major depression and RBD [20].

The Zurich study findings indicate that RBD is as stable a diagnosis as major depression: approximately 20 percent of people with RBD develop major depressive episodes when followed up, and a similar proportion show a change in the opposite direction (Angst, [15, 17]). The term *combined depression* has been suggested as suitable to describe the group of patients whose depressive episodes vary in length, typically with prolonged (i.e., more than 2 weeks) episodes becoming "superimposed" on a background of intermittent brief depressive episodes. It is therefore possible to compare individuals with RBD alone to those individuals with major depression alone, and to those with combined depression [17].

The 1-year prevalence of RBD is approximately 7 percent, somewhat greater than that for major depression. Both RBD and combined depression are more common in women. The prevalence of RBD may be greater in younger people (aged 14–24 years) than in the general population [21, 22]. There are few differences between RBD and major depression in terms of social class, although the social class of the father and level of education of the proband were found to be higher among those with combined depression. Adults with RBD report a significantly greater number of childhood emotional (especially anxiety) and behavioural problems than that described by adults with major depression. More than 50 percent of individuals with RBD and 70 percent of individuals with combined depression described themselves as being more anxious and fearful than their peers throughout childhood. All three groups report a similarly increased number of somatic disorders, when compared to the general population, with increased rates of gastro-intestinal, cardiac and circulation syndromes, and sexual and eating problems [17].

The clinical features of RBD and major depressive episodes are broadly similar: the mean age of onset, rates of family history of depression, and the proportion presenting for treatment are not different [17] although "difficulty in thinking" may be more common in individuals with major depression. RBD may have greater co-morbidity with panic disorder than is seen with major depression, but less co-morbidity with dysthymia [15]. A small Japanese case series suggests psychotic symptoms are not uncommon during brief depressive episodes in adolescence [23]. The lifetime risk of suicidal behaviour (11.4 percent) in RBD is similar to that seen in major depression; the risk being even greater in those with combined depression, where approximately 30 percent of individuals had attempted suicide by the age of 28 years [17].

Recurrent brief depression in clinical studies

Despite its prevalence, burden, and risk, the features of RBD in clinical populations have not been studied extensively. Regular and frequent assessments of a large number of psychiatric outpatients in London, performed over 2 years, reveal that the duration of brief depressive episodes shows an approximately "normal" distribution, around a median length of 3–4 days [24]. Around 90 percent of episodes resolve within 14 days, and hence do not fulfill diagnostic criteria for major depression. Some individuals may experience depressive episodes that last no more than 24 hours: a questionnaire survey of the "general population" (in fact, health professionals working in a teaching hospital) found that approximately one-half of individuals experiencing brief episodes had depressive symptoms which lasted for 1 day [25]. The severity of depressive episodes, assessed with the Montgomery-Asberg Depression Rating Scale (MADRS [26]) is high, with a mean MADRS score of around 30, though with substantial variation in symptom intensity between episodes. This severity is similar to that seen in outpatients with major depression [24]. The recurrence rate (i.e., the time from onset of one episode to the onset of the next) is highly variable, but with a median interval of around 18 days. The periodicity is irregular, with approximately 95 percent of episodes occurring more frequently than every 8 weeks, though with only two-thirds showing a monthly recurrence [24, 27].

RBD has a number of "troublesome disguises." Depressive episodes in people with RBD tend to have an abrupt onset, last a few days, and then resolve swiftly, and this rapidly changing picture suggests a possible link with "rapid cycling" bipolar disorder. Longitudinal studies indicate that short-lived (2–4 days) depressive episodes are common in both bipolar I and bipolar II disorder [28] and bipolar spectrum disorder [29], but data from epidemiological and clinical studies suggest that any connection of RBD to bipolar disorder is not certain. For example, the Zurich study findings indicate that individuals with RBD had lower rates of mania/hypomania (2.2 percent) than individuals with either major depression (5.9 percent) or no depressive disorder (5.0 percent) [15, 17]. Furthermore, in the London clinical sample only a small minority (3.0 percent) of patients developed mania/hypomania during follow-up, the rate being somewhat higher in patients with combined depression [30]. However, in a Norwegian sample, approximately 47 percent of individuals with RBD described a history of brief hypomanic episodes [31].

Other differential diagnoses include cyclothymia, dysthymia, or persistent depressive disorder, premenstrual dysphoric disorder (PMDD), and personality disorder. In the ICD-10 system, cyclothymia is described as a persistent instability of mood involving numerous periods of mild depression and mild elation: this instability develops in early adult life and persists for many years, despite long periods of normal mood. However, in clinical samples there is minimal overlap with cyclothymia, as even over long periods few individuals experience periods of elation; and the brief depressive episodes are too severe to be considered mild, in contrast to cyclothymia, where underlying mood changes are often inconspicuous: RBD should be regarded as a serious and disruptive illness [30]. RBD shows little overlap with dysthymia (and presumably, with persistent depressive disorder) in epidemiological and clinical samples, as depressive symptoms are present for only 15–20 percent of the time in prospective studies, so failing to meet the criteria for these conditions [24, 27]. RBD is not uncommon in men, having a 1-year prevalence of 4.2 percent compared to 10.3 percent in women, and in women is no more linked to the menstrual cycle than is major depression [17]; furthermore prospective studies find no obvious relationship to menstruation [24, 27]. Detailed characterisation of mood ratings finds significant differences between patients with RBD and PMDD [32]. Finally, the overlap between RBD and certain personality disorders includes affective instability, impulsivity, and repeated non-fatal self-harm. These phenomena could be understood as manifestations of persistent underlying maladaptive personality traits, or as features arising from an intermittent affective disorder. Many patients with RBD probably receive the diagnosis of personality disorder, where the possibility of an underlying mood disorder is easily overlooked.

The association of both RBD and combined depression with an increased risk of suicidal behaviour seen in epidemiological studies is also apparent in clinical samples. Two early double-blind placebo-controlled investigations of the effects of psychotropic drugs in the secondary prevention of suicidal behaviour demonstrated that the reappearance of brief but severe depressive episodes was significantly associated with subsequent deliberate self harm [33, 34]. In a longitudinal study, patients with combined depression had higher scores on measures of suicidal behaviour, when compared to patients with RBD or major depression alone [35].

Underlying causes

There have been few explorations of the potential underlying neurobiology of RBD. The syndrome of RBD has been reported in association with Prader-Willi syndrome (a chromosomal abnormality) [36], Fabry disease (an inborn error of metabolism) [37], and agenesis of the corpus callosum [38]. The reported association with both celiac disease [22] and chronic hepatitis C [39] suggests immunological mechanisms may be important in its etiology. The observation of a seasonal clustering of brief depressive episodes in some patients suggests circadian rhythms may be disturbed in a sub-group of individuals with RBD, and should encourage investigation of the effects of phototherapy [40, 41].

An early study found that patients with RBD did not differ from patients with major depression with respect to dexamethasone non-suppression, blunting of the thyroid-stimulating hormone response to challenge with thyrotrophin-releasing hormone, or shortening of rapid eye movement latency in sleep [42]. Comparison of individuals with RBD to inpatients with borderline personality disorder and patients with major depression suggests that RBD has neuroendocrine similarities to both conditions [43], and an investigation of sleep architecture found no significant differences between patients with RBD or borderline personality disorder [44]. A recent investigation suggests RBD patients with or without a history of brief hypomanic episodes differ in their performance in measures of attention and working memory [45].

Like other mood disorders, temperament and personality traits may be important in RBD; early data from the Zurich study suggest that "negative affectivity" is an antecedent for RBD (and other depressive disorders) [46]. Antisocial, dependent, and histrionic traits were found to be common in patients with RBD and a history of suicide attempts [47]. More recently, when compared to controls, primary care patients with RBD were found to have high trait anxiety, high neuroticism, and low extraversion [48]. A series of reports from a Norwegian cohort of patients with RBD suggest it is associated with impairments in working memory, processing speed, verbal and visual memory, and various measures of executive function [49], and, like bipolar II disorder, with higher harm avoidance and lower self-directedness [50].

Could RBD be treatable with psychotropic drugs?

Despite its prevalence, burden, and official recognition within classificatory schemes, RBD remains "an illness in search of a treatment" [51]. Most patients seem to recognise and tolerate the intermittent nature of the condition but some present to doctors while acutely depressed, demanding treatment. There is no evidence that acute brief depressive episodes can be treated effectively, and it is probably misguided to attempt treatment, as symptoms will usually have resolved before any prescribed drug has the chance to become effective. However, it is probably sensible for patients to avoid alcohol or benzodiazepines, in view of the reported (though disputed) ability to "disinhibit" reckless behaviour.

Only few investigations of long-term treatment of patients with RBD have been undertaken, although the findings of a number of randomised placebo-controlled studies of the secondary prevention of suicidal behaviour offer some guidance. Lithium is effective in reducing impulsivity and self-harm across a range of diagnoses [52], and was found beneficial in prophylaxis in an individual with RBD [53]. A case series suggests the selective serotonin reuptake inhibitor fluoxetine could be beneficial [54], although the findings of a large randomised controlled trial indicate fluoxetine was no different to placebo in preventing brief depressive episodes and associated suicidal behavior [55]. Treatment studies with paroxetine have also provided disappointing results [56]. The monoamine oxidase inhibitor (MAOI) tranylcypromine was found helpful in reducing affective instability and impulsivity in patients with borderline personality disorder [57] and beneficial in two patients with RBD [58], but the MAOI moclobemide was not found efficacious in a subsequent imipramine- and placebo-controlled study in patients with RBD (Baldwin et al., 2014 Baldwin DS, Green M, Montgomery SA. Lack of efficacy of moclobemide or imipramine in the treatment of recurrent brief depression: results from an exploratory randomized, double-blind, placebo-controlled treatment study. International Clinical Psychopharmacology 2014. E-pub ahead of print - PMID:24859491). Further case reports suggest potential benefit from treatment with the antidepressant drugs mirtazapine [60] and reboxetine [61], the antipsychotic drug olanzapine [62], the anticonvulsant and mood-stabilising drug lamotrigine [64], and the calcium channel antagonist nimodipine [64], but none of these compounds appear to have been subject to more detailed controlled investigation.

Could RBD be treatable with psychological interventions?

In the absence of proven effective pharmacological treatments, it seems likely that potentially beneficial psychological approaches involve strengthening of individual coping mechanisms, and acceptance of the condition.

Table 8.4 Proposed criteria for efficacy studies in recurrent brief depression (from Montgomery et al. [27]).

1. Three or more short-lived (1 week or less) depressive episodes in the previous 3 months
2. Recurrent pattern (unspecified) of intermittent short episodes of depression over the previous year
3. At least two of the episodes in the previous 3 months should satisfy criteria for major depression according to the DSM system, but without the 2-week duration criterion
4. At least two of the episodes in the previous 3 months should be of at least moderate severity
5. No episode of major depression in the previous 6 months

Non-directive psychodynamic or confrontational behavioural approaches may be considered vague and unhelpful, or intrusive and counter-therapeutic [55]. Supportive approaches and non-intrusive advice seem sensible, and patients may be wise to avoid important meetings or emotionally charged situations, given the irritability and sensitivity to criticism that often appear during brief depressive episodes [55]. Simply making patients aware of the concept of RBD and what is known about the condition may be helpful in terms of managing the condition.

The inclusion of RBD within the group of mood disorders in both ICD-10 and DSM-5 should encourage further research into the treatment of the condition. There is a particular need for well-designed randomised double-blind placebo-controlled long term studies, involving lithium or other mood stabilising drugs, or antipsychotic drugs. However the diagnostic criteria within ICD-10 and DSM-5 are not especially suitable for treatment studies, and a set of criteria for efficacy studies in patients with RBD have been proposed (Table 8.4).

Conclusion

The findings of detailed epidemiological investigations and often painstaking clinical studies together have influenced decisions to include RBD within the two major internationally recognised classificatory schemes. These investigations emphasize that RBD should be regarded as a common and serious disorder, associated with significant co-morbidity and suicide risk. However, there is still no proven efficacious treatment for this damaging and disruptive condition. Without advances in treatment, brief depressive episodes will remain "nasty, brutish, and short" and patients with RBD will continue to experience a burdensome, disruptive, and often dangerous condition. Brief depressive episodes may indeed "pass" from severe symptoms into states of unremarkable mood without medical intervention, but when present can be highly hazardous and when frequently recurrent are typically distressing, disabling, and disruptive.

Acknowledgments

Many thanks to Professor Dinesh Bhugra of the Institute of Psychiatry, and Miss Magda Nowak of the University Department of Psychiatry in Southampton for secretarial assistance. Explanatory note: "This too shall pass" is a Persian Sufi proverb indicating that all conditions—positive or negative—are temporary. Versions of the proverb appear in Jewish folklore and colloquial Turkish. Commenting on the phrase, Abraham Lincoln stated, "How much it expresses . . . how consoling in the depths of affliction."

References

1 Feighner JP, Robins E, Guze SB, et al. Diagnostic criteria for psychiatric research. *Archives of General Psychiatry.* 1972;26:57–63.
2 Spitzer RL, Endicott J, Robins E. Research diagnostic criteria: Rationale and reliability. *Archives of General Psychiatry.* 1978;35(6):773–782.
3 World Health Organisation. *ICD-10 Classification of Mental and Behavioural Disorders.* 1992.
4 American Psychiatric Association. *Diagnostic and Statistical Manual of Mental Disorders (DSM-5).* 5th ed. Washington DC: American Psychiatric Pub; 2013.
5 Shepherd M, Cooper B, Brown AC, Kalton G. *Psychiatric Illness in General Practice,* 2nd ed. London: Oxford University Press; 1981.
6 Kraepelin E. Manic depressive insanity and paranoia. In: Kraepelin E (ed.) 8th German ed. *of Textbook of Psychiatry.* 3 and 4. Edinburgh: E & S Livingstone; 1921.
7 Strohmeyer W. *Manisch-Depressive Irresein.* Wiesbaden: Bergman; 1914.
8 Gregory MS. Transient attacks of manic-depressive insanity. *Medical Record* (New York). 1915;88:1040–1044.
9 Paskind HA. Brief attacks of manic-depressive depression. *Archives of Neurology and Psychiatry.* 1929;22:123–134.
10 Read CF. Discussion. *Archives of Neurolo and Psychiatry (Chicago).* 1929;22:133.
11 Buzzard EF, Miller HE, Riddoch G, et al. Discussion on the diagnosis and treatment of the milder forms of the manic-depressive psychosis. *Proceedings of the Royal Society of Medicine.* 1930;23:881–895.
12 Angst J, Doblermikola A, Binder J. The Zurich study: A prospective epidemiological study of depressive, neurotic and psychosomatic syndromes. 1. Problem, methodology. *European Archives of Psychiatry and Clinical Neuroscience.* 1984;234(1):13–20.
13 Illes P. *Validierung des Fragebogens SPIKE an Diagnosen der Krankengeschichten des Sozialpsychiatrischen Dienstes Oerlikon.* Med. Diss. Zurich: University of Zurich; 1991.
14 American Psychiatric Association. *Diagnostic and Statistical Manual of Mental Disorders,* 3rd (DSM-III) ed. Washington, DC: American Psychiatric Association; 1980.
15 Angst J, Hochstrasser B. Recurrent brief depression: The Zurich Study. *Journal of Clinical Psychiatry.* 1994;55:3–9.
16 Angst J, Dobler-Mikola A. The Zurich study: A prospective epidemiological study of depressive, neurotic and psychosomatic syndromes. 4. Recurrent and nonrecurrent brief depression. *European Archives of Psychiatry and Clinical Neuroscience.* 1985;234(6):408–416.
17 Angst J, Merikangas K, Scheidegger P, Wicki W. Recurrent brief depression: A new subtype of affective disorder. *Journal of Affective Disorders.* 1990;19(2):87–98.

18 Weiller E, Lecrubier Y, Maier W, Ustun TB. The relevance of recurrent brief depression in primary care: A report from the WHO project on Psychological Problems in General Health Care conducted in 14 countries. *European Archives of Psychiatry and Clinical Neuroscience.* 1994;244(4):182–189.

19 Maier W, Herr R, Gansicke M, Lichtermann D, Houshangpour K, Benkert O. Recurrent brief depression in general practice: Clinical features, comorbidity with other disorders, and need for treatment. *European Archives of Psychiatry and Clinical Neuroscience.* 1994;244(4):196–204.

20 Altamura AC, Carta MG, Carpiniello B, Piras A, Maccio MV, Marcia L. Lifetime prevalence of brief recurrent depression (results from a community survey). *European Neuropsychopharmacology.* 1995;5:99–102.

21 Pezawas L, Wittchen HU, Pfister H, Angst J, Lieb R, Kasper S. Recurrent brief depressive disorder reinvestigated: A community sample of adolescents and young adults. *Psychological Medicine.* 2003;33(3):407–418.

22 Carta MG, Hardoy MC, Usai P, Carpiniello B, Angst J. Recurrent brief depression in celiac disease. *Journal of Psychosomatic Research.* 2003;55(6):573–574.

23 Abe K, Ohta M. Recurrent brief episodes with psychotic features in adolescence: Periodic psychosis of puberty revisited. *Psychiatry and Clinical Neurosciences.* 1998;52:S313–S316.

24 Montgomery SA, Montgomery D, Baldwin D, Green M. The duration, nature and recurrence rate of brief depressions. *Progress in Neuro-Psychopharmacology & Biological Psychiatry.* 1990;14(5):729–735.

25 Snaith RP. An enquiry into recurrent brief depressive episodes in the general population. *European Psychiatry.* 2000;15(4):261–263.

26 Montgomery S, Asberg M. A new depression scale designed to be sensitive to change. *British Journal of Psychiatry.* 1979;134:382–389.

27 Montgomery SA, Montgomery D, Baldwin D, Green M. Intermittent 3-day depressions and suicidal behaviour. *Neuropsychobiology.* 1989;22(3):128–134.

28 Bauer M, Glenn T, Grof P, Pfennig A, Rasgon NL, Marsh W, et al. Self-reported data from patients with bipolar disorder: Frequency of brief depression. *Journal of Affective Disorders.* 2007;101(1–3):227–233.

29 Shabani A, Zolfigol F, Akbari M. Brief major depressive episode as an essential predictor of the Bipolar Spectrum Disorder. *Journal of Research in Medical Sciences.* 2009;14(1):29–35.

30 Montgomery SA, Montgomery DB, Bulloch T. Brief unipolar depressions: Is there a bipolar component? *Encephale.* 1992;18(1):41–43.

31 Lovdahl H, Andersson S, Hynnekleiv T, Malt UF. The phenomenology of recurrent brief depression with and without hypomanic features. *Journal of Affective Disorders.* 2009;112(1–3):151–164.

32 Pincus SM, Schmidt PJ, Palladino-Negro P, Rubinow DR. Differentiation of women with premenstrual dysphoric disorder, recurrent brief depression, and healthy controls by daily mood rating dynamics. *Journal of Psychiatric Research.* 2008;42(5):337–347.

33 Montgomery SA, Montgomery DB, McAuley R, Rani DH, Shaw PJ. Maintenance therapy in repeat suicidal behaviour: A placebo controlled trial. *Proceedings of the 10th International Congress for Suicide Prevention and Crisis Intervention, Ottawa, Canada.* 1979. p. 222–227.

34 Montgomery SA, Roy D, Montgomery DB. The prevention of recurrent suicidal acts. *British Journal of Clinical Pharmacology.* 1983;15:S183–S188.

35 Pezawas L, Stamenkovic M, Jagsch R, Ackerl S, Putz C, Stelzer B, et al. A longitudinal view of triggers and thresholds of suicidal behavior in depression. *Journal of Clinical Psychiatry.* 2002;63(10):866–873.

36 Watanabe H, Ohmori O, Abe K. Recurrent brief depression in Prader-Willi syndrome: A case report. *Psychiatric Genetics.* 1997;7(1):41–44.

37 Mueller MJ, Fellgiebel A, Scheurich A, Whybra C, Beck M, Mueller K-M. Recurrent brief depression in a female patient with Fabry disease. *Bipolar Disorders.* 2006;8(4):418–419.

38 Bhattacharyya R, Sanyal D, Chakraborty S, Bhattacharyya S. A case of corpus callosum agenesis presenting with recurrent brief depression. *Indian Journal of Psychological Medicine.* 2009;31(2):92–95.

39 Carta MG, Angst J, Moro MF, Mura G, Hardoy MC, Balestrieri C, et al. Association of chronic hepatitis C with recurrent brief depression. *Journal of Affective Disorders.* 2012; 141(2–3):361–366.

40 Kasper S, Ruhrmann S, Haase T, Moller HJ. Recurrent brief depression and its relationship to seasonal affective disorder. *European Archives of Psychiatry and Clinical Neuroscience.* 1992;242(1):20–26.

41 Kasper S, Ruhrmann S, Haase T, Moller HJ. Evidence for a seasonal form of recurrent brief depression (RBD-seasonal). *European Archives of Psychiatry and Clinical Neuroscience.* 1994;244(4):205–210.

42 Staner L, Delafuente JM, Kerkhofs M, Linkowski P, Mendlewicz J. Biological and clinical features of recurrent brief depression: A comparison with major depressed and healthy subjects. *Journal of Affective Disorders.* 1992;26(4):241–246.

43 De la Fuente JM, Bobes J, Vizuete C, Mendlewicz J. Biological nature of depressive symptoms in borderline personality disorder: Endocrine comparison to recurrent brief and major depression (vol. 36, p. 137, 2002). *Journal of Psychiatric Research.* 2002;36(4): 267–268.

44 De la Fuente JM, Bobes J, Morlan I, Bascaran MT, Vizuete C, Linkowski P, et al. Is the biological nature of depressive symptoms in borderline patients without concomitant Axis I pathology idiosyncratic? Sleep EEG comparison with recurrent brief, major depression and control subjects. *Psychiatry Research.* 2004;129(1):65–73.

45 Korsnes M, Lövdahl H, Andersson S, Björnerud A, Due-Tönnesen P, Endestad T, et al. Working memory in recurrent brief depression: An fMRI pilot study. *Affective Disorders.* 2013;149(1–3):383–392.

46 Ernst C, Schmid G, Angst J. The Zurich study. XVI. Early antecedents of depression. A longitudinal prospective study on incidence in young adults. *European Archives of Psychiatry and Clinical Neuroscience.* 1992;242(2–3):14251.

47 Pretorius HW, Bodemer W, Roos JL, Grimbeek J. Personality traits, brief recurrent depression and attempted suicide. *South African Medical Journal.* 1994;84(10):690–694.

48 Williams WR, Richards JP, Ameen JRM, Davies J. Recurrent brief depression and personality traits in allergy, anxiety and premenstrual syndrome patients: A general practice survey. *Medical Science Monitor.* 2007;13(3):CR118–CR124.

49 Andersson S, Lovdahl H, Malt UF. Neuropsychological function in unmedicated recurrent brief depression. *Journal of Affective Disorders.* 2010;125(1–3):155–164.

50 Lovdahl H, Boen E, Falkum E, Hynnekleiv T, Malt UF. Temperament and character in patients with bipolar II disorder and recurrent brief depression. *Comprehensive Psychiatry.* 2010;51(6):607–617.

51 Baldwin DS. Recurrent brief depression - more investigations in clinical samples are now required. *Psychological Medicine.* 2003;33(3):383–386.

52 Wickham EA, Reed JV. Lithium for the control of aggressive and self-mutilating behaviour. *International Clinical Psychopharmacology.* 1987;2(3):181–190.

53 Corominas A, Bonet P, Nieto E. Recurrent brief depression successfully treated with lithium. *Biological Psychiatry.* 1998;44(9):927–929.

54 Stamenkovic M, Blasbichler T, Riederer F, Pezawas L, Brandstatter N, Aschauer HN, et al. Fluoxetine treatment in patients with recurrent brief depression. *International Clinical Psychopharmacology.* 2001;16(4):221–226.

55 Montgomery DB, Roberts A, Green M, Bullock T, Baldwin D, Montgomery SA. Lack of efficacy of fluoxetine in recurrent brief depression and suicidal attempts. *European Archives of Psychiatry and Clinical Neuroscience.* 1994;244(4):211–215.

56 Kasper S, Stamenkovic M, Fischer G. Recurrent brief depression: Diagnosis, epidemiology and potential pharmacological options. *CNS Drugs.* 1995;4(3):222–229.

57 Cowdry RW, Gardner DL. Pharmacotherapy of borderline personality disorder. Alprazolam, carbamazepine, trifluoperazine, and tranylcypromine. *Archives of General Psychiatry.* 1988;45(2):111–119.

58 Joffe RT. Tranylcypromine in recurrent brief depression: Two case reports. *International Clinical Psychopharmacology.* 1996;11(4):287–288.

59 Baldwin DS, Green M, Montgomery SA. Lack of efficacy of moclobemide or imipramine in the treatment of recurrent brief depression: Results from an exploratory randomized, double-blind, placebo-controlled treatment study. *International Clinical Psychopharmacology.* 2014. E-pub ahead of print - PMID:24859491.

60 Stamenkovic M, Pezawas L, de Zwaan M, Aschauer HN, Kasper S. Mirtazapine in recurrent brief depression. *International Clinical Psychopharmacology.* 1998;13(1):39–40.

61 Pezawas L, Stamenkovic M, Aschauer N, Moffat R, Kasper S. Successful treatment of recurrent brief depression with reboxetine: A single case analysis. *Pharmacopsychiatry.* 2002;35(2):75–76.

62 De la Fuente JM. Case report: Excellent response to long-term higher dose single olanzapine in a case of recurrent brief depression. *Pharmacopsychiatry.* 2008;41(4): 156–158.

63 Ravindran LN, Ravindran AV. Lamotrigine in the treatment of recurrent brief depression. *International Clinical Psychopharmacology.* 2007;22(2):121–123.

64 Pazzaglia PJ, Post RM, Ketter TA, George MS, Marangell LB. Preliminary controlled trial of nimodipine in ultra-rapid cycling affective dysregulation. *Psychiatry Research.* 1993; 49(3):257–272.

CHAPTER 9

Conversion disorders

Santosh K. Chaturvedi[1] and Soumya Parameshwaran[2]

[1] *Department of Psychiatry, National Institute of Mental Health and Neurosciences, Bangalore, India*
[2] *Department of Psychiatry, Kasturba Medical College, Mangalore, India*

Introduction

Conversion disorders have existed for many centuries, called by different names, and its nosology has changed at regular intervals. In clinical practice, these are rather common disorders in some countries and considered to be less frequent or rare in other countries. People might have conversion symptoms and when these symptoms form a predominant clinical presentation, a conversion disorder is diagnosed. Conversion symptoms may be reported in other psychiatric disorders as well. The common presentation of conversion disorders is through bodily or neurological symptoms or in loss of function of any particular system or part of body, or occurrence of sensation or pain in relation to psychological or emotional stress. The term *conversion* has a psychodynamic connotation, wherein the conflict or psychic anxiety was considered to be "converted" into a loss of function of a bodily part.

Historical aspects

The first description of conversion disorders is found in ancient times of Hippocrates and Galen. Greek physicians, who considered the symptoms to be specific to women, called it hysteria, which meant "a wandering uterus, *hustera*." The term *conversion* was first used by Freud and Breuer to refer to the substitution of a somatic symptom for a repressed idea. This introduced the psychological concept of primary gain, (i.e., psychological anxiety is converted into a somatic symptom), and secondary gain of such a reaction is the subsequent benefit that a patient may derive from being in the "sick role" [1]. Conversion disorder has always remained at the interface between neurology and psychiatry since the days of Charcot, Breuer, and Freud.

Troublesome Disguises: Managing Challenging Disorders in Psychiatry, Second Edition.
Edited by Dinesh Bhugra and Gin S. Malhi.
© 2015 John Wiley & Sons, Ltd. Published 2015 by John Wiley & Sons, Ltd.

Like any poorly understood phenomenon or disorder, there are many theories explaining the development of conversion disorders, namely, psychodynamic, behavioural, learning, sociocultural, philosophical, and neurobiological. Conversion disorder is conceptualised as a disorder of the brain associated with disordered emotions, in those with certain personality traits and inappropriate coping to stress, which helps the person avoid the stress rather than face it [2].

Epidemiology: Where are the conversion disorders of yesteryear?

Conversion disorders are universal in their presentation. These are one of the common presentations of common mental disorders or neurosis. In the last five or six decades, conversion disorders have been reported less commonly in the Western and developed countries. It was considered that conversion disorders are a common form of presentation of reaction to the stress in some traditional societies. One Indian epidemiological survey repeated 10 years and 15 years later in the same settings, which confirmed that the prevalence of conversion disorders or hysteria is on the wane [3]. The decline in hysteria was probably due to the improved socioeconomic status of women, because of greater economic power in the younger age group [4]. and increasing psychological sophistication of the population . The proportion of patients diagnosed as dissociative disorders during a decade in a psychiatric hospital ranged between 1.5 and 15.0 per 1000, reiterating the fact that dissociative disorders continue to exist and form a sizable proportion of mental disorders [5]. Of these, two-thirds of the cases were dissociative motor disorders and dissociative convulsions (conversion disorders) and were the most frequent [5]. The total incidence of conversion disorder has been estimated at 2.5–500 per 100,000 in the general population and at 20–120 per 100,000 among hospital inpatients [6]. In clinical practice, psychiatrists come across both conversion symptoms in depressive or anxiety disorders, as well as conversion disorders. Somatoform disorders are a common differential diagnosis for conversion, discussed later in the chapter.

In this chapter dissociative disorders would also be considered under conversion disorders.

Terminology: There's a lot in a name!

It is not an easy task to provide suitable names for symptoms unexplained by underlying organic pathology; hence, these have to meet certain criteria and description. The preferred term should be acceptable and of use to patients and doctors in a way that facilitates appropriate treatment. Despite being in official nomenclature since 1935, "conversion" has not achieved the dominance as a term among clinicians and researchers that might have been hoped for [7]. The term should also reflect etiological neutrality about the nature of a problem that we still do not properly understand. The term *conversion disorder* implies a specific psychological etiology in which intrapsychic distress is "converted" into "somatic" symptoms, thereby reducing the distress. Thus, it is not etiologically neutral. While not necessarily wrong, the conversion hypothesis is as yet unproven and must compete with other plausible psychological and biopsychosocial theories [7].

In clinical practice, a wide variety of terminology is used between countries and between physicians, neurologists, psychiatrists, and other health care providers (see below).

Stone and colleagues [7] have suggested, like many others, that the name conversion disorder should be changed. According to them, conversion disorder is not a useful term for this group of symptoms. Functional neurological symptom disorder, dissociative neurological symptom disorder and psychogenic neurological symptom disorder are possible alternatives suggested by them. One could take these suggestions with a pinch of salt. The term "functional" is poorly understood: Does it mean loss of function of a body part (as in monoparesis) or defect in function of the brain in the lack of anatomical and pathological evidences for the symptom. It perhaps implies a lack of morphological or biochemical abnormality; nevertheless the functions are impaired. With the growing use of functional magnetic resonance imaging fMRI, the term *functional* would add to the confusion, that functional disorders need a functional MRI. The term *dissociative,* like *conversion,* has its roots in psychodynamic defense mechanism. *Psychogenic* would imply the role of psychological factors and confirm their role in causing the symptoms and being an etiological term.

The arguments [8, 9] for abandoning the term *conversion disorder,* summarised by Reynolds [10], reiterate that the concept of conversion is based on a questionable psychoanalytical concept, and it is not widely used by general physicians and neurologists, and some assume it is not liked by patients. The current conversion diagnostic criteria require a psychosocial association with onset of symptoms, which is difficult to find in a minority of patients, and when present is sometimes of questionable relevance; and the exclusion of malingering, which is difficult, if not impossible. Neurologists tend to use their own terminology and concepts, commonly "functional" but with a variety of meanings, most often "non-organic" [11]. The heterogeneity of conversion disorders does not make it any easier to select a suitable, acceptable name for such disorders.

Difficulties in diagnosing conversion disorders

Conversion, as a disorder, has been a condition difficult to understand, explain, and manage. No wonder it is difficult to diagnose confidently and reliably. As the ages have gone by, different explanations have been propounded; the most popular were psychoanalytical explanations a few decades back. However, the term *hysteria* went into disrepute and has been replaced by conversion and dissociation symptoms, which unfortunately are also rather inadequate. Hysteria is also considered a form of abnormal illness behavior [12], and current biological research is desperately exploring the pathophysiology underlying hysteria. The varied presentations, course, and outcome make hysteria a rather charmingly difficult condition to treat.

There are a number of difficulties in diagnosing conversion disorders, mainly due to their varied presentations, heterogeneity, fluctuating course, sudden appearance and disappearance of symptoms, and a lack of concern shown by the patient and absence of any confirmatory method of diagnosis. The common reasons for these difficulties are:

Due to the attitude of health professionals. Many professionals and physicians may not feel competent in identifying conversion disorders and symptoms and manage the distress symptomatically in a medical form. There are others who consider conversion as something produced voluntarily by the person and as a form of malingering or "just acting." This attitude makes it difficult to confirm the diagnosis as these patients are brushed aside.

Most patients with conversion disorders are probably never referred to specialists, but are managed by the general practitioner. Many are not diagnosed or even identified. This may be because symptoms are minor, short-lived, or self-limiting or because the disorder is recognised as clearly having a psychological etiology. General practitioners are happier to work with the concept of nondiagnosis and may simply describe the symptoms, after any appropriate investigation, as "medically unexplained" or see the sociological concept of "abnormal illness behaviour" as being the most appropriate way of understanding these patients [12].

It has been reported that in clinical practice, neurologists use a wide variety of terms for diagnosing patients lacking a neurological basis for their symptoms, such as *functional, psychogenic,* and *hysteria.* However, when talking informally, the terms *neurotic, "malingering,* and *supratentorial"* become more common, whereas the terms *somatoform* and *conversion,* which are among the preferred official terms, were used by fewer than 30 percent of respondents in a survey of British neurologists [13].

Due to socio cultural factors. It is noted that in traditional societies expression of stress and emotional distress is prohibited or discouraged. Some cultures may lack adequate expressions or vocabulary for such emotions. In such societies, conversion symptoms form a method of expression of distress. Traditional societies willingly "accept" this physical and bodily presentation of stress rather than accepting emotional distress.

Case vignette

A teenaged girl was brought in with history of episodes of possession, in which she believed she was a goddess, and that the goddess was speaking through her and giving her orders to punish others. She heard the goddess's voices (a religious experience or pseudohallucinations) only in the temple and when she prayed to the goddess's idol. She had three such episodes, following a religious practice. She felt good about the episodes and did not want to lose these. She requested us to explain to her family that it was God's work and not to blame her. After treatment, 1 month later she denied belief of the goddess. Psychological tests showed no psychotic features but a possibility of conversion hysteria. There were no clear-cut stressors identified on sentence completion tests. After medications were stopped, she was seen 3 months later without any symptoms. She maintained improvement without any medications, and a final diagnosis was one of dissociative possession syndrome.

Due to the nature of presentation. This is a common reason for the difficulties in diagnosing conversion disorders. Since the investigations and evaluations of the loss of bodily function turn out to be normal, these symptoms are considered "medically unexplained." These symptoms are also considered to be "functional" as there is a loss of function without any anatomical or morphological abnormality. Due to the presence of perceived stress and a psychological precipitant, these disorders are considered to be psychogenic. These are methods of exclusion (of medical cause or identifiable abnormality), and hence, could be rather temporary situations till the medical cause is identified. This also depends on the sensitivity of the medical examination or investigations.

The current classifications do not provide a method for clinicians to express diagnostic uncertainty. There are patients in whom the clinician suspects conversion disorder but is uncertain of the diagnosis, perhaps because of a co-existing neurological or medical disorder or because they have insufficient clinical evidence [7]. Some patients have both a conversion symptom and a neurological disease (e.g., about 15 percent of patients with non-epileptic seizures [NES] also have epilepsy [14]) and some patients with cancer have been reported to have unexplained physical or bodily symptoms, unrelated to the underlying disease, but considered as somatoform symptoms or a form of abnormal illness behaviour [15].

Case vignette

An 18-year-old female, an undergraduate student of a professional course, was brought with a history of stammering since 4 days earlier. She reported that 5 days ago her father had an argument with her boyfriend and disapproved of their relationship. While listening to their argument, the girl had an attack characterized by falling on the bed and jerky movements of all her limbs; this lasted for nearly an hour until she was hospitalized. On waking up she couldn't speak. She was examined and investigated by a physician and given feedback that no neurological abnormality was found and she was normal. She gave a history of not being able to speak fluently 2 years earlier, following the death of her grandmother, to whom she was attached, and the condition improved gradually. After counseling parents and cutting down the secondary gains by parents, including their attention, and brief therapy sessions with patient, significant recovery was noticed.

Difficulty in understanding conversion disorders

In the absence of definitive explanations about the occurrence of conversion symptoms and disorders, clinicians struggle to understand the pathogenesis of these disorders. Over the last half century, the common mechanisms that are considered to underlie conversion disorders are as follows.

Psychodynamic mechanisms. Conversion is a neurotic psychodynamic defense mechanism. Mental health professionals may be in a position to explain any bodily symptom or conversion symptom, whether medically explained or not, by psychodynamics. Symbolism, a model for symptom (identification), and histrionic personality were reported to be important features of conversion symptoms [16].

Neurobiological mechanisms. Recent biochemical and imaging studies have pointed toward certain abnormalities in the localization and neurochemical mechanisms.

Studies in conversion disorder have demonstrated decreased activity of the primary motor or sensory cortex, and increased activation of the right orbitofrontal and cingulate cortices, as well as altered basal ganglia function [17]. As all these structures are involved in sensorimotor function and are interconnected with the limbic system, further investigations would help in understanding their role in the pathophysiology of somatisation, as well as the neural basis of gender differences. A role of the corpus callosum has been hypothesised, based on studies showing a larger anterior corpus callosum in subjects with high hypnotisability, a status linked to conversion [18], and activation of brain areas associated with traumatic recall has been reported in a woman experiencing motor conversion [19].

The study by Stone and colleagues [20] suggested that fMRI can help in studying the neural basis of conversion disorder. They noted consistent reductions in the activation of the motor cortex in cases with conversion disorder and control subjects simulating weakness. Cases but not controls showed activations in the basal ganglia, insula, lingual gyri, and inferior frontal cortex in association with movement of the weak limb, indicating that the cases were attempting to move with greater mental effort than occurred in controls.

Other functional imaging studies suggest that patients with conversion disorder have an abnormal pattern of cerebral activation in which limbic areas (or areas richly connected to the limbic system) override the activation of the motor and sensory cortices [21]. The exact mechanism is unclear, but one theory holds that specific regions of the cingulate cortex may function in a mutually exclusive way by "reciprocal inhibition," which allows each region to shut off the other during the processing of information. This is relevant to conversion disorder in that the caudal segment, responsible for willed action, may be deactivated or suppressed by the pregenual anterior cingulate cortex as it processes intense emotion [22].

Magico religious mechanisms or explanatory models. In many traditional societies, conversion symptoms are easily removed by magico religious methods. Similarly, some conversion symptoms are also produced by magico religious methods. The explanatory model of black magic and magico religious mechanism makes it difficult for a mental health professional to diagnose and treat such conversion disorders. Many a time persons with such explanations do not accept psychiatric intervention and insist on alternative traditional healing methods.

Case vignette

A 20-year-old unmarried male reported hearing voices of God talking to him, and being possessed by God, following a liking for a girl. He was religious and felt cheerful and energetic, attributing his energy to being possessed by God. With treatment, the possession attacks stopped and the voices of God stopped. He later admitted having experienced them, but on remission felt these were his "imaginations."

As discussed above, the diagnosis is difficult to make due to lack of confirmatory method. Reliability of diagnosis is poor, and as patients deny psychological stress, it is even more difficult to understand the occurrence of conversion symptoms. Most current views on conversion are either over- or under-inclusive, due to which defining boundaries is difficult. They even include certain normal phenomena that do not have any structural disintegration as an underlying mechanism. This has led to blurring of the boundaries in the conversion and dissociative disorders [23].

Diagnosing conversion disorders

The diagnosis of conversion disorders is highly dependent on the presentation, and lack of evidence of medical or organic features. The presence of psychological stressor has a subjective bias of the examiner, which limits the reliability of the diagnosis.

Signs and symptoms. There are a variety of different signs and symptoms, many which cannot be easily correlated with one another. Invariably, these are sudden in onset and dramatic in their presentations. These are preceded by an identifiable stressor or a presumed unidentifiable conflict or stressor. The conversion symptoms might be pain, weakness of limbs, loss of sight or vision, loss of speech, or loss of hearing. Loss of functions of other bodily systems may also happen. The symptoms are usually short lasting, and may be replaced by other similar or different symptoms. Psychological tests may give a hint of possible conflict and psychological stressor.

Presentations. The presentations are mainly in the form of physical or bodily symptom with denial of psychological stressor. The presentation is usually dramatic, demonstrative, and highly attention seeking. The unconcern for the loss of function is easily noticed and is termed *la belle indifference*. Though *la belle indifference* was once considered of diagnostic value, it was subsequently found to have no diagnostic validity [16].

Medically unexplained and functional somatic symptoms. When the routine and special investigations turn out be normal, the bodily symptom is considered "medically unexplained." Needless to say, this depends on the sensitivity of the investigative procedures. Many medically unexplained symptoms of the preimaging era have proved to be explained by technologically sophisticated investigations.

Comorbid medical and psychological symptoms. Known medical disorders may also have psychological distress and conversion symptoms. Conversion symptoms may coexist with comorbid medical illness, for example, seizures with pseudo seizures.

Some of the behaviours and features described above that are considered diagnostic features of conversion disorders have been found to lack diagnostic specificity [16]. Secondary gain, once a key feature, has been noted in other medical disorders as well. Similarly, attention seeking behaviour, is a personality trait, nonspecific to any illness. Persons who do not receive due attention to their symptoms and suffering try to draw the attention of their health professionals. *La belle indifference* was considered diagnostic of hysteria for a long time, but was found to be a nonspecific feature, and a way of coping and response to stress. *La belle indifference* could also be considered a dissociative phenomenon. There was a lack of evidence that symbolism could explain the hysterical symptoms, since the psychodynamic formulations became less popular. As mentioned above, histrionic personality does not always lead to hysterical symptoms, and persons with this personality could develop other disorders, and persons with other personality traits could develop conversion symptoms [24]. Whether there is a possible shift of gradual reduction in conversion disorders with increasing prevalence of eating disorders, BDD, deliberate self-harm, or the like (i.e., shift in abnormal coping mechanisms) is an interesting area of epidemiological research.

Making a reliable diagnosis

There is ongoing debate about making a reliable diagnosis of conversion disorders. In practice, professionals make a diagnosis by exclusion, which is not really a scientific way. The diagnosis needs to be a positive diagnosis, which is many times difficult to confirm confidently. In the past, when fewer investigations were possible, the diagnosis of conversion hysteria was made on the basis of a set of certain features such as those described by Lazare [16], such as the presence of other unexplained somatic symptoms, the presence of a model or stressor prior to onset, associated psychopathology, *la belle indifference*, secondary gain, disturbed sexuality, symptom symbolism, hysterical personality, and sibling position. Although these symptoms have been implicitly accepted as the key to diagnosis, little effort has been made to validate them except by a follow-up study [24], of hysteria. The report concluded that although a cluster of these features had some predictive validity, several of them, such as *la belle indifference* and the presence of a model, were of little value. Furthermore, these signs have been found to be present often in patients with acute organic neurological disease [25].

Case vignette

A 35-year-old female presented with a 1-year history of dissociative attacks. During these attacks, she would show childish behaviour and play with toys; she would talk like a child, sometimes go out of the house and wander, and even try to smoke a cigarette. She had undergone a hysterectomy 3 years earlier due to fibroids in the uterus. She denied any psychosocial stresses. Neurological examination was normal and there were no indications of any other medical disorder. She revealed that she used to practice and perform "black magic" therapy on distressed people in her village. The family considered these attacks to be due to supernatural forces and had gotten her treated by an "expert traditional healer." Since this did not help, they suspected some problem in her brain and got an MRI done on their own, but there was no abnormality. Projective tests indicated sexual conflicts, which the woman denied on interview. A number of psychotherapeutic sessions, aimed at dealing with her stressors, led to only partial improvement.

Table 9.1 Clinical subtypes of conversion disorders.

Clinical subtype	Presentations
Seizure or convulsion like	Non-epileptic seizures (pseudoseizures), hystero-epilepsy, hysterical convulsions
Motor weakness	Functional weakness, hysterical paralysis, conversion hysteria
Sensory losses	Loss of any sensation, loss of pain, touch etc.
Gait disturbances	Fluctuation of gait, giving way without fall/injury, dragging of a foot
Movement disorders	Bizarre and flailing movements, inconsistent tone, reflexes

One should consider conversion symptoms as a cry for help. Conversion symptoms could also be considered idioms of distress. This means that there may be conflict or anxiety that a person is unable to verbalize. Hence, appropriate communication skills and interview skills are necessary to explore the stressor.

Pentothal interviews, used a few decades back to elicit psychological or psychosexual stresses, are no longer popular and are not used to aid revealing stress or for producing catharsis. Psychological tests can be of assistance in some cases.

Some of the clinical subtypes of conversion disorders and their presentations are given in Table 9.1.

The subtypes can be differentiated by a meticulous neurological examination [26], as discussed below.

Non-epileptic seizures (pseudoseizures, hystero-epilepsy, hysterical convulsions, non-epileptic attack disorder) are triggered by stressors, and characterized by duration of greater than 2 minutes, partial responsiveness, and bizarre movements, such as sideways head movement or pelvic thrusts or resistance to eye opening. The episodes may be very brief or very prolonged, with flexor plantar reflexes, synchronous motor movements, and "limp" muscles.

Conversion disorders presenting with weakness (functional weakness, hysterical paralysis, conversion hysteria) exhibit varying power of the limb, sudden collapsing weakness, Hoover's sign, hemiparesis without facial weakness, and normal tone and reflexes. If there is a sensory loss, the distribution does not have any anatomical or dermatomal conformity.

Conversion disorders with gait disturbances (astasia-abasia) are characterized by fluctuation of gait disturbance, giving way without fall/injury, inconsistent Romberg's test, dragging an inverted/everted foot, but with normal cerebellar/sensory systems. Movement disorders (dissociative motor disorder, psychogenic movement disorder) are bizarre and flailing movements, with inconsistent findings of tone, reflexes, and varying site of movements.

Case vignette

A 30-year-old male, married for 1 year, presented with odd walking style. He would take three steps forward, turn right, turn around and walk. He reported anxiety and felt forced to walk this way. There was no evidence of any identifiable movement disorder or neurological illness. There were no psychological stresses preceding the difficulty in walking. This was neither preceded by any obsession, nor was it a compulsion. This movement did not appear to be an indecision or ambitendence.

Differential diagnosis

The common differential diagnosis that should also be considered are somatoform disorders, which are characterized by bodily symptoms, usually multiple, including pain, fatigue and sensory symptoms, and hypochondriasis. Conversion disorders are clearly distinguished from hypochondriasis, which is thought to be more common in men, having a less sudden onset and being accompanied by anxiety and multiple somatic complaints.

Conversion disorders also need to be differentiated from other forms of abnormal illness behaviour [12], other psychiatric disorders, undetected medical disorder, or neurological disease.

Nosological issues

Diagnosis of conversion disorders has been facilitated by the modern diagnostic systems. ICD-9 had the diagnostic category of hysterical neuroses, which were of two types: conversion and dissociation. In ICD-10, conversion disorders have been included partly under somatoform disorder and partly under dissociative disorder and called dissociative motor disorder.

In the DSM system, conversion disorders have been placed under somatoform disorders to emphasize the importance of considering neurological or other general medical conditions in the differential diagnosis. In the DSM-5, newer criteria have been described for conversion disorder (functional neurological symptom disorder); the criteria for conversion disorder (functional neurological symptom disorder) are modified to emphasize the essential importance of the neurological examination, and in recognition that relevant psychological factors may not be demonstrable at the time of diagnosis [27]. The DSM-5 classification defines disorders on the basis of positive symptoms (i.e., distressing somatic symptoms plus abnormal thoughts, feelings, and behaviors in response to these symptoms). Medically unexplained symptoms do remain a key feature in conversion disorder because it is possible to demonstrate definitively in such disorders that the symptoms are not consistent with medical pathophysiology [27].

The working group of ICD-11 has been considering newer criteria for diagnosis of conversion disorders, but these are not yet declared. Diagnostic systems have increasingly discouraged the use of the term *hysteria* because of its ambiguity, and current systems have dropped the term altogether.

Challenges in management and outcome

The management can be easy or difficult and frustrating. First of all, it is difficult to arrive at a diagnosis. Second, it is difficult to identify the psychological stressor, and finally, to understand the presentation of the disorder. Some professionals look for symbolism, which is quite subjective and not quite reliable.

The management is made difficult due to the treatment-seeking behaviours. The pathway to care expectedly finds its way to the mental health professional, through portals of faith healing and traditional healers. Religious interventions in conversion disorder highlighted a spectrum of approaches. The studies relating to patients attending the Mehandipur Balaji temple [28] and the description of religious healing in the southern Indian state of Tamil Nadu illustrate the use of places of Hindu communal worship in the treatment of patients [29]. Patients with conversion symptoms heading first to a psychiatrist is not a common observation.

Investigations focus on an endless search for an abnormality, the absence of which is unfortunately considered as evidence for conversion disorder. Many psychiatrists rely on their interviewing skills to unravel psychological or psychodynamic conflicts; others resort to psychological tests or psychometry, or commonly projective tests, like the thematic apperception test, sentence completion tests, or Rorschach inkblot tests.

Symptom removal is one of the key objectives of management. Sometimes this happens rather easily. A few decades back symptom removal was attempted with pinching the nose or with an ether swab on the nose, which would terminate the stupor, and restore function of the part having weakness or loss of function, including muteness or monoparesis, in the absence of neurological deficit or etiology.

The management consists of clinical and medical assessment, psychometric investigations, symptom removal, and psychotherapeutic intervention. Pharmacological management would involve a judicious use of antidepressants and anti-anxiety medications. The non-pharmacological managements are of more importance to understand the personal and interpersonal dynamics and use of psychotherapeutic interventions.

While acute presentations may show a benign course, conversion disorders presenting to specialist or tertiary services tend to run a chronic course

[26]. In the study by Mace and Trimble [13], over 50 percent of patients were rated as improved, and about 30 percent were considered to be in remission; however, a sizeable number also developed the features of somatisation disorder. Certain symptom subtypes, such as non-epileptic seizures, may be associated with a worse prognosis; factors predicting a poorer outcome include a longer duration of illness, the use of non-psychotropic medications, and psychiatric co-morbidity [26].

Psychological interventions, though difficult and time consuming, are still popular in many places. Therapies are either supportive or dynamic, and many times include family therapies.

Conclusion

Conversion disorders continue to fox the clinicians and are both a charm and a challenge to manage. However, there are no signs that conversion disorders will disappear from clinical practice. Hence, it is important to understand the significance of these disorders. The challenges in diagnosing and managing conversion disorders would need extra attention to the presentation, and understanding the phenomenology. A neurobiological understanding, when found, would perhaps make the diagnosis easier, but one cannot say the same about the management. It needs to be seen whether high technological investigations in future may explain the medically unexplained symptoms, and whether that could change the management or the outcome.

References

1 Owens C, Dein S. (2006). Conversion disorder: The modern hysteria. *Advances in Psychiatric Treatment* 12, 152–157.
2 Chaturvedi SK, Desai G. (2007). Neurosis. In Bhui K, Bhugra D (eds.) *Textbook of Cultural Psychiatry*. Cambridge: Cambridge University Press; 193–206.
3 Nandi DN, Banerjee G, Nandi S, Nandi P. (1992). Is hysteria on the wane? A community survey in West Bengal, India. *British Journal of Psychiatry* 160, 87–91.
4 Nandi DN, Banerjee G, Mukherjee SP, Ghosh A, Nandi PS, Nandi S. (2000). Psychiatric morbidity of a rural Indian community over 20 years. *British Journal of Psychiatry* 176, 351–356.
5 Chaturvedi SK, Desai G, Shaligram D. (2010). Dissociative Disorders in a Psychiatry Institute in India: A selected review and patterns over a decade. *International Journal of Social Psychiatry* 56, 533–539.
6 Krem MM. (2004). Motor conversion disorders reviewed from a neuropsychiatric perspective. *Journal of Clinical Psychiatry* 65, 783–790.

7 Stone J, LaFrance Jr WC, Brown R, Spiegel D, Levenson JL, Sharpe M. (2011). Conversion disorder: Current problems and potential solutions for DSM-5. *Journal of Psychosomatic Research* 71, 369–376.

8 Stone J, Lafrance WC, Levenson JL, Sharpe M. (2010). Issues for DSM-5: Conversion disorder. *American Journal of Psychiatry* 167: 626–627.

9 Kanaan RA, Carson A, Wessely SC, Nicholson TR, Aybek S, David AS. (2010). What's so special about conversion disorder? A problem and a proposal for diagnostic classification. *British Journal of Psychiatry* 196: 427–428.

10 Reynolds EH. (2012). Hysteria, conversion and functional disorders: A neurological contribution to classification issues. *British Journal of Psychiatry* 201, 253–254.

11 Kanaan RA, Armstrong D, Wessely SC. (2012). The function of "functional": A mixed methods investigation. *Journal of Neurology, Neurosurgery & Psychiatry* 83, 248–250.

12 Pilowsky I. (1996). From conversion hysteria to somatisation to abnormal illness behaviour. *Journal of Psychosomatic Research* 40, 345–350.

13 Mace CJ, Trimble MR. (1991). 'Hysteria', 'functional' or 'psychogenic'? A survey of British neurologists' preferences. *Journal of Royal Society of Medicine* 84, 471–475.

14 Widdess-Walsh P, Nadkarni S, Devinsky O. (2010). Comorbidity of epileptic and psychogenic nonepileptic seizures: Diagnostic considerations. In Schacter SC, LaFrance Jr WC (eds.) *Gates and Rowan's Nonepileptic Seizures*. Cambridge: Cambridge University Press; 51–61.

15 Chaturvedi SK, Maguire P, Somashekhar BS. (2006). Somatization in cancer. *International Review of Psychiatry* 18, 49–54.

16 Lazare A. (1981). Current concepts in psychiatry: Conversion symptoms. *New England Journal of Medicine* 305, 745–748.

17 Vuilleumier P, Chicherio C, Assal F. (2001). Functional neuroanatomical correlates of hysterical sensorimotor loss. *Brain* 124, 1077–1090.

18 Nash, MR. (2005). Salient findings: A potentially groundbreaking study on the neuroscience of hypnotizability, a critical review of hypnosis' efficacy, and the neurophysiology of conversion disorder. *Journal of Clinical and Experimental Hypnosis* 53, 87–93.

19 Kanaan RAA, Craig TKJ, Wessely SC, David AS. (2007). Imaging repressed memories in motor conversion disorder. *Journal of Psychosomatic Medicine* 69, 202–205.

20 Stone J, Zeman A, Simonotto E, Meyer M, Azuma R, Flett S, Sharpe M. (2007). fMRI in patients with motor conversion symptoms and controls with simulated weakness. *Psychosomatic Medicine* 69, 961–969.

21 Feinstein A. (2011). Conversion disorder: Advances in our understanding. *CMAJ* 183, 915–919.

22 van Beilen M, Vogt B, Leenders K. (2010). Increased activation in cingulate cortex in conversion disorder: What does it mean? *Journal of Neurological Sciences* 289, 155–158.

23 Isaac MK, Chand PK. (2006). Dissociative and conversion disorders: Defining boundaries. *Current Opinion in Psychiatry*, 19, 61–66.

24 Sharma P, Chaturvedi SK. (1995). Conversion disorder revisited. *Acta Psychiatrica Scandinavica* 92, 301–304.

25 Crimlisk HL, Ron MA. (1999). Conversion hysteria: History, diagnostic issues, and clinical practice. *Cognitive Neuropsychiatry* 4(3), 165–180.

26 Chaturvedi SK, Rajkumar RP. (2009). Somatisation and dissociation. In Chandra PS, Herrman H, Fisher J, Kastrup M, Niaz U, Randon MB, Okasha A. *Contemporary Topics in Women's Mental Health: Global Perspectives in a Changing Society*. London: Wiley; 65–96.

27 American Psychiatric Association. (2013). Highlights of changes from DSM IV TR to DSM 5. Accessed from www.dsm5.org/Documents/changes%20from%20dsm-iv-tr%20to%20dsm-5.pdf, September 1, 2013.

28 Satija, DC, Nathawat SS, Singh D, Sharma A. (1982). A study of patients attending Mehandipur Balaji temple: Psychiatric and psychodynamic aspects. *Indian Journal of Psychiatry* 24, 375–379.

29 Somasundaram O. (1973). Religious treatment of mental illness in Tamil Nadu. *Indian Journal of Psychiatry* 15, 38–48.

CHAPTER 10

ADHD controversies: More or less diagnosis?

Florence Levy

School of Psychiatry, University of New South Wales and Prince of Wales Hospital, Sydney, Australia

Introduction

Attention deficit hyperactivity disorder (ADHD) remains a controversial diagnosis despite being one of the most, if not the most, researched conditions in child psychiatry. Why might this be? Some of the reasons relate to a lack of agreement among professionals and the public in the degree of activity and distractibility that should be regarded as normal in childhood and at what age overactivity should be regarded as abnormal. In other words, ADHD is a developmental condition and developmental norms are difficult to establish, particularly when there are no gold standard objective measures. In addition, there may be cultural and geographical differences in diagnostic conventions.

Rutter and Sroufe [1] outlined three key issues for developmental psychiatry: (1) The understanding of causal processes, (2) the concept of development, and (3) continuities between normality and pathology. Rutter and Sroufe also described the rising influence of behaviour genetics on our understanding of causality as well as issues in the progressive reorganisation of behaviour as the organism transacts with the environment during development. Finally, the delineation of what is involved in the continuities and discontinuities between normality and pathology is a central concern of developmental psychopathology. They point out that that regardless of whether the underlying liability to psychopathology is dimensional with a continuum spanning normality and pathology, categorical decisions will often be required for practical decision-making purposes.

Historically, a lecture by George Still [2] described a group of children who manifested a deficit in "volitional inhibition" or moral control. Still described an overrepresentation of males, increased alcoholism, and

---

criminality, as well as a familial disposition to the disorder. He also observed the possibility of acquired injury giving rise to the disorder. The latter idea was reenforced by the pandemic of encephalitis lethargica that swept Europe in 1917–18, which was followed by a syndrome of overactivity and distractibility. Subsequent inability to demonstrate "hard" neurological signs gave rise to theories of minimal brain dysfunction (MBD) [3, 4]. A further important historical milestone was the finding by [5] that Benzedrine, a central nervous system stimulant, had a controlling effect on the overactive behaviour of children treated for spina bifida. This serendipitous discovery brought the syndrome into the arena of psychopharmacology, with subsequent controversies and public concerns that are still current despite numerous effectiveness studies [6, 7].

Genetic influences

Some of the underlying issues that contribute to the ADHD dilemmas relate to genetics, gender differences, comorbidity, and classification systems. There are at least two disparate approaches to analysis of behaviour, one focused on discrete behavioural categories, and the other on continua throughout the population [8]. For example, Levy and colleagues [9] showed that the heritability of DSM-III-R defined ADHD was not statistically different whether ADHD was defined as a continuum or a category. That is, the DSM-III-R (8/14) and DSM-IV (6/9) cut-offs are arbitrary points along dimensions of inattention and hyperactivity-impulsivity that we all share, and studies may reflect the initial classification methods.

Despite the above findings, the issue of ADHD subtype definition remains clinically important. For example, Rasmussen and colleagues [10] investigated familial clustering of latent class and DSM-IV defined attention-deficit/hyperactivity (ADHD) subtypes. The investigators utilised logistic regression to assess the clustering of same and different subtype combinations among twin and twin-sibling pairs and whether genetic influences contributed significantly to the observed patterns of subtype combinations the same and different subtype combinations among siblings. They concluded that with the exception of the DSM-IV hyperactive-impulsive subtype and the severe hyperactive-impulsive latent class, all other sibling DSM-IV and latent class ADHD subtypes consistently exhibited same-subtype clustering with MZ probands, DZ probands, and their siblings in both samples. The overall pattern of findings in both samples was thought to indicate significant genetic influences contributing to patterns of subtype concordance, and in general provided empirical validity for DSM-IV subtypes.

Classification issues and ADHD: DSM-IV versus DSM5

The fifth edition of the *Diagnostic and Statistical Manual of Mental Disorders (DSM5)* was released in May 2013 [11]. A number of issues have relevance for ADHD. These include the removal of the multi-axial assessment while not directly involving ADHD does affect the context in which the diagnosis is made. The apparent reasoning is that there was no evidence of its use by U.S. clinicians, despite some concerns that a broad assessment is useful for treatment planning and teaching. According to Frances [9], this change "would result in the loss of much valuable clinical information. Multi-axial diagnosis provides a disciplined approach to distinguishing between state and trait (Axis I versus Axis II) and to determining the contributions of medical conditions (Axis III) and of stressors (Axis IV) to the diagnosis and treatment of psychiatric disorders" [12].

A second question relates to preschool ADHD and whether ADHD is a valid diagnosis, and at the other end of the spectrum whether fewer symptoms should be required for a diagnosis of adult ADHD. A related question is the age at which first symptoms need to be observed and whether this should be increased. The broad question of whether a separate childhood classification of disorders should be retained rather than a combination with appropriate adult diagnoses is combined with the suggestion that ADHD should be classified as a neuro-developmental disorder. ADHD is classified as a neuro-developmental disorder and there is no separation of childhood and adult sections in the DSM5, with childhood qualifications in the appropriate sections. DSM5 has changed the requirement for onset to below 12 years rather than 7 years, and above age 17 requires a threshold of only 4 symptoms of inattention and hyperactivity. Also for the impulsivity section, additional items "acting without thinking," "uncomfortable doing things slowly," and "difficulty resisting temptation" were considered but ultimately not included. In general, these changes reflect the greater emphasis of DSM5 on spectra rather than categorical diagnoses and also a greater emphasis on developmental disorders. While these changes do not appear to be major, their implications for diagnostic epidemiology and treatment approaches to ADHD are for future determination. It remains to be seen whether the more "dimensional" approach will continue to give rise to questions about the boundary for treatment versus non-treatment. It is also unclear whether future revision of the ICD-10 [13] will follow the somewhat more dimensional DSM5 changes or maintain a more categorical approach.

According to Frances [9], "The greatest general impact would come from the suggestion to eliminate the 'clinical significance' criterion required in DSM-IV for each disorder that has a fuzzy boundary with normality (about two-thirds of them)." "These were included to ensure the presence of clinically significant distress or impairment when the symptoms of the disorder in mild form might be compatible with normality" [12]. Frances maintains, "Removing this requirement would reduce the role of clinical judgment as a gatekeeper in determining the presence or absence of mental disorders and thus would increase the already swollen rates of psychiatric diagnosis." He also suggests, "It has been widely accepted for several decades that adding dimensions would help to solve the categorical system's problem with fuzzy boundaries—thus improving the accuracy and precision of psychiatric diagnosis. Unfortunately, however, the field has never achieved consensus on which dimensions to choose and how best to measure them. Moreover, and most crucial, clinicians find dimensional ratings far too unfamiliar and cumbersome for use in everyday practice and all efforts to include even a few simple dimensional ratings into previous DSM's have been met by clinician resistance and neglect" [12].

Gender differences in ADHD

Gaub and Carlson [14] reported a meta-analysis of gender differences in ADHD, which found that non-referred girls with ADHD displayed lower levels of inattention, internalising behavior, and peer aggression than boys with ADHD, while clinic-referred samples displayed similar levels of impairment and comorbidity. Gershon reported a meta-analysis comparing results with the Gaub and Carlson study and to examine potential moderators of effect size estimates [15, 16]. The results indicated that females manifested significantly less externalizing problems, but significantly more internalising problems than ADHD males (the latter in contrast with Gaub and Carlson). ADHD females performed worse on Full Scale and Verbal IQ. Teachers rated ADHD females as less inattentive and having fewer externalising problems than ADHD males. Clinically referred samples tended to manifest more severe symptoms than community samples. They also found a possible gender bias in rating scales, but despite this there were large gender differences in the manifestation of ADHD symptoms and correlates.

Levy and colleagues investigated patterns of comorbidity in the three DSM-IV [15] subtypes of ADHD—predominantly inattentive (I), predominantly hyperactive impulsive (HI), and combined (C)—with oppositional defiant disorder (ODD), conduct disorder (CD), separation disorder (SA), and speech and reading problems in a large sample of twins and siblings (2173 males, mean age 10.69 years, and 2197 females, mean age 10.75 years) [17, 18]. The findings showed significant between-group differences in males and females for inattention and hyperactivity-impulsivity symptom count with higher ODD and CD in males, and higher SA in females. Separation anxiety was higher in females in the inattention subtype.

While the above studies suggest greater comorbid internalizing disorders in girls, and more externalizing disorders in boys, there is no clear understanding of etiological factors in these differences. It is possible that hormonal differences in utero and/or genetic and environmental factors are important, but this remains an area for further research.

Comorbidity and ADHD

Between 50 and 80 percent of children with ADHD also meet diagnostic criteria for other disruptive behaviour disorders, namely oppositional defiant disorder (ODD) and conduct disorder (CD) or for learning disorders and communication disorders [19–21]. There are also higher rates for internalising problems such as anxiety [22]. Kraemer [23] has described the greater vulnerability of males to developmental and social problems, but he says that this "biological fragility" is little understood. He discusses the observations that girls have better literary skills and are more aware of and explicit about their feelings and boys lack an emotional vocabulary.

A report from the NIMH Collaborative Multisite Multimodal Treatment Study of children with ADHD (MTA study) related comorbidity of ADHD with ODD/CD and anxiety disorders [24]. The investigators found that ADHD children with comorbid ODD/CD were more impulsive, according to parent and teacher ratings, than children with ADHD only and /or children with ADHD and anxiety. They also found that girls with ADHD were generally less symptomatic than boys, particularly in levels of impulsivity, underlining the need for further studies of gender differences. The authors point out that although the MTA provided an excellent opportunity to evaluate the effects of comorbidity and gender, the study related to clinically referred children only, and subdividing by gender and comorbidity resulted in some cells being smaller than optimal.

ADHD and bipolar disorder

A further controversial issue relates to the phenomenology of a group of children who tend to be diagnosed as having ADHD when they are young (under 5 or 6), but when their non-compliant or defiant behaviour, impulsivity, aggression, and mood problems continue, clinicians add diagnoses of ODD/CD or mood disorder, and in some cases pediatric bipolar disorder. These children can sometimes receive medication for many years without getting any significant treatment benefit. It is postulated that while ADHD is primarily a developmental/cognitive disorder, bipolar disorder is primarily a mood disorder, but in either case comorbid symptoms may phenocopy the alternate diagnosis. Thus pediatric bipolar disorder has been described as showing clinical features of irritability, rapid cycling with little inter-episode recovery, and high comorbidity with ADHD and ODD, while ADHD is described as age-inappropriate inattention, motor overactivity, and impulsivity observed before 7 years, often accompanied by ODD and sometimes CD. The comorbidity of bipolar mania and ADHD: (1) chance, (2) artifact of overlapping criteria, (3) a common predisposition to separate illnesses, and (4) symptoms of ADHD that precede the onset of bipolar disorder may represent a prepubertal illness antecedent to the development of a full affective episode. While these hypotheses require further investigation, the lack of a definitive distinction has given rise to the criticism of overmedication and inappropriate use of psychotropic medications at an early age range with possible adverse effects [12]. As a result of these concerns, the pediatric bipolar disorder diagnosis has been removed, and replaced with Disruptive Mood Dysregulation Disorder (DMDD) with the following features: Severe recurrent temper outbursts that manifest verbally and /or behaviourally in rages, or aggression toward people or property, with reaction grossly out of proportion, and occurring 3 or more times a week on average [25]

Mood between outbursts is persistently irritable or angry most of the day, nearly every day, and is observable by others (e.g. parents, teachers, peers).

Above criteria present at least 12 or more months.

Occurs in at least two of three settings (i.e. at home, at school, with peers).

Age at least 6 or equivalent developmental level

Exclude if more than 1 day of abnormally elevated mood, grandiosity, inflated self-esteem, decreased need for sleep, pressured speech, flight of ideas

While this change may reduce inappropriate use of medication at a young age, DSM5 allows co-diagnosis with ADHD, conduct disorder and/or oppositional defiant disorder (ODD) and it remains unclear how the ODD diagnosis in particular as well as ADHD treatment will be affected by this change.

Learning problems and ADHD

Wilcutt and Pennington investigated the association between reading disability (RD) and internalising and externalising psychopathology in a large community sample of twins (N=209) [26]. They found that RD was not significantly associated with symptoms of aggression, delinquency, oppositional defiant disorder, or conduct disorder, after controlling for a significant relation between RD and ADHD. Logistic regression analyses indicated that RD was not significantly associated with symptoms of aggression, delinquency, oppositional defiant disorder, or conduct disorder after controlling for the significant relation between RD and ADHD. In contrast, relations between RD and symptoms of anxiety and depression remained significant even after controlling for comorbid ADHD, suggesting that internalizing difficulties may be specifically associated with RD. Analyses of gender differences indicated that the significant relation between RD and internalizing symptoms was largely restricted to girls, whereas the association between RD and externalizing psychopathology was stronger for boys. Finally, preliminary etiological analyses suggested that common familial factors predispose both probands with RD and their non-RD siblings to exhibit externalizing behaviors, whereas elevations of internalizing symptomatology are restricted to individuals with RD.

Levy and colleagues reported on a study of ADHD and learning comorbidity in twins and siblings from the Australian Twin ADHD Project aged 6–18 years [27]. Analysis of the mean reading disorder scores in children with and without ADHD showed that children with conduct disorder had significantly more reading problems, as did children with multiple comorbid disorders, separation anxiety disorder, generalised anxiety disorder, depression, conduct disorder, and oppositional defiant disorder. Both age and ADHD diagnosis were associated with variations in these comorbid disorders, and multiple comorbid disorders were associated with greater reading impairment. A regression analysis of ADHD diagnostic subtypes by age and reading disorder showed that only generalized anxiety disorder remained significant after controlling for ADHD subtypes.

While reading problems have been consistently described in children with externalising disorders, Wilcutt and colleagues studied a sample of 313 8–16 year old same-sex twin pairs (183 monozygotic and 130 dizygotic twins), utilising the DSM-III version of the Diagnostic Interview for Children and Adolescents to assess ADHD symptoms and the Peabody Individual Achievement test [28]. They demonstrated that children with reading disorders are more likely than those without to meet criteria for ADHD and this relationship is stronger for symptoms of inattention than for symptoms of hyperactivity.

Raskind and colleagues have comprehensively reviewed the genetics of reading disabilities, from phenotypes to candidate genes [29]. They conclude that it is increasingly clear that genes are involved not only in neural migration in brain development, but also in the functioning of the brain throughout development. According to the authors, studies of genetic polymorphisms with inter-individual variability in brain activation and functional asymmetry in frontal and temporal cortices revealed that SNP's rs6980093 and rs7799109 in FOXP2 were associated with variations of activation in the left frontal cortex [30]. fMRI studies of developmental language and reading disorders suggest a "genetic risk" factor in a temporo-parietal area involved in phonological processing.

Inattentive ADHD

The question has been raised of whether a subgroup of inattentive ADHD symptoms represents a separate subtype, sometimes referred to as sluggish cognitive tempo (SCT) [31]. Adams and colleagues have pointed out, "clinical observations suggest that inattention often occurs in the absence of hyperactivity" [32]. They also describe empirical evidence supporting the validity of a group with significant symptoms of inattention, but not hyperactivity or impulsivity [33, 34]. Proponents of ADHD-PI (predominantly inattentive) have questioned the empirical and theoretical rationale for continuing to include ADHD-PI in the same category as disruptive disorders despite clinical and empirical evidence suggesting a lack of disruptive behavior in this group of children. Adams and colleagues [32] have recommended the creation of a new diagnosis, with its own code characterised by inattention without hyperactivity or impulsivity, somewhat reminiscent of DSM-III, which described a similar subtype.

A problem with the "inattentive" categorisation relates to the absence of clear psychometric or pathological underpinnings for a definitely separate subtype, as well as quantitative genetic data indicating covariation with hyperactive subtypes [10]. A further issue, often neglected in the U.S. literature, is the relationship demonstrated above by Levy and colleagues of ADHD subtypes to reading (and language) disorders [27]. Stevenson discusses evidence from twin studies for co-segregation of reading and spelling disorders and ADHD, despite different results from a family study by Faraone and colleagues [35, 36].

Molecular genetic studies may help resolve this question. Loo and colleagues have published a genome-wide scan supporting the existence of genetic factors that have pleiotropic effects on ADHD and reading ability—as suggested by shared linkages on 16p, 17q, and possibly 10q—but also those that appear to be unique to reading, as indicated by linkages on 2p, 8p, and 15q that coincided with those previously found in studies of RD [37]. Their study also suggested that reading measures might represent useful phenotypes in ADHD research. Stevenson and colleagues reported evidence of an association of alpha 2A adrenergic receptor (ADRA2A) polymorphism with the G allele in a study of one 152 children (140 boys, 12 girls) of British Caucasian origin, aged between 6 and 13 years and with a diagnosis of ADHD, demonstrating preferential transmission in those with ADHD plus RD [38].

These studies suggest that further behavior and molecular genetic studies of reading, spelling, and ADHD may help provide a useful understanding of attention-related ADHD subtypes, particularly in relation to reading and inattention. In this regard, the classification in DSM5 of ADHD as a neuro-developmental disorder could be a useful development in studying these relationships, which can be overlooked by a purely categorical approach. On the other hand, classificatory separation from other comorbid disruptive disorders such as ODD and CD may or may not be useful.

Conclusion

While the diagnosis of ADHD has been controversial since first described in the early 1900s, this intriguing condition continues to challenge clinicians and researchers, in terms of etiology, diagnosis, and treatment boundaries. Preschool and adult phenotypes, as well as degree of comorbidity with mood and learning disorders, are not well understood, and attitudes to treatment vary culturally and geographically. The advent of DSM5 continues to pose important questions, while future phenotypic studies will need to combine genetic, psychometric and brain imaging technologies.

References

1 Rutter M, Sroufe LA. (2000). Developmental psychopathology: Concepts and challenges. *Development and Psychopathology,* 12: 265–96.
2 Still GF. (1902). Some abnormal psychical conditions in children. *Lancet,* 1: 1008–12.
3 Laufer E, Denhoff MW. (1957). Hyperkinetic behavior syndrome in children. *Journal of Pediatrics,* 50(4): 463–74.
4 Kessler JW. (1980). History of minimal brain dysfunction. In Rie H, Rie E (eds.), *Handbook of Minimal Brain Dysfunctions: A Critical View.* New York, NY: Wiley (pp. 18–52).
5 Bradley C. (1937). The behavior of children receiving Benzedrine. *American Journal of Psychiatry,* 94: 577–585.
6 Faraone SV, Buitelar J. (2010). Comparing the efficacy of stimulants for ADHD in children and adolescents using meta-analysis. *European Journal of Child and Adolescent Psychiatry,* 19: 353–64.
7 Kavale K. (1982). The efficacy of stimulant drug treatment for hyperactivity: A meta-analysis. *Journal of Learning Disabilities,* 15(5): 280–89.
8 Hay DA, McStephen M, Levy F. (2001). Introduction to the genetic analysis of attentional disorders. In, Levy F. & Hay D. (eds). *Attention, Genes and ADHD.* Brunner-Routledge, Hove, East Sussex, UK: Taylor and Francis, Philadelphia, PA (pp 7–34).
9 Levy F, Hay DA, McStephen M, Wood C, Waldman I. (1997). ADHD: A category or a continuum? Genetic analysis of a large-scale twin study. *Journal of the American Academy of Child and Adolescent Psychiatry,* 36(6): 737–44.
10 Rasmussen E, Neuman R, Heath A, Levy F, Hay DA, Todd R. (2002). Replication of the latent class structure of attention-deficit/hyperactivity disorder (ADHD) subtypes in a sample of Australian twins. *Journal of Child Psychology and Psychiatry and Allied Disciplines,* 43(8): 1018–28.
11 American Psychiatric Association: Diagnostic and Statistical Manual of Mental Disorders, Fifth Edition. Arlington, VA, *American Psychiatric Association,* 2013.

12 Frances A. (2010). Opening Pandora's box: The 19 worst suggestions for DSM5. *Psychiatric Times,* February 11, 2010.

13 WHO. (1992). *International Classification of Disease,* 10th revision (ICD-10). World Health Organisation (WHO).

14 Gaub M, Carlson CL. (1997). Gender differences in ADHD: A meta-analysis and critical review. *Journal of the American Academy of Child and Adolescent Psychiatry,* 36: 1036–45.

15 Gershon J. (2002). A meta-analytic review of gender differences in ADHD. *Journal of Attention Disorders,* 5: 143–54.

16 Gershon J (2002). Gender differences in ADHD. *ADHD Report,* 10, 8–9, 14–16.

17 Levy F, Hay DA, Bennett K, McStephen M. (2005). Gender differences in ADHD subtype comorbidity. *Journal of the American Academy of Child and Adolescent Psychiatry,* 44(4): 368–76.

18 American Psychiatric Association. (1994). *Diagnostic and Statistical Manual of Mental Disorders (DSM-IV).* Washington DC: Author.

19 Waldman ID, Lilienfeld SO. (1991). Diagnostic efficiency of symptoms for oppositional defiant disorder and attention-deficit hyperactivity disorder. *Journal of Consulting and Clinical Psychology,* 59(5): 732–38.

20 Thapar A, Harrington R, McGuffin P. (2001). Examining the comorbidity of ADHD-related behaviours and conduct problems using a twin study design. *British Journal of Psychiatry,* 179: 224–29.

21 Tannock R, Martinussen R, Fritjers J. (2000). Naming speed performance and stimulant effects indicate effortful, semantic processing deficits in attention-deficit/hyperactivity disorder. *Journal of the American Academy of Child and Adolescent Psychiatry,* 28: 237–52.

22 Jensen PS, Hinshaw SP, Kraemer HC, Lenora N, Newcorn JH, Abikoff HB, March JS, et al. (2001). ADHD comorbidity findings from the MTA study: Comparing comorbid subgroups. *Journal of the American Academy of Child & Adolescent Psychiatry* 40(2): 147–58.

23 Kraemer S. (2000). The fragile male. *British Medical Journal,* 321: 1609–12.

24 Newcorn JH, Halperin JM, Jensen PS, Abikoff HB, Arnold LB, Cantwell DP, Conners CK, et al. (2001). Symptom profiles in children with ADHD: Effects of comorbidity and gender. *Journal of the American Academy of Child & Adolescent Psychiatry,* 40(2): 137–46.

25 Liebenluft E. (2011). Severe mood dysregulation, irritability, and the diagnostic boundaries of bipolar disorder in youths. *American Journal of Psychiatry,* 168: 129–42.

26 Wilcutt EG, Pennington BF. (2000). Psychiatric comorbidity in children and adolescents with reading disability. *Journal of Child Psychology and Psychiatry,* 41(8): 1039–48.

27 Levy F, Young DJ, Bennett KS, Martin NC, Hay DA. (2012). Comorbid ADHD and mental health disorders: Are these children more likely to develop reading disorders? *ADHD Attention Deficit Hyperactivity.* doi:10.1007/s12402-012-0093-3.

28 Wilcutt EG, Pennington BF, DeFries JC. (2000). Twin study of the etiology of comorbidity between reading disability and attention-deficit/hyperactivity disorder. *American Journal of Medical Genetics (Neuropsychiatric Genetics),* 96: 293–301.

29 Raskind WH, Beate P, Richards T, Eckert MM, Berninger VW. (2013). The enetics of reading disabilities: From phenotypes to candidate genes. *Frontiers in Psychology.* Doi: 10.3389/fpsyg.2012.00601.

30 Pinel P, Fauchereau F, Moreno A, Barbot A, Lathrop M, Zelenika D, et al. (2012). Genetic variants of FOXP2 and KIAA0319/TTRAP/THEM2 locus are associated with altered brain activation in distinct language: Related regions. *Journal of Neuroscience,* 32: 817–25.

31 McBurnett K, Pfiffner L, Frick P. (2001). Symptom properties as a function of ADHD type: An argument for continued study of sluggish cognitive tempo. *Journal of Abnormal Child Psychology,* 29(3): 207–13.

32 Adams ZW, Milich R, Fillmore MT. (2010). A case for the return of attention-deficit disorder in DSM5. *ADHD Report,* 18(3): 1–5.

33 Lahey BB, Carlson CL. (1991). Validity of the diagnostic category of attention deficit disorder without hyperactivity. *Journal of Learning Disabilities,* 24: 110–20.

34 Milich R, Balentine AC, Lineham DR. (2001). ADHD combined type and ADHd inattentive type are distinct and unrelated disorders. *Clinical Psychology Science and Practise,* 8: 463–88.

35 Stevenson J. (2001). Comorbidity of reading/spelling disability and ADHD. In Levy F, Hay D (eds.), *Attention. Genes and ADHD.* Hove, East Sussex, UK: Brunner-Routledge; Philadelphia, PA: Taylor and Francis (pp. 99–114).

36 Faraone SV, Biederman J, Lehman BK, Keenan K, Norman D, Seidman LJ, Kolodny R, Kraus I, Perrin J, Chen WJ. (1991). Evidence for the independent familial transmission of attention-deficit hyperactivity disorder and learning disabilities: Results from family genetic study. *American Journal of Psychiatry,* 150: 891–95.

37 Loo SK, Fisher SE, Francks C, Ogdie MN, Macphie IL, Yang M, McCracken T, McGough JJ, Nelson SF, Monaco AP, Smalley SL. (2004). Genome-wide scan of reading ability in affected sibling pairs with attention-deficit/hyperactivity disorder: Unique and shared genetic effects. *Molecular Psychiatry,* 9: 485–93.

38 Stevenson J, Langley K, Pay H, Payton A, Worthinton J, Ollier W, Thapar A. (2005) Attention deficit hyperactivity disorder with reading disabilities: Preliminary genetic findings on the involvement of the ADRA2A gene. *Journal of Child Psychology and Psychiatry,* 46(10): 1081–88.

CHAPTER 11

Post-traumatic stress disorder: Biological dysfunction or social construction?

Richard A. Bryant

School of Psychology, University of New South Wales, Sydney, Australia

Introduction

Post-traumatic stress disorder remains one of the more controversial diagnoses. It has tended to polarise opinions since its very early conceptualisations. Despite great advances in our understanding of how humans response to severe stress, it still manages to activate heated discussions in the academic, government, and public domains. This chapter attempts to provide some insight into the major controversies that have plagued the diagnosis since its inception, and hopefully give a balanced view of both sides of the debate.

History of PTSD

Many people trace the historical roots of the PTSD diagnosis back to antiquity. For example, it has been suggested that descriptions of the disturbing nature of traumatic memories can be found in Homer's *Iliad* [1]. Others have found accounts of stress responses in the Napoleonic Wars, Spanish conflicts in the 17th century, and the American Civil War [2]. This is hardly surprising considering that people can be very distressed by traumatic events. How this early recognition has transitioned to a formal diagnosis has been a lengthy process, influenced by many societal and political issues.

The initial conceptualizations of traumatic stress were marked by confusion over whether anxiety arising from trauma reflected organic damage to the brain or emanated from psychological dysfunction. Early debates about the etiology of traumatic stress arose in the 19th century, partly as a result of

Troublesome Disguises: Managing Challenging Disorders in Psychiatry, Second Edition.
Edited by Dinesh Bhugra and Gin S. Malhi.

increasing industrialization. As railways became commonplace across the Western world, accidents among railway workers (and passengers) were very commonplace. These injuries often resulted in conditions characterised by generalized somatic reactions (including dizziness, fatigue, headaches, as well as symptoms of anxiety). Whereas neurologists initially attributed these reactions to spinal damage (hence the term *railway spine* as one of the very early descriptors of traumatic stress), some blamed these responses on psychological factors. For example, Professor Erichsen of University College London wrote in 1875:

> The mental or moral unconsciousness may occur without the infliction of any physical injury, blow or direct violence to the head or spine. It is commonly met with in persons who have been exposed to comparatively trifling degrees of violence, who have suffered nothing more than a general shock or conclusion of the system. It is probably dependent in a great measure upon the influence of fear.

Despite this recognition of psychological factors, the prevailing view at the time by neurologists was that traumatic stress responses were a result of damage to the nervous system.

It is important to understand that the timing of this development occurred in the context of increasing political concerns about the societal costs of railway accidents. In 1846 an act was passed in the UK permitting those who suffered as a result of a railway accident to claim damages from railway companies; this led to many claims for psychological damages and, perhaps because railway companies were most unpopular with the general public, they tended to lose nearly every case [3]. Not surprisingly, this led to a situation in which insurance companies were suspicious that motivational factors were driving these claims, and either consciously or unconsciously, stress responses may be confounded by the lure of compensation. This possibility was even recognized in the *Lancet*, which in 1861 noted:

> the difficulties proverbially attached to the exposure of the tricks of military malingers are as nothing compared with the task of determining the reality of some of the injuries to health, physical or mental, which those interested in recovering substantial damages assign to railway collisions [4].

These debates were fostered by developments in World War I, which saw all sides faced with the most horrendous numbers of casualties. The controversy over the extent to which traumatic stress was a function of organic or psychological disturbance raged throughout the war, as military leaders tried to stem the tide of the hundreds of thousands of troops who showed signs of marked distress, termed "shell shock." Medical figures commonly believed that the reactions (which ranged from inexplicable paralysis, conversion reactions, fatigue, and amnesia to explicit anxiety states) arose from exposure to bomb blasts or mustard gas that adversely affected the central nervous system [5]. As the war progressed, society became increasingly aware of the horrors endured by troops. For the first time, writers and poets expressed the suffering of soldiers rather than portraying them simply as brave warriors. British poet Wilfred Owen (who clearly suffered a form of psychological distress after his experiences in the war) wrote graphic poems of the horrors experienced in the trenches. For example, in his classic poem "Dulce et Decorum Est" he wrote:

> *Gas! Gas! Quick, boys! – An ecstasy of fumbling,*
> *Fitting the clumsy helmets just in time;*
> *But someone still was yelling out and stumbling*
> *And flound'ring like a man in fire or lime . . .*
> *Dim, through the misty panes and thick green light,*
> *As under a green sea, I saw him drowning.*
> *In all my dreams, before my helpless sight,*
> *He plunges at me, guttering, choking, drowning*

Such prose led to far greater societal acceptance of the validity of traumatic stress as a condition. However, military agencies saw the situation differently. Trench warfare resulted in massive loss of manpower that hugely dented the war effort. For example, the Battle of the Somme in 1916 alone saw tens of thousands of men withdraw from the frontline because of shell shock. In his compelling account of wartime psychiatry, Shephard [6] points out that military commanders were apparently personally removed from the trauma faced by troops in the trenches, and presumed that stress responses reflected cowardice. In fact, it was commonly believed that the public attention being given to stress reactions was fostering "soft-hearted" soldiers, which was undermining the war effort. This led to policies on all sides that attempted to discourage people from reporting stress reactions by reducing the possible motivations of removal from the frontline. This resulted in the birth of frontline psychiatry, which held that treating people as soon as possible in relation to the war reduced reinforcement of illness behavior, and encouraged return to normal functioning. In this episode, we can see how cultural, legal, and political issues were shaping the construct of traumatic stress.

One would think the lessons learned from WWI might have led to more sophisticated understanding, and management, of traumatic stress in WWII. Stress factors continued to plague the war effort. Nearly one-third of all medical discharges from the British Army in WWI were because of psychological issues [7]. This situation seems to have increased military commanders' conviction that signs of distress indicated weakness, or even treason. This was exemplified by the infamous slap by General George Patton of a fearful soldier, who complained he was incapable of functioning. Ironically, the widespread attention to this incident led to a public backlash, and further highlighted community awareness of traumatic stress responses in those affected by the horrors of war. This perspective did not alter the prevailing view of authorities that social forces were pivotal in reinforcing trauma survivors' response to the event. For example, British authorities expected massive stress reactions during the Blitz, which was feared would cause massive destruction throughout London (approximately 40,000 were actually killed). The Ministry of Health employed a strong approach of encouraging the "stiff upper lip" attitude by encouraging people to expect quick recovery from stress reactions, which would only be transient in those who experienced them. Subsequent analyses have noted that economic and political concerns during this period dominated policies, and although relatively few cases of traumatic stress were detected, in all probability genuine cases were neglected for the sake of minimizing a feared epidemic of traumatic stress reactions [6].

In considering the history of traumatic stress, we can see that it has oscillated in its professional and societal conceptualizations over time. In earlier times, it was definitely considered a transient response to trauma; this was partly motivated by the political inclination to encourage resilience and downplay the likelihood of people exaggerating their stress reactions. As time progressed, however, it became increasingly accepted that traumatic stress conditions could be long-lasting in some individuals. An undeniable conclusion in this unfolding history of PTSD is the effect of economic, societal, and political influences on the construct.

DSM and PTSD

This changing conceptualization of traumatic stress is seen in the formal diagnostic definitions provided to describe traumatic stress in the DSM. Going back to the initial publication, we can see that in DSM-I, "gross stress reaction" was used to describe those people psychologically affected by traumatic exposure [8]. In the post-war era, this very generic category was seen as clinically useful for initially classifying military veterans, ex-PoWs, rape victims, and survivors of the Holocaust. Consistent with wartime psychiatrists' views of traumatic stress, this diagnosis was considered a temporary state, and if the condition persisted the person would subsequently be described as suffering a "neurotic reaction." DSM-II eliminated the category of "gross stress reaction," replacing it with "situational reaction," an even broader category intended to describe adverse psychological reactions to traumatic and non-traumatic experiences, and still considered a transient state.

The Vietnam era saw a major shift in U.S. perspectives on post-traumatic mental health, with widespread awareness of the difficulties that troops experienced during deployment. Unlike previous wars, this was often an unpopular war and so there was greater sensitivity to those who were forced to fight it. As public attention had increased during prior wars, the media attention and lobby groups that emerged from the Vietnam War led to widespread recognition of the mental health problems arising from deployments. It was in this context that in 1980 DSM-III introduced PTSD as a formal diagnosis [9]. This was the first time that the spectrum of conditions previously termed rape trauma syndrome, post-Vietnam syndrome, prisoner-of-war syndrome, concentration camp syndrome, war sailor syndrome, child abuse syndrome, and battered women's syndrome were all categorized together. The core criteria of the DSM-III diagnosis of PTSD were three major symptom clusters (reexperiencing, numbing, and miscellaneous) that have formed the basis of more recent iterations of the diagnosis. There were shifts in the diagnosis in DSM-III-R [10] and DSM-IV [11], but the major structure of PTSD has remained steady for 20 years, with reexperiencing, avoidance, and arousal forming the basis of the disorder. These symptoms have been based on the notion of fear circuitry, such that the traumatic event creates extremely strong fear reactions that have a cascading effect on neural, behavioural, and cognitive processes. Phenomenologically, this leads to intrusive memories, nightmares, and flashbacks that contribute to the person wanting to engage in avoidance behaviours. It is also hypothesised that it triggers more passive avoidance responses, such as emotional numbing, dissociative amnesia, and social withdrawal. This state of affairs results in elevated anxiety states, involving sleep disturbance, heightened startle reactions, and hypervigilance to threat. To limit overdiagnosis of transient responses, PTSD is only diagnosed after at least 1 month of trauma exposure. Importantly, in addition to the symptoms being present, it is imperative that the person suffers impairment or clinically significant distress as a result of the symptoms.

What was the impact of DSM formally recognising the condition? Some considered that it merely summarised a human condition that has remained stable over hundreds of years, and the new diagnosis simply formalised this with a new name [12]. Others disagreed. For example, Summerfield [13] wrote of the diagnosis:

> the mental health field rapidly accorded it the status of scientific truth, supposedly representing a universal and essentially context-independent entity. This was to say that from the beginning of history people exposed to shocking experiences had been liable to a psychiatric condition which only in 1980 had been fully discovered and named. (p. 1450).

In an attempt to address the question as to whether the notion of PTSD is a timeless construct, the British historian Jones studied military records of UK personnel who served from 1854 up to the 1991 Persian Gulf War [14]. The interesting finding was that whereas flashback memories were virtually unreported in the early wars, they were reported by 9 percent of troops in 1991.

Conversely, somatic symptoms decreased markedly over this time. It is difficult to explain the exact reasons for this shift; however, it does appear that manifestations of stress conditions after trauma evolve, and the advent of PTSD represents the latest step in this evolution.

Impact of DSM-5

In 2013 DSM-5 was published. This marked a number of changes for the PTSD diagnosis, with the number of symptoms increasing from 17 in DSM-IV to 20 in DSM-5. The most salient change was the addition of a fourth cluster of symptoms, termed "Alterations in Cognition and Mood." This addition was motivated by a number of factors. Led predominantly by concerns about military personnel returning from Middle East conflicts and victims of crime, many believed that the traditional focus on fear in PTSD was too narrow. Accordingly, this new cluster added an item that recognised "pervasive negative emotional state," including guilt, shame, and anger. On the basis that exaggerated appraisals about the traumatic experience strongly predict PTSD [15], two additional symptoms reflecting cognitive biases were added. Finally, numerous factor analytic studies of DSM-IV criteria demonstrated that the previous avoidance cluster was more accurately conceptualised as two factors: active avoidance (including avoidance of trauma-related thoughts and situations) and passive avoidance (including emotional numbing, social withdrawal, and disinterest in activities) [16, 17]. Accordingly, DSM-5 separated the active avoidance symptoms into a single cluster and integrated passive avoidance symptoms with the new symptoms in the cluster of alterations in cognitions and mood,

Heterogeneity of PTSD

One of the interesting fallouts of the DSM-5 diagnosis was its impact on the potential heterogeneity of the diagnosis. PTSD has always been one of the most heterogeneous disorders because of the need to satisfy different numbers of symptoms in different clusters. For example, in DSM-IIIR there were 84,645 possible presentations of the disorder because it was required that the person satisfies 1 of 4 reexperiencing symptoms, 3 of 7 avoidance symptoms, and 2 of 6 arousal symptoms. In contrast, in DSM-IV there 227 permutations of major depression, 3 of obsessive compulsive disorder, 7,814 of panic disorder, 1 of specific phobia, and 1 of social phobia. In DSM-5, however, PTSD requires 1 of 5 reexperiencing symptoms, 1 of 2 avoidance symptoms, 3 of 7 negative alterations in cognition, and 3 of 6 arousal symptoms. This results in a staggering 636,120 possible ways that PTSD can manifest itself [18]. This situation has arisen, in part, because of the desire to make the diagnosis more amenable to a broader range of post-traumatic mental health problems. The potential cost of this, however, is that the definition of the phenotype has become very difficult to identify. From a researcher's perspective, this is problematic because the attempt to understand etiology and treatment of the disorder is hindered by the broad range of ways that people may have the disorder. For example, meta-analyses of risk factors for PTSD have highlighted massive variability in effect sizes; whereas extent of trauma severity is regarded as one of the strongest predictors of PTSD; effect sizes range from 0.02–58 percent [19]. There are also many examples of non-replications in the field of PTSD, and the heterogeneity of the disorder is one possible explanation. Enormous effort has been allocated in recent years to discovering biological markers of PTSD, with remarkably little success. It is likely that the increasing broadening of the phenotype being studied will only hinder this venture.

Role of impairment

One of the key debates about the PTSD diagnosis has centered on the role of impairment. Underpinning this issue is the extent to which we distinguish between common stress reactions following trauma and "disorder." Many commentators have argued that society has become too sensitive to stress reactions and psychiatry has been too keen to label reactions that in yesteryear were considered part and parcel of life as psychopathology [20]. One of these criticisms is that PTSD is too quickly diagnosed in the absence of thorough assessment of impairment (which is one of the required criteria for the diagnosis). DSM has been repeatedly criticized for not operationalizing functional impairment adequately, which results in poor conceptualization of the distinction between mild (and normative stress) and problematically persistent responses [21]. The resulting confusion was highlighted a number of years ago in a major re-analysis of the National Vietnam Veteran Readjustment Study, which in its original form was an epidemiological survey of men who served in the Vietnam War [22]. This study initially found that 30.9 percent of those who had served had developed PTSD at some point and 15.2 percent had current PTSD in the late 1980s. In the re-analysis adjustments were made such that prevalence required onset related to war activities, corroboration of traumatic events, and at least "mild impairment" (the initial figures did not require the impairment criterion). These changes reduced lifetime prevalence to 18.7 percent and current PTSD to 9.1 percent [23]. When another analysis was conducted with a slightly stricter definition of moderate impairment, current prevalence further reduced to 5.4 percent [24]. This highlights that the actual definition of PTSD can varying markedly according to the impairment level one requires. It also points to the potential tendency of some researchers to set a very low bar for impairment, thereby potentially artificially elevating the prevalence of the condition.

The issue of caseness

Inherent in all psychiatric diagnoses is the issue of justifying the demarcation between those who satisfy the criteria and those who do not. Perhaps this is a more vexed question in the case of PTSD than other disorders because there is much evidence that many people experience many of the symptoms of PTSD to varying degrees following trauma, including nightmares and sleep disturbance [25]. Many commentators have proposed that post-traumatic stress is better described as a single dimension of severity rather than adopting a taxon approach. Taxometric analyses have suggested that PTSD does not form a distinct taxon, and that PTSD symptoms are different in severity rather than in kind [26, 27]. Underscoring this point is the evidence that people who do not meet full criteria for PTSD, but display subsyndromal PTSD levels, nonetheless experience marked social and occupational impairment [28–31], and help-seeking behaviour [32].

Compensation and PTSD

PTSD has always held a special place in psychiatric compensation law because it is rare that the diagnosis itself contains the cause of the resulting symptoms and impairment. That is, by linking the PTSD symptoms with the Criterion A stressor, attorneys can strongly make the case that a plaintiff's impairment is directly attributable to a given event, and this brings into legal play the issue of liability for either preventing the event from occurring or adequately managing the reactions subsequently. As we have seen, this situation was a major social issue in the 1800s when governments and insurance companies were grappling with the issue of inordinate numbers of claimants presenting with psychological injuries. In more recent times, this situation has caused much concern about the motivations of people claiming a PTSD diagnosis when compensation is available [33]. Summarizing this situation in the U.S. (arguably the hotbed of compensation law internationally), it has been noted, "No diagnosis in the history of American psychiatry has had a more dramatic and pervasive impact on law and social justice than post-traumatic stress disorder" (p. 23) [34].

This issue has become very contentious in recent years in the context of deployments to warzones over the past few decades. For example, by 2012 45 percent of U.S. veterans had claimed service-related disability compensation [35], and 35 percent of these were for PTSD [36]. It is interesting to note that rates of compensation seeking have apparently increased over time. For example, the proportions of veterans receiving disability compensation (for any reason) in the context of World War II, Vietnam, and the Persian Gulf War were 11 percent, 16 percent, and 21 percent, respectively. It is also interesting to compare the relative trends of casualties across wars. The annual death rate in Afghanistan and Iraq was 270 troops per 100,000 troops deployed. When compared with other wars, it has been documented that the fatality rate was 2.5, 9, and 61 times greater in Vietnam, World War II, and the U.S. Civil War, respectively, relative to Afghanistan [37]. That is, whereas fatality rates are dropping progressively in warzones, the rates for seeking disability appears to be increasing [38].

Much debate has emerged in recent years, in both civilian and military contexts, over the extent to which increases in compensation-seeking may be a function of malingering or exaggeration of symptoms. The inherent problem in this regard is assessment of PTSD is largely reliant on self-report because there are no biomarkers or other objective indicators that reliably indicate the presence of the disorder. To date the best objective marker of PTSD is psychophysiological reactivity to trauma reminders; however, this does not have the capacity to distinguish between those experiencing genuine and simulated PTSD [39].

Critics have put forward some evidence indicating that PTSD claims are commonly driven by malingering, relying on validity scales on psychological instruments and interviews designed to detecting salient symptom exaggeration [40, 41]. One meta-analysis of over 100 studies found that most studies reported poorer outcomes in individuals involved in compensation [42]. In the context of the military, the U.S. Veterans' Affairs Office of the Inspector General studied claims and found that whereas there was an increase of 12.2 percent in veterans receiving compensation for all health condition between 1999 and 2004, the increase in those being compensated for PTSD increased by 79.5 percent [43]. Highlighting how the diagnosis of PTSD is susceptible to the influences of the compensation process, the Veterans' Affairs system in the U.S. will only confer compensation on the condition of a veteran having the diagnosis of PTSD, and payments will only continue as long as they continue to display the condition. This is hardly a constructive diagnostic label to motivate treatment-response.

Biological dysfunction or social construction?

We can see that underpinning much of the debate over the PTSD construct is the extent to which it is regarded as a biological disturbance or a social construction motivated by contextual factors. The former perspective highlights the evidence that people with diagnosed PTSD show certain characteristics, including disturbed neural fear circuitry and HPA axis activity [44, 45]. The extreme biological position holds that trauma memories are encoded in a fundamental way such that they are "hard-wired" in subcortical networks that function very differently from other forms of declarative memory. This account suggests that PTSD is universally consistent because this biological response is inherent across time and culture [46]. The opposite point of view holds that social forces play a key role in the definition and conceptualization of the condition, and accordingly varies according to culture and context. Exemplifying this perspective, anthropologist Alan Young states:

> The disorder is not timeless. . . . Rather, it is glued together by the practices, technologies, and narratives with which it is diagnosed, studied, treated, and represented and by the various interests, institutions, and moral arguments that mobilised these efforts and resources [47].

Perusing the evidence indicates that an extreme view in either direction is probably incorrect. On the one hand, there do seem to be certain universal characteristics of PTSD [48], and on the other hand there are distinctive cultural manifestations of the disorder [49]. The social, political, and financial factors that can influence how PTSD is understood and reported suggest PTSD may always be a controversial diagnosis. Nonetheless, overwhelming evidence that people with the core characteristics of PTSD suffer social, personal, and occupational impairment indicate that despite this controversy, its functional utility in identifying people in need after trauma and its capacity to direct them to evidence-based interventions suggests its longevity is guaranteed.

References

1 Shay J. Learning about combat stress from Homer's Iliad. *Journal of Traumatic Stress* 1991;4(4):561–79.

2 Jones E. Historical approaches to post-combat disorders. *Philosophical Transactions of the Royal Society B-Biological Sciences* 2006;361(1468):533–42.

3 Harrington R. The railway accident: trains, trauma, and technological crisis in nineteenth-centry Britain. In: Lerner A, Micale MS (eds.) *Traumatic Pasts: History, Psychiatry, and Trauma in the Modern Age, 1870–1930.* Cambridge: Cambridge University Press; 2001. p. 31–56.

4 *Lancet.* 14 September, 1861.

5 Mott FW. *War Neuroses and Shell Shock.* London: Oxford Medical Publications; 1919.

6 Shephard B. *A War of Nerves: Soldiers and Psychiatrists in the Twentieth Century.* London: Johnathan Cape; 2000.

7 Ahrenfeldt RH. *Psychiatry in the British Army in the Second World War.* London: Routledge & Kegan Paul; 1958.

8 American Psychiatric Association. *Diagnostic and Statistical Manual of Mental Disorders.* 1st ed. Washington, DC: American Psychiatric Association; 1952.

9 American Psychiatric Association. *Diagnostic and Statistical Manual of Mental Disorders,* 3rd ed. Washington, DC: American Psychiatric Association; 1980.

10 American Psychiatric Association. *Diagnostic and Statistical Manual of Mental Disorders,* 3rd ed. rev. Washington, DC: American Psychiatric Association; 1987.

11 American Psychiatric *Association. Diagnostic and Statistical Manual of Mental Disorders,* 4th ed. Washington, DC: American Psychiatric Association; 1994.

12 Trimble MR. Post-traumatic stress disorder: history of a concept. In: Figley C (ed.) *Trauma and Its Wake,* vol 1. New York: Brunner/Mazel; 1985. p. 5–14.

13 Summerfield D. A critique of seven assumptions behind psychological trauma programmes in war-affected areas. *Social Science and Medicine* 1999;48(10):1449–62.

14 Jones E, Vermaas RH, McCartney H, Beech C, Palmer I, Hyams K, et al. Flashbacks and post-traumatic stress disorder: the genesis of a 20th-century diagnosis. *British Journal of Psychiatry* 2003;182:158–63.

15 Ehring T, Ehlers A, Glucksman E. Do cognitive models help in predicting the severity of posttraumatic stress disorder, phobia, and depression after motor vehicle accidents? A prospective longitudinal study. *Journal of Consulting and Clinical Psychology* 2008;76(2):219–30.

16 King DW, Leskin GA, King LA, Weathers FW. Confirmatory factor analysis of the clinician-administered PTSD Scale: evidence for the dimensionality of posttraumatic stress disorder. *Psychological Assessment* 1998;10(2):90–6.

17 Asmundson GJ, Frombach I, McQuaid J, Pedrelli P, Lenox R, Stein MB. Dimensionality of posttraumatic stress symptoms: a confirmatory factor analysis of DSM-IV symptom clusters and other symptom models. *Behaviour Research and Therapy* 2000;38(2):203–14.

18 Galatzer-Levy I, Bryant, RA. 636,120 ways to have posttraumatic stress disorder: the relative merits of categorical and dimensional approaches to posttraumatic stress. *Perspectives in Psychological Science* 2013;8:651–62.

19 Brewin CR, Andrews B, Valentine JD. Meta-analysis of risk factors for posttraumatic stress disorder in trauma-exposed adults. *Journal of Consulting and Clinical Psychology* 2000;68(5):748–66.

20 Joseph S. *What Doesn't Kill Us: A Guide to Overcoming Adversity and Moving Forward.* New York: Basic Books; 2011.

21 Wakefield JC. Disorder as harmful dysfunction: a conceptual critique of DSM-III-R's definition of mental disorder. *Psychological Review* 1992;99(2):232–47.

22 Kulka RA, Schlenger WE, Fairbank JA, Hough RL, Jordan BK, Marmar CR, et al. *The National Vietnam Veterans Readjustment Study: Table of Findings and Technical Appendices.* New York: Brunner/Mazel; 1990.

23 Dohrenwend BP, Turner JB, Turse NA, Adams BG, Koenen KC, Marshall R. The psychological risks of Vietnam for US veterans: a revisit with new data and methods. *Science* 2006;313(5789):979–82.

24 McNally RJ. Revisiting Dohrenwend et al.'s revisit of the National Vietnam Veterans Readjustment Study. *Journal of Traumatic Stress* 2007;20(4):481–86.

25 Bonanno GA, Galea S, Bucciarelli A, Vlahov D. Psychological resilience after disaster: New York City in the aftermath of the September 11th terrorist attack. *Psychological Science* 2006;17(3):181–6.

26 Broman-Fulks JJ, Ruggiero KJ, Green BA, Kilpatrick DG, Danielson CK, Resnick HS, et al. Taxometric Investigation of PTSD: data from two nationally representative samples. *Behavior Therapy* 2006;37(4):364–80.

27 Ruscio AM, Ruscio J, Keane TM. The latent structure of posttraumatic stress disorder: a taxometric investigation of reactions to extreme stress. *Journal of Abnormal Psychology* 2002;111(2):290–301.

28 Norman SB, Stein MB, Davidson JRT. Profiling posttraumatic functional impairment. *Journal of Nervous and Mental Disease* 2007;195(1):48–53.

29 Stein MB, Walker JR, Hazen AL, Forde DR. Full and partial posttraumatic stress disorder: findings from a community survey. *American Journal of Psychiatry* 1997;154:1114–49.

30 Breslau N, Lucia VC, Davis GC. Partial PTSD versus full PTSD: an empirical examination of associated impairment. *Psychological Medicine* 2004;34(7):1205–14.

31 Walker EA, Katon W, Russo J, Ciechanowski P, Newman E, Wagner AW. Health care costs associated with posttraumatic stress disorder symptoms in women. *Archives of General Psychiatry* 2003;60(4):369–74.

32 Stein MB, Walker JR, Hazen AL, Forde DR. Full and partial posttraumatic stress disorder: findings from a community survey. *American Journal of Psychiatry* 1997;154(8):1114–49.

33 Lees-Haley PR, Dunn JT. The ability of naive subjects to report symptoms of mild brain injury, post-traumatic stress disorder, major depression, and generalized anxiety disorder. *Journal of Clinical Psychology* 1994;50(2):252–56.

34 Stone AA. Post-traumatic stress disorder and the law: critical review of the new frontier. *Bulletin of the American Academy of Psychiatry and the Law* 1993;21(1):23–36.

35 Marchione M. *Almost half of new vets seek disability*. Associated Press; May 27, 2012. Retrieved from http://news.yahoo.com/ap-impact-almost-half-vets-seek-disability-160656481.html.

36 Veterans for Commonsense. Iraq and Afghanistan impact report, January 2012. Retrieved from: http://veteransforcommonsense.org/wp-content/uploads/2012/01/VCS IAIR JAN 2012.pdf.

37 Leland A, Oboroceanu M-J. *American war and military operations casualties: lists and statistics*. Washington, DC: Congressional Research Service; 2010 [July 24, 2010]. Retrieved from: www.crs.gov RL32492.

38 McNally RJ, Frueh BC. Why are Iraq and Afghanistan War veterans seeking PTSD disability compensation at unprecedented rates? *Journal of Anxiety Disorders* 2013;27(5):520–26.

39 Orr SP, Kaloupek DG. Psychophysiological assessment of posttraumatic stress disorder. In: Wilson JP, Keane TM (ed.) *Assessing Psychological Trauma and PTSD*. New York: Guilford; 1997. pp. 69–97.

40 Frueh BC, Hammer MB, Cahill SP, Gold PB, Hamlin K. Apparent symptom overreporting in combat veterans evaluated for PTSD. *Clinical Psychological Review* 2000;20:853–85.

41 Freeman T, Powell M, Kimbrell T. Measuring symptom exaggeration in veterans with chronic posttraumatic stress disorder. *Psychiatry Research* 2008;158(3):374–80.

42 Harris I, Mulford J, Solomon M, van Gelder J, Young J. Association between compensation status and outcome after surgery: a meta-analysis. *JAMA* 2005;293(13):1644–52.

43 Veterans Affairs Office of Inspector General. Review of state variances in VA disability compensation payments. VA Office of Inspector General report no. 05-00765-137 2005. Retrieved from: www.va.gov/foia/err/standard/requests/ig.htm.

44 Patel R, Spreng RN, Shin LM, Girard TA. Neurocircuitry models of posttraumatic stress disorder and beyond: a meta-analysis of functional neuroimaging studies. *Neuroscience Biobehavioral Review* 2012;36(9):2130–42.

45 Yehuda R, Flory JD. Differentiating biological correlates of risk, PTSD, and resilience following trauma exposure. *Journal of Traumatic Stress* 2007;20(4):435–47.

46 van der Kolk BA. The body keeps the score: memory and the evolving psychobiology of posttraumatic stress. *Harvard Review Psychiatry* 1994;1(5):253–65.

47 Young A. *The Harmony of Illusions: Inventing Post-traumatic Stress Disorder*. Princeton, NJ: Princeton University Press; 1995.

48 Stein DJ, Koenen KC, Friedman MJ, Hill E, McLaughlin KA, Petukhova M, et al. Dissociation in posttraumatic stress disorder: Evidence from the world mental health surveys. *Biological Psychiatry* 2013;73(4):302–12.

49 Hinton D L-FR. The cross-cultural validity of posttraumatic stress disorder: Implications for DSM-5. *Depression and Anxiety* 2011;28:783–801.

CHAPTER 12

Bipolar disorder: A troubled diagnosis

Gin S. Malhi[1] and Michael Berk[2]

[1] Professor and Chair, Department of Psychiatry, Sydney Medical School, University of Sydney, Sydney, Australia
[2] IMPACT Strategic Research Centre, Deakin University, Department of Psychiatry, Orygen Research Centre, and The Florey Institute for Neuroscience and Mental Health, University of Melbourne, Australia

Introduction

Bipolar disorder is one of the most interesting and talked about psychiatric diagnoses of our times, and the stories of its inception and its current positioning within psychiatric classification serve to highlight a number of fundamental problems with psychiatric taxonomy [1].

Despite assiduous efforts to better delineate and understand bipolar disorder, especially over the past two decades, it remains poorly defined and some would argue that its boundaries have become less well delimited and that it has become a more nebulous concept. Consequently, advances in the management of bipolar disorder have been stilted and slow, and patients who attract this diagnosis continue to face the prospect of a chronic illness with often-unsatisfactory outcomes. This chapter briefly traces the history of this troublesome diagnosis and examines those aspects that continue to cause confusion and concern.

Manic-depressive illness

Early observations

When considering the history of an illness, it is important to recognize that the views of many ancient physicians and philosophers concerning mental phenomena, although they may appear to correspond to our contemporary understanding of an illness, almost certainly referred to symptoms, signs, and behaviours associated with diseases of very varied and altogether different origin. For example, a large variety of infections, left unchecked, can

Troublesome Disguises: Managing Challenging Disorders in Psychiatry, Second Edition.
Edited by Dinesh Bhugra and Gin S. Malhi.

cause marked fever and delirium, which often mimic symptoms of both mania and depression.

Some of the earliest written descriptions of melancholia were penned in ancient Greece by Hippocrates of Cos (460–377 BC) and members of his school who alluded, for example, to irritability, despondency, and an inability to sleep or eat. Interestingly, these writers argued strongly that mental illnesses, such as mania and melancholia, stemmed from organic causes and reflected brain dysfunction, in opposition to the prevailing view of the time, which explained mental illnesses in magical or supernatural terms. Hippocrates considered the brain to be pivotal to the generation of emotions and rejected the role of divine forces [2]. Unfortunately, these ideas, which seem at first sight to correspond to our own modern-day thinking, were based on wholly inaccurate biological models that survive metaphorically. Plato's (428–348 BC) theory of ideas incorporated rationalism, which has many parallels with modern thinking. He postulated that non-material abstract forms or ideas possess the highest and most fundamental kind of reality. Plato gave psychological importance to childhood trauma and asserted that the psychological significance that people assign to events is more important than the actual events themselves.

The *humoral theory*, adopted by physicians from Hippocrates until the 19th century, attributed health and disease to a delicate balance between the four humours: blood, phlegm, yellow bile, and black bile. Mania was thought to occur because of excess yellow bile, whereas an over-secretion of black bile (*melaina chole*) from the liver was thought to culminate in melancholia. As with modern physicians, ancient thinkers and great philosophers did not always agree: Aristotle (himself a student of Plato and tutor to Alexander the Great) assigned much more importance to the heart than he did to the brain. Nonetheless, when considering causality, he too believed that melancholia was a consequence of excess black bile. It was Aristotle who developed the quite visionary concept that some individuals are somehow *predisposed* to melancholia. He further linked this concept to temperament and, with this coruscating insight, anticipated much of our current ideas regarding biomarkers, vulnerability, and the role of personality and functioning in relation to the mental illnesses of today [3, 4].

Following on from these early concepts, subsequent observers tentatively linked mania and melancholia, suggesting that both either followed similar trajectories or were in fact the same illness, happening to present in varied forms or at different stages of disease. Aretaeus of Cappadocia, who suggested that mania was the end stage of melancholia, made the first definitive link between the two conditions [5]. A physician in Rome during the second century AD, he viewed "mania as a variety of melancholia" and described it as an alternating pattern of illness in which an individual could oscillate between the two forms. Remarkably, he also alluded to cyclothymia and described how personality could, perhaps, contribute to intermittent presentations of manic symptoms. Aretaeus' rich descriptions of mania detailed a spectrum that overlapped with psychosis, but he only associated the classical form of mania with melancholia. Prophetically, Aretaeus regarded mania as a disorder of the brain, and thus linked it, both phenomenologically and etiologically, to melancholia, which was also of endogenous origin [6].

Other aspects of the mood disorders, as we know them today, were successively added over time as physicians continued to observe patients with mental illness. Galen of Pergamon (AD 131–201), for example, drew out the recurrent nature of melancholia and established it as a chronic condition. But despite these many early insights, the concepts of mania and depression failed to develop further as medicine, and indeed science as a whole, fell prey to religious and spiritual thinking. During these "dark ages," divinity dominated and mental signs and symptoms were blamed on any number of evil forces, supernatural events, or black magic. Despite the Renaissance, not until the 19th century did a more informed discussion regarding melancholia and mania resume [7].

Great minds thinking alike

In the middle of the 19th century, two French physicians had the same idea at the same time. Both linked mania to depression and, in essence, created the concept of manic-depressive illness. Jean-Pierre Falret termed his interpretation *la folie circulaire* (circular disorder), which he used to describe a regular continuous succession of mania and depression [8]. Simultaneously, Jules Baillarger described *la folie double forme* (double insanity), a single illness in which both mania and depression could be manifested [9]. Wilhem Griesinger echoed this union although, more in tune with Aretaeus' thinking, he formulated mania as the end stage of a progressively worsening melancholia, and thus viewed the two presentations as manifestations of the same entity occurring at different epochs of the illness. Griesinger regarded the illness as having a chronic course that invariably eventuated in a poor outcome. In contrast, Ludwig Kahlbaum and Ewald Hecker identified much milder forms of "circular disorders," which also manifest an alternating pattern, but which do not develop a chronic course or culminate in dementia [10, 11]. Again, the descriptions by these early observers are prescient of today's mood disorder subtypes, such as bipolar II disorder and cyclothymia. However, it is noteworthy that not everyone was in concordance with these ideas: many physicians still regarded mania and melancholia as quite separate illnesses with distinct trajectories.

It was at this juncture that Emil Kraepelin synthesized the observations and insights of his predecessors and contemporaries by creating a model that remains with us today [12]. Kraepelin gave definition to manic-depressive illness by separating it from dementia praecox. As it gradually crystallized and took form as a diagnosis, its boundaries underwent gradual successive expansion until manic-depressive illness eventually consumed all forms of melancholia. Kraepelin's differentiation of manic-depressive illness from dementia praecox (subsequently known as schizophrenia) was predicated on the former being more likely to: (1) have a family history of manic-depressive illness, (2) run a relatively benign course and have a benign prognosis, and (3) manifest an episodic or cyclical pattern of illness. Kraepelin's model was widely adopted and remains a principal driver in psychiatric classification today. One reason for its success is its relative simplicity, along with the fact that it arose from empirical observations and therefore resonated strongly with clinicians. Another advantage that perhaps also contributed to its popularity and longevity is that it allowed the inclusion of additional causal factors, both psychological and social. It was, therefore, a relatively holistic model, and one that provided an accessible framework for interrogating mental phenomena [13].

Despite a common ancestry, ideas concerning manic-depressive illness developed along different lines in Europe and the United States [14]. In the latter, psychoanalysis played a significant role, along with social and psychological factors, partly because of Adolf Meyer's influence and emphasis on bio-psychosocial factors, which he termed "ergasiology" [15], and partly because, at the beginning of the 20th century, treatments that were derived from the disease model were largely ineffective. In contrast, European psychiatry maintained allegiance to the medical model of disease, and concepts of manic-depressive illness grew independently from both psychoanalytical and psychosocial schools of thought.

Bipolar disorder

Birth and adoption

In 1957 Karl Leonhard (1904–1988) noted that patients with manic-depressive illness could be separated into those that experienced *only* depression and those that experienced *both* mania and depression. He called these two groups monopolar and bipolar, respectively, and thus in effect coined the bipolar descriptor [16]. This separation was subsequently validated by studies based on family history [17, 18]. However, it is important to note that the terms actually refer to two kinds of *recurrent* affective disorders. This nuance was lost in the DSM classification of bipolar disorder, which adopted this nosology but which, instead of prioritizing cyclical recurrence, emphasized polarity.

The term *bipolar disorder* appeared in DSM-III in 1980. This edition of DSM was the first to recognize the unipolar–bipolar distinction proposed by Leonhard two decades earlier. However, use of the term failed to permeate into clinical practice for quite some time, and the diagnosis of manic-depressive illness remained in use, alongside bipolar disorder, until 1992, when the publication of ICD-10 finally led to its more widespread adoption [7].

Within DSM, bipolar and depressive disorders are partitioned on the basis of manic symptoms; but this classification fails to accommodate the many unipolar depressed individuals who have a recurrent form of affective illness. For example, in DSM-IV, two episodes over a lifetime qualify for the description of "recurrent unipolar depression" but because "two or more" is a very broad range, and one that encompasses virtually all depressed patients encountered in clinical practice, it is in effect a meaningless descriptor. These and other problems remain in the latest edition of DSM.

DSM-5

Published in 2013, the most dramatic change in DSM-5 in relation to bipolar disorder is its repositioning relative to other groups of disorders [19]. In DSM-IV the chapter on mood disorders contained both depressive and bipolar disorders [20]. However, in DSM-5, bipolar and related disorders are assigned a separate chapter, between depressive disorders and schizophrenia spectrum and other psychotic disorders, purportedly to reflect its genetic and phenomenological linkages to both sets of disorders. This displacement in classification is significant because it suggests that bipolar disorders are fundamentally distinct from depressive disorders, but in reality this may not be the case.

Hypomania: Hype or mania

Within bipolar and related disorders in DSM-5, bipolar I disorder remains the archetype, characterized by a sustained period of recognizable mania. The latter, known colloquially as a "high," features a range of symptoms among which elevated or irritable mood and increased energy or goal-directed activity are key, along with additional features such as a decreased need for sleep and marked impairment in functioning. An episode of depression is not necessary for a diagnosis of bipolar disorder, even though, for the majority of patients, this is the predominant phase of the illness and the guise in which the illness usually emerges for the first time. Therefore, in practice, mania defines and equates to bipolar disorder, but such pristine separation of bipolar and depressive disorders is lacking with respect to further definition of bipolar-related disorders. For instance, bipolar I disorder is separated from bipolar II, quiet arbitrarily, on the basis of duration and severity of manic symptoms. The upper and lower limits of 7 and 4 days, respectively, that are used to define periods of manic symptoms in bipolar II disorder (termed hypomania), do not reflect any phenomenological trend breaks in frequency or severity of symptoms and have not been found to correlate with any biological characteristics of the two subtypes [21]. The term *hypomania* was first used by

Emanuel E. Mendel to describe a mental state featuring moderated symptoms of mania [22], but it took more than a century and the development of an operational definition [23] for it to appear in the DSM. In DSM, hypomania equates to bipolar II disorder.

Clinically, bipolar II disorder is more common than bipolar I disorder and, by definition, periods of hypomania are shorter in duration and less severe than periods of mania. DSM-5 also stipulates that hospitalization is only necessary for mania and subtypes bipolar disorder on the basis of these characteristics. In practice, bipolar II disorder is at least as disabling as bipolar I, and more likely to result in suicide. Whether or not an individual is hospitalized is contingent on many additional factors (for example, bed availability within developed countries) and is particularly sensitive to availability of care and the diverse service systems within developing countries. Similarly, psychotic symptoms occur more commonly in mania as compared to hypomania but, again, they are not exclusive to this subtype and can of course also occur in "mixed states" and in the depressive phase of bipolar disorders. Thus the arbitrary separation of bipolar disorder subtypes on the basis of symptom duration and severity has resulted in decades of inconsistent diagnostic subtyping.

In reality, the timely and accurate definition of hypomania poses many challenges for a host of reasons. First, the natural course of bipolar disorder is such that depression usually precedes the onset of hypomania, and therefore 30–60 percent of patients with bipolar II disorder are diagnosed initially as having major depression [24] and this diagnosis is only revised many years later [25]. As an exemplar, data exists to show that, on aggregate, depressive symptoms precede hypomanic symptoms by 2 years, and a similar gap separates hypomania and mania [26]. Secondly, hypomanic symptoms are often missed or overlooked and individuals are frequently unaware that their experiences are abnormal. This is partly because the symptoms of hypomania (by definition) do not cause marked impairment and may in fact be somewhat desirable. For example, increased drive and energy, elevated mood, and feeling happy are intrinsically attractive states of mind and rarely perceived as abnormal. Thirdly, there are few sensitive and specific means for detecting hypomania, and the many self-report screening instruments that have been widely distributed on the Internet have encouraged self-assessment and amplified incorrect diagnosis [27, 28]. Many of these instruments have item structures that overlap considerably with affective dysregulation in disorders such as borderline personality disorder. These tend to have poor sensitivity and specificity, particularly in community studies [29].

Switching diagnosis

Compounding this situation further, hypomania, or even mania, can be precipitated by treatment with either antidepressants or ECT; a phenomenon termed switching. These treatment-emergent symptoms of mania are thought to reflect the unmasking of a latent bipolar diathesis and their presentation has been dubbed bipolar III disorder [30]. Apart from further complicating the diagnosis of hypomania, this syndrome can be easily confused with the side effects of treatment such as agitation and irritability [31]. Furthermore, characterizing these treatment-emergent symptoms retrospectively is often difficult, even with careful elicitation of symptoms. However, for prognostic purposes, it is important to clearly identify such episodes, because the triggering of bipolar disorder by antidepressants or ECT is thought to be possible only in true bipolar disorder. Thus such patients should be treated similarly to those with spontaneous episodes of mania/hypomania [32]. In a similar vein, symptoms akin to bipolar disorder can also occur because of the effects of substances (e.g., stimulants) or other medications (e.g., corticosteroids); however, the timing of the emergence of these symptoms in relation to exposure to these agents usually allows the cause to be determined, and the avoidance of an erroneous diagnosis of bipolar disorder.

Subsyndromal manifestations

Another subtype of bipolar disorder now included in section III of DSM-5 under "conditions for further study" is depressive episodes with short-duration hypomania [19]. In this instance, the duration of manic symptoms is between 2 and 4 days. This new category highlights once again the key problem with extant classifications: the cut-offs, although based on informed judgments, correlate poorly with functional impairment and biological responses to treatments. One of the reasons for this is that the severity of bipolar symptoms appears to be dimensional, with seemingly no trend breaks, whereas DSM classification necessitates the creation of diagnostic categories, which is only achievable by specifying a beginning and end-point for each disorder [33]. In practice, categorical diagnoses are needed to confer illness status and to decide whether treatment should be commenced; but a fundamental problem remains: how can we determine where normalcy ends and bipolar disorders begin?

At a basic level, normal emotional experience is a product of changes in mood and cognition and is subject to personality factors. An abnormal personality or temperament can produce subclinical bipolar symptoms, which may then attract the diagnosis *cyclothymic disorder*. To qualify, the illness has to be chronic (2 years in adults and 1 year in children) and, during this time, the individual must experience many periods of change characterized by either hypomanic or depressive symptoms, none of which ever meet the criteria for an episode. Interestingly, but perhaps not surprisingly given that personality is a core substrate of human experience, the concept of cyclothymia preceded that of bipolar disorder. As mentioned earlier, working closely in the latter half of the 19th century, Kahlbaum and his junior associate, Hecker, spawned a reclassification of psychiatric illness. In particular, Kahlbaum regarded "illness course" to be of paramount importance for identifying patterns of change that may ultimately reveal etiology. Together with Hecker, he described cyclothymia as "recurrent episodes of hyperthymia or hypomania which punctuated recurrent episodes of depression or dysthymia," a definition that essentially still holds today. However, a diagnosis of cyclothymia is seldom made nowadays, because of: (1) the difficulty of excluding the possibility of a mood episode earlier in the course of illness, and (2) the difficulty of demarcating abnormal from normal personality traits.

Bipolar personality

The potential role of personality in bipolar disorder is fascinating, but our understanding of this association remains rudimentary and a cause of considerable frustration. Creative traits are undoubtedly overrepresented among the personalities of bipolar individuals and, in opportune circumstances, "symptoms" of bipolar disorder, such as heightened confidence, often go unnoticed and are overlooked, especially if they confer an advantage. Other symptoms, such as irritability and impulsivity, may also go undetected and instead be regarded as character flaws. These symptoms, residing as they do in an ill-defined zone that spans personality and disorder, are often described as subsyndromal. A key difficulty in this regard is the perceived overlap between borderline personality disorder and bipolar disorder [34]. This overlap occurs across the whole spectrum of bipolar disorder, but disentangling the two entities is particularly troublesome for bipolar II disorder and subsyndromal presentations of bipolar symptoms [35]. In reality, the two constructs are very different, both with respect to their clinical histories and clinical features [36]. They share impulsivity and mood lability, but even these superficial similarities likely stem from differential neurobiological processes [37], such that they are fundamentally different.

Featuring mixed symptoms

The clinical pictures of mania and depression are also very different—indeed they are poles apart—prompting the question of whether this is an accurate model for bipolar disorder. The existence of mixed states has once again brought the limitations of our model into sharp relief. Mixed states have long been recognized as part of manic-depressive illness and are defined as depressive and manic features occurring coterminously within the same mood episode. From earlier editions of DSM to DSM-IV the concept narrowed to mixed episodes, which required the criteria for both a manic and depressive episode to be fulfilled concurrently for at least 1 week. This was a high threshold, which in reality was rarely satisfied, and hence mixed episodes were seldom described in either clinical practice or research studies. Hence the changes in DSM-5 are welcome, but have inadvertently created a new set of problems. Mixed episodes as defined in DSM-IV no longer exist; instead, we have "mixed features specifiers," which indicate the presence of at least three symptoms from the opposite pole of illness within a depressive, manic, or hypomanic episode [19]. One problem with this approach is that it perhaps broadens the concept excessively and allows even transient perturbations of mood to be labeled as "mixed features." Irritability, for example, is common within the context of bipolar depression and may reflect underlying anxiety or personality. Another key issue with the DSM-5 diagnosis of mixed features is that the classification has dispensed with its core elements. Features such as psychomotor agitation and distractibility have been excluded as mixed features because they fail to discriminate between depression and mania per se. However, early studies show that this may not be the case [38], and indeed these features may be the defining elements of mixed states. In this case, the current definition of mixed state features is akin to defining migraine without the mention of headache. Such diagnostic imprecision is likely to inflate further the diagnosis of bipolar disorder.

Diagnosing bipolar disorder in children

One area in which diagnostic confusion and impulsive maneuvering has already led to dire consequences is that of pediatric bipolar disorder. With the dawn of the new millennium, the diagnosis of bipolar disorder increased, especially in children [39]. The expansion in diagnosis occurred so rapidly that it took the field by surprise, and it took considerable time to catch up and fully appreciate what was happening. The increase in diagnosis was found to be occurring predominantly in North America and appeared to be driven by a small number of centres in the U.S. At its peak, the diagnosis of pediatric bipolar disorder was fortyfold that occurring anywhere else.

Two main factors led to this phenomenon. First, diagnosing changes in mood, behavior, and thinking in children is inherently difficult, because it is typical for emotions to "run high" in childhood. Secondly, the criteria for diagnosing bipolar disorder have gradually become less stringent. For example, affective instability, which is not a defining characteristic of bipolar disorder per se, has disproportionately influenced the diagnosis of bipolar disorder both in adults and in adolescents/children, and diagnoses such as ADHD, which have similarly struggled to find definitions, have often been confused with bipolar disorder [40]. There is no doubt that some of the observed increase in the diagnosis of bipolar disorder has occurred because of heightened awareness, but such a dramatic increase cannot be explained on this basis alone. Prodromal research in first-episode mania has failed to find the common occurrence of prototypical pediatric bipolar disorder [41, 42]. The final critical issue is that of medication. One could argue that response to therapy may be a biomarker of an underlying biological diathesis; if all cases of "cough disorder" responded to antibiotics, this might suggest a common root. However, unlike in adult disorder, the response of pediatric bipolar disorder to standard agents such as lithium in clinical trials has been disappointing [43].

DSM-5 has consequently attempted to tackle this problem, but the solution is rather puzzling. To reduce the diagnosis of pediatric bipolar disorder, DSM-5 has created an altogether new category called disruptive mood dysregulation disorder (DMDD). The onset of this disorder is between 6 and 10 years of age and it can be diagnosed until adulthood. For classification purposes, it has been placed within the depressive disorders in DSM-5, because preliminary studies indicated that clinically it is more likely to eventuate in the development of depression as opposed to bipolar disorder. Colocation of DMDD with depressive disorders also emphasizes its distinction from bipolar disorder; however, it should be noted that the data to support this new diagnostic category is at best tentative. This has prompted concerns that it will not solve the problem and may instead add to it [44].

Clinical and neurobiological signals point to early origins of emotional symptoms, which may be antecedents of bipolar disorder; but only in adolescence are there discernable brain changes that underpin clinical symptoms [45]. However, until the mechanisms of these changes are understood, trying to identify and differentiate those with early "bipolar" in childhood and adolescence remains a fraught exercise with considerable risks. Diagnostic difficulties and uncertainty are worrying, but the real concern is the initiation of treatment that usually follows diagnosis. In bipolar disorder this invariably involves the administration of medications, the actions of which remain largely unknown. Indeed there is still total mystery about the effects of most psychotropic medications on the growing and developing brain. Consequently, administering medications to young people—extrapolating from modest evidence in adults—is a tremendous risk that may result in more harm than good.

Conclusion

This chapter highlights some of the diagnostic dilemmas bedeviling bipolar disorder. Of all the disorders within psychiatry, bipolar disorder is arguably the cleanest and most discrete, making this state of affairs troubling for the entire field. Mania occurs only in bipolar disorder, and agents such as lithium have arguably greater specificity for bipolar disorder than any other pharmacological class exhibits for any particular disorder [46]. The existing diagnostic classifications represent the efforts of researchers struggling to distill a meaningful answer from an evidence base lacking a pathophysiological foundation. To paraphrase Churchill, perhaps our current classification is the worst possible system, except for all the alternatives. Thus, this chapter serves to illustrate the critical importance of clinicians using these diagnoses with caution and judgment. We know, for example, that the efficacy of core bipolar treatments decreases as one's use of them strays further along the spectrum from the phenomenological core of the disorder. As well as a critical appraisal of the available state of the art, clinical judgment and caution are required.

Acknowledgments

Gin S. Malhi is funded by a NHMRC Program Grant and Michael Berk is supported by a NHMRC Senior Principal Research Fellowship.

References

1 Malhi GS. DSM-5: Ordering disorder? *Aust NZJ Psychiatry*. 2013. 47:7–9.

2 Hippokrates. *Sämtliche Werke*. München: H. Lüneburg, 1897.

3 Georgotas A. Evolution of the concepts of depression and mania. In: Georgotas A, Cancro R (eds.), *Depression and Mania*. New York: Elsevier, 1988: 3–12.

4 Angst J, Marneros A. Bipolarity from ancient to modern times: Conception, birth and rebirth. *J Affect Dis*. 2001. 67:3–19.

5 Aydemir O, Malhi GS. Aretaeus of Cappadocia. *Acta Neuropsychiatrica*. 2007. 19(1):62–63.

6 Kotsopoulos S. Aretaeus the Cappadocian on mental illness. *Compr Psychiatry*. 1986. 27:171–179.

7 Goodwin FK, Jamison KR. *Manic-Depressive Illness. Bipolar Disorders and Recurrent Depression*. 2nd ed. Oxford: Oxford University Press; 2007.

8 Falret JP. Mémoire sur la folie circulaire, forme de maladie mentale caractérisée par la reproduction sucessive et réguliäre de l'état maniqaue, de l'état mélancolique, et d'un intervalle lucide plus or moins prolongé. *Bull Acad Med* (Paris). 1854. 19:382–415.

9 Baillarger J. De la folie à double-forme. *Ann Med Psychol* (Paris). 1854. 6:367–391.

10 Baethge C, Salvatore P, Baldessarini RJ. "On cyclic insanity" by Karl Ludwig Kahlbaum: A translation and commentary. *Harv Rev Psychiatry*. 2003. 11:78–90.

11 Malhi G, Allwang C, Keshavan MS. Kahlbaum's katatonie and Hecker's hebephrenia. *Acta Neuropsychiatrica*. 2007. 19:314–315.

12 Kraepelin E. *Psychiatrie*. 5th ed. Leipzig: Barth; 1896.

13 Henderson S, Malhi GS. Swan song for schizophrenia? *Aust NZJ Psychiatry*. 2014. 48(4):302–305.

14 Pichot P. European perspectives on the classification of depression. *BJ Psych*. 1988. 153(supp3):11–15.

15 Malhi G, Keshavan MS. Biology to psychobiology. *Acta Neuropsych*. 2007. 19:211–212.

16 Leonhard K. *The Classification of Endogenous Psychoses*. New York: Irvington Publishers; 1957.

17 Angst J. *Zur Ätiologie und Nosologie endogener depressiver Psychosen. Eine genetische, soziologische und klinische Studie*. Berlin, Heidelberg, New York: Springer; 1966.

18 Perris C. A study of bipolar (manic-depressive) and unipolar recurrent depressive psychoses. *Acta Psychiatr Scand*. 1966. 194(suppl):1–89.

19 American Psychiatric Association. *Diagnostic and Statistical Manual of Mental Disorders*. 5th ed. (DSM-5). Arlington, VA: American Psychiatric Publishing; 2013.

20 American Psychiatric Association. *Diagnostic and Statistical Manual of Mental Disorders*. 4th ed. (DSM–IV). Washington DC: American Psychiatric Association; 1994.

21 Malhi GS, Berk M. Depolarizing bipolar disorder: Both the illness and our views. *Aust NZJ Psychiatry*. 2011. 45(11):909–910.

22 Mendel E. *Die Manie. Eine Monographie*. Vienna: Urban & Schwarzenberg; 1881.

23 Feighner JP, Robins E, Guze SB, et al. Diagnostic criteria for use in psychiatric research. *Arch Gen Psychiatry*. 1972. 26:57–63.

24 Angst J, Gamma A, Benazzi F, et al. Atypical depressive syndromes in varying definitions. *Eur Arch Psychiatry Clin Neurosci*. 2006. 256(1):44–54.

25 Ferrier IN, MacMillan IC, Young AH. The search for the wandering thymostat: A review of some developments in bipolar disorder research. *British Journal of psychiatry*. 2001. 178:103–106.

26 Berk M, Dodd S, Callaly P, et al. History of illness prior to a diagnosis of bipolar disorder or schizoaffective disorder. *J Affect Disord*. 2007. 103(1–3):181–186.

27 Zimmerman M, Ruggero CJ, Chelminski I, Young D. Is bipolar disorder overdiagnosed? *J Clin Psych*. 2008. 69:935–940.

28 Hadjipavlou G, Mok H, Yatham LN. Bipolar II disorder: And overview of recent developments. *Can J Psych*. 2004. 49: 802–812.

29 Dodd S, Williams LJ, Jacka FN, et al. Reliability of the mood disorder questionnaire: Comparison with the structured clinical interview for the DSM-IV-TR in a population sample. *Aust N Z J Psychiatry*. 2009. 43(6):526–530.

30 Akiskal HS, Pinto O. The evolving bipolar spectrum. Prototypes I, II, III, and IV. *Psychiatr Clin North Am*. 1999. 22(3):517–534.

31 Frye MA, Helleman G, McElroy SL. Correlates of treatment-emergent mania associated with antidepressant treatment in bipolar depression. *Am J Psychiatry*. 2009. 166(2):164–172.

32 Perlis RH, Ostacher MJ, Goldberg JF, et al. Transition to mania during treatment of bipolar depression. *Neuropsychopharmacology*. 2010. 35:2545–2552.

33 Malhi GS. DSM-5: Il buono, il cattivo, il brutto. *Aust NZJ Psychiatry*. 2013. 47(7): 595–598.

34 Coulston C, Tanious M, Mulder RT, et al. Bordering on bipolar: The overlap between borderline personality and bipolarity. *Aust NZJ Psychiatry*. 2012. 46:506–521.

35 Bassett D. Borderline personality disorder and bipolar affective disorder. Spectra or spectre? A review. *Aust NZJ Psychiatry*. 2012. 46:327–339.

36 Ghaemi SN, Dalley S. The bipolar spectrum: Conceptions and misconceptions. *Aust NZJ Psychiatry*. 2014. 48(4):314–324.

37 Malhi GS, Tanious M, Fritz K, et al. Differential engagement of the fronto-limbic network during emotion processing distinguishes bipolar and borderline personality disorder. *Mol Psychiatry*. 2013. 18(12):1247–1248.

38 Malhi GS, Lampe L, Coulston CM, et al. Mixed state discrimination: A DSM problem that won't go away? *J Affect Disord*. 2014. 158:8–10.

39 Morano C, Laje G, Blanco C, et al. National trends in the outpatient diagnosis and treatment of bipolar disorder in youth. *Arch Gen Psych*. 2007. 64(9):1032–1039.
Cahill CM, Green MJ, Jairam R, Malhi GS. Bipolar disorder in children and adolescents: Obstacles to early diagnosis and future directions. *Early Interv Psychiatry*. 2007. 1(2): 138–149.

40 Martin DJ, Smith DJ. Is there a clinical prodrome of bipolar disorder? A review of the evidence. *Expert Rev Neurother*. 2013. 13(1):89–98.

41 Correll CU, Hauser M, Penzner JB, et al. Type and duration of subsyndromal symptoms in youth with bipolar I disorder prior to their first manic episode. *Bipolar Disord.* 2014. Doi:10.1111/bdi.12194. Epub ahead of print.

42 Peruzzolo TL, Tramontina S, Rohde LA, Zeni CP. Pharmacotherapy of bipolar disorder in children and adolescents: An update. *Rev Bras Psiquiatr.* 2013. 35(4):393–405.

43 Frances A. ANZJP ICD, DSM and the Tower of Babel. *Aust NZJ Psychiatry.* 2014. 48(4): 371–373.

44 Das P, Coulston C, Bargh D, et al. Neural antecedents of emotional disorders: A functional magnetic resonance imaging study of subsyndromal emotional symptoms in adolescent girls. *Biol Psychiatry.* 2013. 74(4):265–272.

45 Malhi GS. Cade's lithium: An extraordinary experiment with a not-so-ordinary element. *Med J Aust.* 2014. 201(1):24–25.

PART II
Rare psychotic disorders

CHAPTER 13

Misidentification delusions

Michael H. Connors[1,2], Robyn Langdon[1], and Max Coltheart[1]

[1] ARC Centre of Excellence in Cognition and Its Disorders, and Department of Cognitive Science, Macquarie University, Sydney, Australia

[2] Dementia Collaborative Research Centre, School of Psychiatry, University of New South Wales, Sydney, Australia

Introduction

Misidentification delusions involve an incorrect belief about the identity of other people, oneself, animals, objects, or places. To meet the definitional criteria of a delusion, this belief needs to be fixed and resistant to counterevidence. In some patients, however, the delusional belief may appear at different times or fluctuate in intensity. Although encompassing many different types of beliefs, misidentification delusions share two common elements: (1) a misidentified entity, and (2) an incorrect belief about the identity of that entity. In the case of Capgras delusion, for example, patients believe that a known person (the misidentified entity) has been replaced by a visually similar impostor (the incorrect belief). In the case of reduplicative paramnesia for place, patients believe that a location (the misidentified entity) has been duplicated (the incorrect belief).

These two elements—a misidentified entity and an incorrect belief about the identity of the entity—distinguish misidentification delusions from other types of delusions. Unfortunately, though, the term *misidentification delusion* has sometimes been used rather loosely in the psychiatric literature. Some authors [1, 2], for example, have referred to Cotard delusion—the belief that one is dead—as a misidentification delusion. In this case, however, there is no misidentified entity, only the ascription of an incorrect property to the correctly identified entity. The belief thus does not constitute a misidentification delusion. In a similar way, the phantom boarder delusion—the belief that there are uninvited strangers living in one's house—and sex change delusion—the belief that one has changed sex—are not strictly misidentification delusions, even though they have been referred to as such, because there is no misidentified entity.

Troublesome Disguises: Managing Challenging Disorders in Psychiatry, Second Edition.
Edited by Dinesh Bhugra and Gin S. Malhi.
© 2015 John Wiley & Sons, Ltd. Published 2015 by John Wiley & Sons, Ltd.

Other authors have used the term *misidentification delusion* to refer exclusively to delusions that involve misidentification of *other people* [3, 4]. These authors have tended to focus on four main delusions—namely, Capgras, Frégoli (the belief that strangers are known people in disguise), intermetamorphosis (the belief that some person has changed into another person), and subjective doubles (the belief in a physical or psychological double). Although misidentification delusions certainly include these four well-known person misidentification delusions, the term itself is broader and need not exclude other forms of misidentification. Misidentification delusions can also apply to oneself, pets, inanimate objects, and places. Indeed, other authors [5] have even applied the term to delusions involving misattribution of body parts, such as somatoparaphrenia (the belief that one's limb is owned by someone else). For the purposes of simplicity, however, the current chapter restricts attention to delusions focused on the identity of an entity in its entirety, rather than just a part of it. Delusions such as somatoparaphrenia, nevertheless, occupy an intermediate area for the purposes of classification and highlight some of the challenges for a complete taxonomy.

Variety of misidentification delusions

Misidentification delusions can be classified according to the type of misidentified entity. There are four broad subtypes: other people and other sentient beings; oneself; inanimate objects; and places. Within each subtype, delusions differ in their belief about the misidentified entity (see Table 13.1). Common beliefs include that the entity has been duplicated, replaced, or transformed into another entity.

Other people and other sentient beings
Capgras delusion
Capgras delusion is the belief that a known other person has been replaced by an impostor of similar appearance [6]. The delusion usually centres on people familiar to the patients whom the patients believe have been replaced by unfamiliar yet similar-looking impostors. Patients often point out what they take to be subtle differences in physical appearance and behaviour between the person and the supposed impostor as confirming their belief. In an early case [7], for example, a 53-year-old woman with schizophrenia believed that her husband, children, police chief, and neighbours had been replaced by visually similar impostors. This patient reported that she could distinguish these impostors by such features as "a little mark on the ear . . . a thinner face . . . the way of speaking . . . the way of walking" [8] (p. 129). In some patients, the delusion is limited to a single impostor of a known person. In most patients, though, the delusion involves multiple impostors of known people. This may include objects and animals that patients believe have similarly been replaced by visual

Table 13.1 Common misidentification delusions.

Misidentified entity	Belief about misidentified entity	Delusion
Other person	Replaced by impostor	Capgras
	Duplicated without replacement	Reduplicative paramnesia
	Transformed into another person	Intermetamorphosis
	Another person in disguise	Frégoli
	The misidentified person is simply another person, physically and psychologically	Generic misidentification of other people
Self	Duplicated	Subjective doubles
	Changed into another person	Reverse intermetamorphosis
	Changed into an animal	Lycanthropy
(Mirror reflection)	Mirror reflection is not oneself	Mirrored-self misidentification
Inanimate object	Replaced by impostor	Inanimate doubles
	Objects are animate companions	Delusional companions
(Television image)	Television image is physical reality	Misidentification of television
(Photograph)	Photograph is three-dimensional reality	Misidentification of photograph
Place	Duplicated	Reduplicative paramnesia

look-alikes [9–12]. The number of impostors may also increase over time. In some cases, the belief can result in violence. In a typical case involving violence [13], for example, a 19-year-old male patient stabbed his mother under the belief that she had been replaced by an evil robot of identical appearance.

Reduplicative paramnesia

Reduplicative paramnesia for people is the belief that a person has been duplicated (reduplicative paramnesia can also apply to places and objects). Unlike Capgras, there is no sense of the original person being replaced or of the duplicate being an impostor look-alike. In one case [14], a 76-year-old female patient, who had recently suffered a right parietal stroke, believed that there were two versions of her husband. The patient correctly reported that her husband was dead but also maintained that her husband was currently a patient in the same hospital as her. The "patient husband" was a duplicate of the "dead husband," albeit alive. The patient did not offer an explanation of how this was possible, but insisted that she was certain in her convictions. The patient also reported that other members of her family—including her two daughters, a grandson, and the father-in-law of one of her daughters—worked at the hospital or were patients there. In many patients, the delusion may co-occur with belief in the duplication of places and objects as well as people.

Intermetamorphosis

Intermetamorphosis is the belief that a person has changed into another person. Patients typically believe the new identity differs both physically and psychologically from the original person. In an early case [15], for example, a 49-year-old woman believed that her husband and her son had both transformed into other people, including neighbours and cousins. The patient described the change: "In a second my husband is taller, smaller or younger" [8, p. 140]. The patient pointed to physical characteristics and behaviour that she believed had changed with the transformation, and other characteristics that she believed had not changed and that indicated her husband's true identity. Unlike her husband, whom she believed transformed radically in appearance, the patient believed that her son transformed into people of similar appearance to himself and that she could only identify him by his large and dirty shoes. The patient came to believe that all inhabitants in the area—with the exception of herself—could change themselves into one another.

Frégoli delusion

Frégoli delusion is the belief that a stranger is a known person in disguise. Patients are thus aware of physical differences between the known person's usual appearance and what they take to be their disguise (i.e., the stranger's appearance), yet maintain that the two people are the same person. In an early case [16], a 27-year-old woman in Paris believed that two actresses of the time (Sarah Bernhardt and Robine) were following her in different disguises "taking the form of people she knows or meets" [8, p. 134]. In particular, the patient believed the actresses disguised themselves as strangers in the street, doctors, friends, and previous employers. The patient believed that she was being persecuted by the actresses and even attacked a woman on the street whom she believed was Robine. The delusion was named after the Italian actor and mimic Leopoldo Frégoli because of his ability to impersonate other people. The delusion is often seen in the context of paranoia and the belief that one is being persecuted [17–19]. Cases not involving paranoia or persecution have been reported, though, such as a patient who believed that friends of her family were disguising themselves as strangers in order to protect her [20] and another patient who believed that family members were disguising themselves for their own personal non-threatening reasons [21].

Generic misidentification of other people

Generic misidentification of other people involves the belief that one person is simply another person, without any notion of transformation or disguise. In one case, a 74-year-old female patient with Alzheimer's disease believed that her daughter was her sister and resisted attempts by both her daughter and her doctors to convince her otherwise [22]. When shown photographs of her family, this patient would also misidentify her other daughter as her sister and misidentify her husband as her father.

Oneself
Subjective doubles
The delusion of subjective doubles is the belief that one has a double, or doppelganger. In a well-known case [23], an 18-year-old female patient, following a febrile episode, believed that a neighbour and at least two other female patients were capable of transforming themselves into her doubles. The patient believed the doubles had the "same face, same build, same clothes, same everything" (p. 250) as herself and that the perpetrators used special makeup, a wig, and a mask to effect the transformation. She later attacked one of the patients whom she believed was impersonating her; as she was pulled away, she begged her doctor to "pull the mask" (p. 250) from the patient's face. Although this particular patient reported that specific people were her double, other patients with this delusion may not specify this and simply indicate that their double exists and is elsewhere [24]. The delusion can involve both physical and psychological doubles. Most cases involve physical doubles in which the patient believes that another person is almost indistinguishable from themselves in appearance, as in the example of the 18-year-old female patient described above. Some cases, however, involve psychological doubles in which the patient believes that people with dissimilar physical bodies hold minds identical to that of the patient [25]. Cases of both physical and psychological duplicates also exist [26]. In some complicated cases, the patient may even believe that they themselves are the impostor [24]. The delusion of subjective doubles often co-occurs with Capgras delusion and persecutory beliefs [24].

Reverse intermetamorphosis
Reverse intermetamorphosis is the belief that one has changed into another person. In one case [14], for example, a 40-year-old female patient with schizophrenia believed that she was her father or, occasionally, her grandfather. The patient would only respond to her father's name and signed her father's name. The patient gave her father's history when questioned about her personal history and described herself as she would her father. Other patients may believe that they have become a person of high status or of particular importance [27]. A complicated variant of reverse intermetamorphosis is the belief that one's mind resides in another person's body [24]. The patient believes that their mind has replaced the mind of the person whose body they are using. The patient thus does not recognise their physical body as their own [28, 29].

Lycanthropy

Another variant of reverse intermetamorphosis is lycanthropy, the belief that one has transformed into an animal [30]. The delusion has been reported for over 2000 years and is referred to in some of the earliest medical writings [31]. Although the delusion may be more common in rural areas and pre-industrialised countries, it is still found in modern Western cities. One study [32], for example, reported 12 cases in a major Boston psychiatric hospital over a 12-year period. The delusion is often associated with wolves or werewolves, but patients may believe they are other animals such as dogs, pigs, birds, rabbits, cats, gerbils, frogs, bees, lions, tigers, hyenas, sharks, and crocodiles. Although some patients may verbally insist that they are a particular animal, others may not speak (since they are animals) and simply behave as though they were an animal by howling, growling, or crawling on all fours. In one such case [33], a 66-year-old woman with psychotic depression, believing that she was a dog, would get down on her hands and knees and bark.

Mirrored-Self misidentification

Mirrored-self misidentification is the belief that one's reflection is not oneself [34]. Some patients identify their mirrored-reflection as a stranger. In one case [35], for example, a 77-year-old male patient believed that his reflection was a "dead ringer" for himself but that he did not know who this person was. Other patients report that their mirrored reflection is a known person, such as a family member. In one case [36], for example, a 62-year-old female patient believed that her reflection was her sister, who had died 2 years earlier. The delusion can occur despite an intact semantic understanding of mirrors (e.g., being able to define mirrors and reflections) and despite being able to identify other people in the mirror [35]. Some patients can also recognise themselves in photographs [35]. Patients may talk to the "stranger" in the mirror. Whereas some patients are indifferent [35] or treat the "stranger" as a friend [37], others are deeply suspicious and upset by the "stranger" [38]. Patients have been known to throw objects at mirrors or cover up all reflective surfaces to avoid seeing the stranger [38].

Inanimate objects
Delusion of inanimate doubles

The delusion of inanimate doubles involves the belief that an inanimate object has been replaced by an almost identical duplicate. The duplicate is usually, though not always, of inferior quality to the original. The objects are usually personal possessions and can include, for example, furniture, household appliances, clothing, spectacles, jewellery, and even handwritten letters and personal identification cards. In one case [39], for example, a 38-year-old male patient believed that his car, various personal belongings, and some of his clothing had been replaced by duplicate objects. The patient pointed to specific differences between the original object and what he considered to be its duplicate (e.g., a lower dashboard in the car and fewer gears on the gearstick). The delusion of inanimate doubles often occurs in the context of paranoia. The delusion can occur by itself, though it can also occur with other delusions, most frequently Capgras. Between 5 and 14 percent of patients with Capgras delusion also report the delusion of inanimate doubles [10–12].

Delusional companions

Delusional companions is the belief that inanimate objects are sentient companions. Although more common in the later stages of dementia, patients in the early stages of dementia with no other symptoms can also report the delusion [40]. In one case [40], for example, an 81-year-old female patient with relatively preserved cognition (mini-mental state examination score of 28/30) and no other unusual beliefs or symptoms would converse with a teddy bear. The patient would have long conversations with the teddy bear, coax it to read newspapers, and take it on drives with her. The patient also tried to encourage her teddy-bear to eat and drink, and became anxious when it did not respond. When visited by her doctor, the patient removed the teddy from the room in order, she explained, to preserve confidentiality.

Misidentification of television and/or photographs

Delusional misidentification of television (also called the "television sign") involves the belief that events and people depicted on a television are real and physically present in the room. One study [41] reported a variety of reactions to the television in patients with Alzheimer's disease. One patient was concerned about people on television watching her while she undressed and would leave the room to change. Another patient believed that the violence on television was real and was frightened that people were trying to shoot him. A third patient believed that a sports game was occurring in the room with her. Other patients may talk to the people on television or offer them food and drink [42].

Delusional misidentification of photographs (also called the "picture sign") likewise involves the belief that images in photographs are real and physically present in three-dimensional space [42]. The delusion similarly occurs in dementia and produces a variety of reactions in patients. One patient, for example, would prepare meals for photographs of her grandchildren in the belief that they were physically present [43]. Another patient believed that a woman pictured in a magazine was in his house and called the police to evict her [43]. Misidentification of photographs may co-occur with delusional misidentification of television and other forms of misidentification. In misidentification of both television and photographs, the boundary between a temporary illusion (a perceptual misinterpretation) and a delusion (a false belief) is admittedly not always clear. The symptom may constitute a perceptual illusion if it occurs only when the television is on or the photograph is present and the patient has no reason to doubt the belief, as might occur with impaired perceptual processing. Alternatively, the symptom may be classed as a delusion if it is resistant to rational counter-argument concerning the nature of the television or photograph, is maintained over time, or clearly affects patients' other beliefs and actions.

Reduplicative paramnesia

Reduplicative paramnesia for places is the belief that a particular location has been duplicated. In an early case [44], a 67-year-old female patient with dementia believed that there were two hospitals in which she had been staying. She believed that she had been moved from a hospital in Prague, where she had been staying for the last 5 months, to a nearly identical one in her home town, a small village outside Prague. She believed that the doctors and medical staff worked at both hospitals and that some of the other patients had also been moved to the new hospital. Other cases have been reported in the literature with strikingly similar beliefs involving a duplicated hospital that is also incorrectly located to a place of significance from earlier in the patient's life [45–47].

Occurrence of misidentification delusions

Associated diagnoses

Misidentification delusions can occur in many different clinical conditions. These include traditional psychiatric disorders—such as schizophrenia, bipolar disorder, schizo-affective disorder, affective disorders, substance-induced psychotic disorders, and short-lived acute psychotic episodes—and frankly organic disorders—such as dementia, stroke, cerebrovascular disease, epilepsy, traumatic brain injury, brain tumours, and other organic brain diseases. The same type of misidentification delusion can occur in many different clinical conditions. Capgras delusion, for example, has been reported in all conditions listed above. In some cases, the misidentification delusion may be a patient's only psychotic symptom, giving rise to a diagnosis of delusional disorder if no other known organic disorder is present (or schizophrenia according to DSM-IV if the delusion is considered sufficiently bizarre [48]; this criterion for schizophrenia is not included in DSM-V [49]).

Certain misidentification delusions are more likely to be seen in some conditions than others. Reduplicative paramnesia, for example, is most frequently seen after brain injury or dementia. Likewise, mirrored-self misidentification, misidentification of the television, misidentification of photographs, and delusional companions are most frequently seen in dementia (though cases of mirrored-self misidentification have also been reported after stroke [50] and in schizophrenia [38]). In a review of 260 cases of misidentification delusion, Förstl and colleagues [51] found that misidentification of oneself and other people was most frequently associated with schizophrenia, dementia, other organic disorders, and affective disorders (misidentification of oneself was also associated with cerebrovascular disease). In contrast, misidentification of places (e.g., reduplicative paramnesia) was most frequently associated with head trauma or cerebral infarction. These patients who misidentified places also tended to show more evidence of right hemisphere lesions than patients with other misidentification delusions.

Prevalence

Misidentification delusions are relatively rare. In psychiatric inpatient admissions, Capgras delusion is found in 0.14–5.4 percent of patients [52–59]. Variation may be due to the location of the study and the methods of recruitment and diagnosis. The prevalence of other misidentification delusions in psychiatric inpatients has not been widely studied. Other misidentification delusions are reported in the literature less frequently than Capgras, so may be less common [51]. In one study of psychiatric inpatients, one case of Frégoli delusion was found in the same time period as 24 cases of Capgras [52], with an estimated prevalence of Frégoli of 0.2 percent of all the psychiatric patients seen. Another study examined lycanthropy in a Boston psychiatric hospital and found 12 cases of this delusion among 5000 psychiatric inpatient admissions, with an estimated prevalence of 0.2 percent in psychiatric patients [32].

In dementia, misidentification delusions are found in 15–34 percent of patients [41, 60–65]. The most frequently reported misidentification delusions in dementia are Capgras, mirrored-self misidentification, and misidentification of the television. Studies report Capgras in 0.5–12 percent of patients with dementia [41, 60, 61, 66–69], mirrored-self misidentification in 2.6–7 percent of patients [41, 60, 61, 66–68], and misidentification of television as real in 0.9–8 percent of patients [41, 60, 61, 64, 68]. Misidentification of people—akin to intermetamorphosis—is also common and found in 11.8 percent of patients with dementia [61]. The belief that one's home is not one's real home—which may involve reduplication of place or transportation to an impostor home—is found in 1.6–15.2 percent of patients [60, 64, 66]. Other misidentification delusions are less common in dementia. Reduplication of identity is found in 1.8–3.3 percent of patients with dementia [67, 70]. The Frégoli and subjective doubles delusions have also been reported in isolated dementia cases [60, 67], both with an estimated prevalence of around 0.5 percent.

Misidentification delusions—and delusions more generally—become more common with the progression of dementia [71]. It is difficult to predict which patients will develop misidentification delusions because patients with misidentification delusions often do not differ from patients without misidentification delusions in terms of demographics, mental status, or other psychiatric symptoms [67, 72]. Rates of misidentification delusions may be higher, however, in dementia with Lewy Bodies. One study reported that as many as 56 percent of patients with Lewy Bodies dementia had misidentification delusions [69]. In contrast, misidentification delusions—and delusions more generally—may be less frequent in fronto-temporal dementia [73]. In all forms of dementia, the phantom boarder delusion, although not strictly a misidentification delusion, is also common, with a reported prevalence ranging from 8.0 to 23.3 percent [41, 60–62, 64, 74]. Interestingly, this delusion frequently co-occurs with misidentification delusions, such as Capgras delusion, mirrored-self misidentification, and misidentification of television [74]. This suggests that the belief in uninvited strangers may result in some cases from elaboration of a misidentification delusion: The uninvited stranger may also be the impostor, the stranger in the mirror, or a person on television.

Theoretical explanations

A number of theories have been offered to account for misidentification delusions. Jaspers [75], a highly influential early theorist, distinguished between two types of delusions: primary delusions (or "delusions proper") and secondary delusions (or "delusion-like ideas"). According to Jaspers, primary delusions are formed when the content of the delusions spring into consciousness without a meaningful context or basis. These delusions, therefore, cannot be understood in terms of ordinary experience and normal belief formation. In contrast, secondary delusions are formed when the content arises from a meaningful context or basis. These delusions may result, for example, from thinking about fears, affects, or other experiences, and so can be more readily understood in terms of ordinary experience and normal belief formation [76, 77]. It is important to note, however, that Jasper's account does not offer explanations of how the contents of specific misidentification delusions arise.

Psychodynamic theories, in contrast, have proposed explanations for the content of specific misidentification delusions. In the case of Capgras, for example, psychodynamic theories have suggested that the delusion could result from conflicted feelings toward the familiar person believed to have been replaced with an impostor [78] or, alternatively, from regression to archaic modes of thought that involve ideas of impostors and doubles [79]. As psychodynamic theories postulate mechanisms that are neither observable nor introspectable, they have been criticised for being post hoc, unfalsifiable, and untestable [80]. Psychodynamic accounts also have some difficulty accounting for misidentification delusions that are specific to animals and inanimate objects, and delusions that are modality-specific: Cases of Capgras, for example, have been reported in which the patient identifies a familiar loved one as an impostor when looking at them, but not when talking to them over the phone [81]. Finally, psychodynamic theories are less consistent with evidence of organic factors, such as brain trauma and dementia, contributing to many misidentification delusions [4].

An alternative approach is offered by theorists who have attempted to explain delusions in terms of breakdowns in normal cognitive processes and neuropsychological functioning [82, 83]. A number of theorists, for example, have noted that the content of delusions may arise from an attempt to explain unusual experiences [84–87]. Following in this tradition, Ellis and Young [88] noted that the content of misidentification delusions toward other people can be explained in terms of various disruptions to normal face processing and person identification. In the case of Capgras delusion, for example, damage to an autonomic response in face processing can lead patients to lose their heightened arousal to familiar faces. As a result, patients encounter their loved ones without the normal heightened arousal they would expect to experience, which may lead to the idea that a familiar person has been replaced by a look-alike impostor [88–90]. In support of this theory, a number of studies have found that patients with Capgras show reduced autonomic response (indexed by skin conductance recordings) to photographs of familiar faces and similar low levels of autonomic response to familiar and unfamiliar faces [81, 91, 92].

While successfully accounting for the content of Capgras delusion, this face-processing account has difficulty explaining the maintenance of delusions. It also has difficulty accounting for many patients with face-processing deficits who do not develop a delusion. There are, for example, patients with damage to the autonomic response pathway in face processing who do not have Capgras delusion [93]. To account for these non-delusional analogue cases, Langdon and Coltheart [94–96] proposed a two-factor theory. According to this theory, two separate factors are responsible in combination for a delusion's content and maintenance. The first factor (Factor 1) explains the delusion's content and typically involves a neuropsychological anomaly affecting perceptual, emotional, or autonomic processing. The second factor (Factor 2) explains the delusion's maintenance and involves a deficit in belief evaluation and revision. Thus patients who have both Factor 1 and Factor 2 will develop a misidentification delusion.

Adopting this approach, it is possible to specify a Factor 1 to account for the content of many different misidentification delusions. In the case of mirrored-self

Table 13.2 Hypothesised deficits responsible for delusions.

Delusion	Factor 1 (content)	Factor 2 (maintenance)
Capgras (Known person replaced by impostor)	Reduced autonomic responsiveness to familiar faces	
Reduplicative paramnesia for people (Person duplicated without replacement)	Déjà vecu	
Intermetamorphosis (Person transformed into another person)	Deterioration of stored representations of familiar faces, leading to inappropriate activation	
Frégoli (Stranger is a known person in disguise)	Overactive autonomic responsiveness to unfamiliar faces, or normal visual processing of strangers' faces with inappropriate activation of stored representations of known people	
Generic misidentification of other people (A person is simply another person)	Impaired updating of stored representations of familiar faces, leading to inappropriate matches	
Subjective doubles (One has a doppelganger)	Autoscopic phenomena, or depersonalisation, or mirror agnosia	
Reverse intermetamorphosis (One has changed into another person)	Real or imagined physical changes and/ or confabulation	Deficit in Belief Evaluation and Revision
Lycanthropy (One has changed into an animal)	Real or imagined physical deformity	
Mirrored-self misidentification (One's mirrored-reflection is not oneself)	Impaired face processing or mirror agnosia	
Inanimate doubles (Inanimate object replaced by replica)	Loss of autonomic responsiveness in the visual processing of personally familiar objects	
Delusional companions (Inanimate object is sentient companion)	Visuospatial deficits in combination with motivational factors (e.g., loneliness)	
Television misidentification (Television image is real)	Deficit in depth perception	
Photograph misidentification (Photograph is real)	Severe visuospatial deficits, including deficit in depth perception	
Reduplicative paramnesia for places (Place is duplicated)	Déjà vecu	

misidentification, for example, two different deficits can act as Factor 1: Either impaired face processing (and hence a difficulty in recognising oneself in a mirror) or mirror agnosia (an inability to use mirror knowledge when interacting with mirrors) can lead to the idea that the person in the mirror is a stranger. In support of this, Breen and colleagues [35] reported two patients with mirrored-self misidentification, each of whom had one of these deficits. In the case of the delusion of inanimate doubles, impaired autonomic response in the visual-processing of personally familiar objects could lead to the idea that inanimate objects have been replaced [97]. Possible candidates for Factor 1 for different misidentification delusions are summarised in Table 13.2. In contrast to Factor 1, Factor 2 is thought to be common to most, if not all, delusions. Factor 2 may involve damage to specific brain areas, such as the right dorsolateral prefrontal cortex [98], the medial prefrontal cortex [99], or the right inferior frontal gyrus [100].

Conclusion

Misidentification delusions encompass a wide range of different beliefs. When viewed through the lens of the two-factor theory, misidentification delusions that may have once appeared bizarre become more comprehensible. Misidentification delusions may simply represent an attempt to understand and make sense of the world in the face of anomalous perceptual or affective input. When viewed in this way, it may become easier to empathise with patients whose unusual and firmly held beliefs often bring great suffering.

References

1 Debruyne H, Portzky M, Peremans K, et al. (2011) Cotard's syndrome. *Mind & Brain, the Journal of Psychiatry* 2, 67–72.

2 Sno HN. (1994) A continuum of misidentification symptoms. *Psychopathology* 27, 144–147.

3 Christodoulou GN, Margariti MM, Kontaxakis VP, et al. (2009) The delusional misidentification syndromes: Strange, fascinating, and instructive. *Current Psychiatry Reports* 11, 185–189.

4 Christodoulou GN. (1991) The delusional misidentification syndromes. *British Journal of Psychiatry* 159, 65–69.

5 Feinberg TE, Venneri A, Simone AM, et al. (2010) The neuroanatomy of asomatognosia and somatoparaphrenia. *Journal of Neurology, Neurosurgery & Psychiatry* 81, 276–281.

6 Edelstyn NMJ, Oyebode F. (1999) A review of the phenomenology and cognitive neuropsychological origins of the Capgras syndrome. *International Journal of Geriatric Psychiatry* 14, 48–59.

7 Capgras J, Reboul-Lachaux J. (1923) L'Illusion des "sosies" dans un délire systématisé chronique. *Bulletin de la Société Clinique de Médecine Mentale* 11, 6–16.

  8 Ellis HD, Whitley J, Luauté J-P. (1994) Delusional misidentification: The three original papers on the Capgras, Frégoli and intermetamorphosis delusions. *History of Psychiatry* 5, 117–146.

  9 Ramachandran VS. (1998) Consciousness and body image: Lessons from phantom limbs, Capgras syndrome and pain asymbolia. *Philosophical Transactions of the Royal Society B: Biological Sciences* 353, 1851–1859.

 10 Anderson DN, Williams E. (1994) The delusion of inanimate doubles. *Psychopathology* 27, 220–225.

 11 Berson RJ. (1983) Capgras' syndrome. *American Journal of Psychiatry* 140, 969–978.

 12 Kimura S. (1986) Review of 106 cases with the syndrome of Capgras. *Bibliotheca Psychiatrica* 164, 121–130.

 13 Silva JA, Leong GB, Garza-Trevino ES, et al. (1994) A cognitive model of dangerous delusional misidentification syndromes. *Journal of Forensic Sciences* 39, 1455–1467.

 14 Breen N, Caine D, Coltheart M, et al. (2000) Toward an understanding of delusions of misidentification: Four case studies. *Mind & Language* 15, 74–110.

 15 Courbon P, Tusques J. (1994) Illusions d'intermétamorphose et de charme. *History of Psychiatry* 5, 139–146.

 16 Courbon P, Fail G. (1994) Syndrome d'illusion de Frégoli et schizophrénie. *History of Psychiatry* 5, 134–138.

 17 de Pauw KW, Szulecka TK, Poltock TL. (1987) Fregoli syndrome after cerebral infarction. *Journal of Nervous & Mental Disease* 175, 433–438.

 18 Edelstyn NM, Riddoch MJ, Oyebode F, et al. (1996) Visual processing in patients with Frégoli syndrome. *Cognitive Neuropsychiatry* 1, 103–124.

 19 Atwal S, Khan MH. (1986) Coexistence of Capgras and its related syndromes in a single patient. *Australian and New Zealand Journal of Psychiatry* 20, 496–498.

 20 Ellis HD. (1997) Misidentification syndromes. In: Bhugra D, Munro A (eds.) *Troublesome disguises: Undiagnosed psychiatric syndromes*. Blackwell, Oxford, UK, pp. 7–23.

 21 Feinberg TE, Eaton LA, Roane DM, et al. (1999) Multiple Fregoli delusions after traumatic brain injury. *Cortex* 35, 373–387.

 22 Abe N, Ishii H, Fujii T, et al. (2007) Selective impairment in the retrieval of family relationships in person identification: A case study of delusional misidentification. *Neuropsychologia* 45, 2902–2909.

 23 Christodoulou GN. (1978) Course and prognosis of the syndrome of doubles. *Journal of Nervous and Mental Disease* 166, 68–72.

 24 Kamanitz JR, El-Mallakh RS, Tasman A. (1989) Delusional misidentification involving the self. *Journal of Nervous and Mental Disease* 177, 695–698.

 25 Silva JA, Leong GB. (1991) A case of "subjective" Frégoli syndrome. *Journal of Psychiatry and Neuroscience* 16, 103–105.

 26 Nagy A, Tenyi T, Kovacs A, et al. (2009) Clonal pluralization, as an interpretative delusion after a hallucinatory form of autoscopy. *European Journal of Psychiatry* 23, 141–146.

 27 Rokeach M. (1964) *The three Christs of Ypsilanti: A psychological study*. Knopf, New York, NY.

 28 Fialkov MJ, Robins AH. (1978) An unusual case of the Capgras syndrome. *British Journal of Psychiatry* 132, 403–404.

 29 Staton RD, Brumback RA, Wilson H. (1982) Reduplicative paramnesia: A disconnection syndrome of memory. *Cortex* 18, 23–35.

 30 Garlipp P, Gödecke-Koch T, Dietrich DE, et al. (2004) Lycanthropy: Psychopathological and psychodynamical aspects. *Acta Psychiatrica Scandinavica* 109, 19–22.

 31 Fahy TA. (1989) Lycanthropy: A review. *Journal of the Royal Society of Medicine* 82, 37–39.

32 Keck PE, Pope HG, Hudson JI, et al. (1988) Lycanthropy: Alive and well in the twentieth century. *Psychological Medicine* 18, 113–120.

33 Coll PG, O'Sullivan G, Browne PJ. (1985) Lycanthropy lives on. *British Journal of Psychiatry* 147, 201–202.

34 Connors MH, Coltheart M. (2011) On the behaviour of senile dementia patients vis-à-vis the mirror: Ajuriaguerra, Strejilevitch and Tissot (1963). *Neuropsychologia* 49, 1679–1692.

35 Breen N, Caine D, Coltheart M. (2001) Mirrored-self misidentification: Two cases of focal onset dementia. *Neurocase* 7, 239–254.

36 Hemphill RE. (1948) Misinterpretation of mirror image of self in presenile cerebral atrophy. *Journal of Mental Science* 94, 603–610.

37 Phillips ML, Howard R, David A. (1996) "Mirror, mirror on the wall, who…?" Towards a model of visual self-recognition. *Cognitive Neuropsychiatry* 1, 153–164.

38 Gluckman LK. (1968) A case of Capgras syndrome. *Australian and New Zealand Journal of Psychiatry* 2, 39–43.

39 Abbate C, Trimarchi PD, Salvi GP, et al. (2012) Delusion of inanimate doubles: Description of a case of focal retrograde amnesia. *Neurocase* 18, 457–477.

40 Shanks MF, Venneri A. (2002) The emergence of delusional companions in Alzheimer's disease: An unusual misidentification syndrome. *Cognitive Neuropsychiatry* 7, 317–328.

41 Rubin EH, Drevets WC, Burke WJ. (1988) The nature of psychotic symptoms in senile dementia of the Alzheimer type. *Journal of Geriatric Psychiatry & Neurology* 1, 16–20.

42 Berrios GE, Brook P. (1984) Visual hallucinations and sensory delusions in the elderly. *British Journal of Psychiatry* 144, 662–664.

43 Aziz VM, Andrews M, Warner NJ. (2010) When photographs come alive: Visual misinterpretations in Alzheimer's disease. *Old Age Psychiatrist* 51, 8–9.

44 Pick A. (1903) Clinical studies. *Brain* 26, 242–267.

45 Benson DF, Gardner H, Meadows JC. (1976) Reduplicative paramnesia. *Neurology* 26, 147–151.

46 Paterson A, Zangwill OL. (1944) Disorders of visual space perception associated with lesions of the right cerebral hemisphere. *Brain* 67, 331–358.

47 Head H. (1926) *Aphasia and kindred disorders*. Cambridge University Press, London, UK.

48 American Psychiatric Association. (2000) *Diagnostic and statistical manual of mental disorders*, 4th ed., text rev. (DSM-IV-TR). American Psychiatric Association, Washington, DC.

49 American Psychiatric Association. (2013) *Diagnostic and statistical manual of mental disorders*, 5th ed. (DSM-V). American Psychiatric Association, Washington, DC.

50 Villarejo A, Martin VP, Moreno-Ramos T, et al. (2011) Mirrored-self misidentification in a patient without dementia: Evidence for right hemisphere and bifrontal damage. *Neurocase* 17, 276–284.

51 Förstl H, Almeida OP, Owen AM, et al. (1991) Psychiatric, neurological and medical aspects of misidentification syndromes: A review of 260 cases. *Psychological Medicine* 21, 905–910.

52 Dohn HH, Crews EL. (1986) Capgras syndrome: A literature review and case series. *Hillside Journal of Clinical Psychiatry* 8, 56–74.

53 Fishbain DA. (1987) The frequency of Capgras delusions in a psychiatric emergency service. *Psychopathology* 20, 42–47.

54 Frazer SJ, Roberts JM. (1994) Three cases of Capgras' syndrome. *British Journal of Psychiatry* 164, 557–559.

55 Huang T-L, Liu C-Y, Yang Y-Y. (1999) Capgras syndrome: Analysis of nine cases. *Psychiatry and Clinical Neurosciences* 53, 455–460.

56 Joseph AB. (1994) Observations on the epidemiology of the delusional misidentification syndromes in the Boston metropolitan area: April 1983–June 1984. *Psychopathology* 27, 150–153.

57 Kirov G, Jones P, Lewis SW. (1994) Prevalence of delusional misidentification syndromes. *Psychopathology* 27, 148–149.

58 Tamam L, Karatas G, Zeren T, et al. (2003) The prevalence of Capgras syndrome in a university hospital setting. *Acta Neuropsychiatrica* 15, 290–295.

59 Walter-Ryan WG. (1986) Capgras' syndrome and misidentification. *American Journal of Psychiatry* 143, 126.

60 Ballard CG, Saad K, Patel A, et al. (1995) The prevalence and phenomenology of psychotic symptoms in dementia sufferers. *International Journal of Geriatric Psychiatry* 10, 477–485.

61 Burns A, Jacoby R, Levy R. (1990) Psychiatric phenomena in Alzheimer's disease II: Disorders of perception. *British Journal of Psychiatry* 157, 76–81.

62 Förstl H, Burns A, Jacoby R, et al. (1991) Neuroanatomical correlates of clinical misidentification and misperception in senile dementia of the Alzheimer's type. *Journal of Clinical Psychiatry* 52, 268–271.

63 Förstl H, Bisthorn C, Gligen-Kelisch C, et al. (1993) Psychotic features and the course of Alzheimer's disease: Relationship to cognitive, electroencephalographic and computerized tomography findings. *Acta Psychiatrica Scandinavica* 87, 395–399.

64 Hirono N, Mori E, Yasuda M, et al. (1998) Factors associated with psychotic symptoms in Alzheimer's disease. *Journal of Neurology, Neurosurgery & Psychiatry* 64, 648–652.

65 Hwang J-P, Yang CH, Tsai SJ, et al. (1996) Psychotic symptoms in psychiatric inpatients with dementia of the Alzheimer and vascular types. *Zhonghua Yi Xue Za Zhi (Chinese Medical Journal, Taipei)* 58, 35–39.

66 Deutsch LH, Bylsma FW, Rovner BW, et al. (1991) Psychosis and physical aggression in probable Alzheimer's disease. *American Journal of Psychiatry* 148, 1159–1163.

67 Mendez MF, Martin RJ, Smyth KA, et al. (1992) Disturbances of person identification in Alzheimer's disease. *Journal of Nervous & Mental Disease* 180, 94–96.

68 Nagaratnam N, Irving J, Kalouche H. (2003) Misidentification in patients with dementia. *Archives of Gerontology and Geriatrics* 37, 195–202.

69 Nagahama Y, Okina T, Suzuki N, et al. (2007) Classification of psychotic symptoms in dementia with Lewy bodies. *American Journal of Geriatric Psychiatry* 15, 961–997.

70 Pagonabarraga J, Llebaria G, García-Sánchez C, et al. (2008) A prospective study of delusional misidentification syndromes in Parkinson's disease with dementia. *Movement Disorders* 23, 443–448.

71 Devanand DP, Jacobs DM, Tang M-X, et al. (1997) The course of psychopathologic features in mild to moderate Alzheimer disease. *Archives of General Psychiatry* 54, 257–263.

72 Migliorelli R, Petracca G, Tesón A, et al. (1995) Neuropsychiatric and neuropsychological correlates of delusions in Alzheimer's disease. *Psychological Medicine* 25, 505–513.

73 Mendez MF, Shapira JS, Woods RJ, et al. (2008) Psychotic symptoms in frontotemporal dementia: Prevalence and review. *Dementia and Geriatric Cognitive Disorders* 25, 206–211.

74 Hwang J-P, Yang C-H, Tsai S-J. (2003) Phantom boarder symptom in dementia. *International Journal of Geriatric Psychiatry* 18, 417–420.

75 Jaspers K. (1963) *General psychopathology*. University of Chicago Press, Chicago, IL.

76 Cermolacce M, Sass L, Parnas J. (2010) What is bizarre in bizarre delusions? A critical review. *Schizophrenia Bulletin* 36, 667–679.

77 Walker C. (1991) Delusion: What did Jaspers really say? *British Journal of Psychiatry* 159 94–103.

78 Enoch DM. (1963) The Capgras syndrome. *Acta Psychiatrica Scandinavica* 39, 437–462.

79 Todd J. (1957) The syndrome of Capgras. *Psychiatric Quarterly* 31, 250–265.

80 de Pauw KW. (1994) Psychodynamic approaches to the Capgras delusion: A critical historical review. *Psychopathology* 27, 154–160.

81 Hirstein W, Ramachandran VS. (1997) Capgras syndrome: A novel probe for understanding the neural representation of the identity and familiarity of persons. *Proceedings of the Royal Society B: Biological Sciences* 264, 437–444.

82 Halligan PW, David AS. (2001) Cognitive neuropsychiatry: Towards a scientific psychopathology. *Nature Reviews Neuroscience* 2, 209–215.

83 David AS, Halligan PW. (2000) Cognitive neuropsychiatry: Potential for progress. *Journal of Neuropsychiatry and Clinical Neurosciences* 12, 506–510.

84 Maher BA. (1974) Delusional thinking and perceptual disorder. *Journal of Individual Psychology* 30, 98–113.

85 Maher BA. (1988) Delusions as the product of normal cognitions. In: Oltmanns TF, Maher BA (eds.) *Delusional beliefs.* John Wiley & Sons, New York, NY, pp. 333–336.

86 Reed G. (1972) *The psychology of anomalous experience: A cognitive approach.* Hutchinson & Co, London, UK.

87 James W. (1890) *The principles of psychology.* Henry Holt and Company, New York, NY.

88 Ellis AW, Young AW. (1990) Accounting for delusional misidentifications. *British Journal of Psychiatry* 157, 239–248.

89 Ellis HD, Young AW. (1996) Problems of person perception in schizophrenia. In: Pantelis C, Nelson HE, Barnes TRE (eds.) *Schizophrenia: A neuropsychological perspective.* John Wiley & Sons, Chichester, UK, pp. 397–416.

90 Stone T, Young AW. (1997) Delusions and brain injury: The philosophy and psychology of belief. *Mind & Language* 12, 327–364.

91 Ellis HD, Young AW, Quayle AH, et al. (1997) Reduced autonomic responses to faces in Capgras delusion. *Proceedings of the Royal Society B: Biological Sciences* 264, 1085–1092.

92 Brighetti G, Bonifacci P, Borlimi R, et al. (2007) "Far from the heart far from the eye": Evidence from the Capgras delusion. *Cognitive Neuropsychiatry* 12, 189–197.

93 Tranel D, Damasio H, Damasio AR. (1995) Double dissociation between overt and covert face recognition. *Journal of Cognitive Neuroscience* 7, 425–432.

94 Langdon R, Coltheart M. (2000) The cognitive neuropsychology of delusions. *Mind & Language* 15, 184–218.

95 Coltheart M, Langdon R, McKay R. (2011) Delusional belief. *Annual Review of Psychology* 62, 271–298.

96 Coltheart M. (2007) The 33rd Bartlett Lecture: Cognitive neuropsychiatry and delusional belief. *Quarterly Journal of Experimental Psychology* 60, 1041–1062.

97 Ellis HD, Quayle AH, de Pauw KW, et al. (1996) Delusional misidentification of inanimate objects: A literature review and neuropsychological analysis of cognitive deficits in two cases. *Cognitive Neuropsychiatry* 1, 27–40.

98 Coltheart M. (2010) The neuropsychology of delusions. *Annals of the New York Academy of Sciences* 1191, 16–26.

99 Gilboa A. (2010) Strategic retrieval, confabulations, and delusions: Theory and data. *Cognitive Neuropsychiatry* 15, 145–180.

100 Sharot T, Korn CW, Dolan RJ. (2011) How unrealistic optimism is maintained in the face of reality. *Nature Reviews Neuroscience*, 14, 1475–1479.

CHAPTER 14

Delirium

Sean P. Heffernan[1], Esther Oh[2], Constantine Lyketsos[3], and Karin Neufeld[4]

[1] *Schweizer Fellow in Affective Disorders, Johns Hopkins Hospital, Baltimore, Maryland, U.S.*

[2] *Assistant Professor, Division of Geriatric Medicine and Gerontology, Johns Hopkins School of Medicine, Associate Director, the Johns Hopkins Memory and Alzheimer's Treatment Center, Baltimore, Maryland, U.S.*

[3] *Elizabeth Plank Althouse Professor and Chair of Psychiatry, Johns Hopkins Bayview Professor of Psychiatry and Behavioral Sciences, Baltimore, Maryland, U.S.*

[4] *Clinical Director of Psychiatry, Johns Hopkins Bayview Associate Professor of Psychiatry and Behavioral Science, Baltimore, Maryland, U.S.*

Introduction

Delirium is defined as disturbances of consciousness, attention, perception, thinking, memory, psychomotor behavior, emotion, and the sleep-wake schedule. The duration is variable, but the cognitive change is abrupt in onset, usually over the course of hours to days, and ranging in severity from mild to very severe [1]. Delirium is a clinical syndrome indicating underlying pathology; it is not a disease unto itself.

One of the earliest described medical syndromes in ancient writings, delirium is referred to by many names; acute or toxic confusional state, intensive care unit (ICU) psychosis, acute brain failure, and altered mental status are some of the synonyms [2]. Despite its numerous names, it is common and prevalent in all hospital settings. Ten to 42 percent of patients admitted to a general hospital develop delirium during their course [3–5], and 60–85 percent of mechanically ventilated patients admitted to an ICU will have delirium during their stay [6]. Prevalence is high in frail elderly patients; nearly 10 percent of those presenting to the emergency department and 60 percent of those admitted are delirious [7–9]. Prevalence is also high on oncology wards and AIDS services, where rates are 18 percent and 46 percent respectively [10, 11], suggesting that severity of medical illness increases delirium risk.

Delirium is associated with adverse outcomes, most notably with an increased risk of death in the months to years following the episode [12–17]. Delirium is also associated with increased length of hospital stay [17–21], prolonged duration of mechanical ventilation [12], longer ICU stays [17, 18], longer inpatient stays [22, 23], and higher rate of transition to long-term care [24]

Troublesome Disguises: Managing Challenging Disorders in Psychiatry, Second Edition.
Edited by Dinesh Bhugra and Gin S. Malhi.

including nursing homes [25]. Associated poor long-term outcomes following an episode of delirium include decreased functional abilities [26] and persistent cognitive impairment [27, 28]. The effects of delirium are not limited to the patient, as an episode of delirium has been shown to cause severe distress in care providers and family alike [29] and is estimated to cost the United States healthcare system between $38 billion and $152 billion annually [30].

One might conclude that the basic ICD-10 description combined with high incidence would make detection easy. Retrospective analyses indicated that delirium is missed in 65 percent of cases in the emergency department and 72 percent of cases on the inpatient medicine ward [7, 31]. Delirium is a difficult diagnosis to make due in large part to its heterogeneous phenomenology, which can masquerade as other conditions.

Phenomenology

The diagnosis of delirium is based on the presence of an abrupt change in the level of consciousness and ability to focus attention. The presentation fluctuates, frequently described as "waxing and waning," and can have associated changes in cognition, perception, affect, motoric capacity, and prominent sleep-wake cycle disturbances including insomnia, nocturnal exacerbation of symptoms, and disturbing dreams [32]. The phenomenology can include symptoms that are evident in other primary psychiatric illnesses.

Delirium is a disorder of sustained attention and as such can affect a patient's thinking in a number of ways. Attentional deficits result in difficulty with learning and retaining new information and can result in short-term and intermediate recall deficits, inability to perform sequential tasks, and difficulty with orientation to time, place, and person. Given these deficits, delirium can mimic an amnestic syndrome. Attention and memory problems may result in disrupted logical thought formation, tangentiality, or loosening of associations, mimicking psychotic disorders such as schizophrenia or dementing illnesses of Alzheimer's or vascular etiology.

Perceptual disturbances, such as hallucinations and illusions, can be present in delirium. Hallucinations, or perceptions without a stimulus, can be present in all sensory modalities in delirium but are most frequently visual. Illusions, or misperceptions of actual stimuli, such as seeing people in shadows, are also reported in delirium. Patients may also develop delusions, or fixed, false, idiosyncratic beliefs. The content of delusions may vary and can be paranoid, persecutory, or somatic. For example, delirious patients may believe their care providers or family members are conspiring against them. The presence of perceptual disturbances and delusions often drive consultation of a psychiatrist since such experiences are often associated with psychotic disorders such as schizophrenia or severe depression and bipolar disorder.

Affective lability, or quick-changing emotional expression, can be seen in delirium. The patient may present with rapid shifts of emotion, with associated anxiety, irritability, or uncontrollable crying. This instability of mood often prompts the team caring for the patient to seek a psychiatric consultation for assessment of a mood disorder. A small study found that 37 percent of general hospital inpatients over the age of 50 years, diagnosed by the non-psychiatric house officers as having major depression at time of consultation, were found to have hypoactive delirium [33].

Psychomotor activity can vary widely and is the distinguishing feature when describing the subtypes of delirium, which include hyperactive, hypoactive, and mixed type [34]. Psychomotor agitation is a constellation of both intentional and unintentional motions, including pacing around a room, wringing or flapping of hands and limbs, and physical aggression. In severe cases, this activity can be harmful to the patient or others due to violence or removal of indwelling catheters and lines. The hyperactive subtype of delirium is associated with psychomotor agitation and aggression; patients are restless, combative, and can be aroused and vocal. While these patients appear alert, their attention is impaired. The psychomotor agitated delirious patient is the most easily recognized by providers but may be mislabeled as a primary psychiatric disturbance such as schizophrenia or mania due to bipolar disorder [35].

Psychomotor slowing is marked by retardation of thought and activity, reduced physical movement and speech, and abulia, a lack of initiative or motivation. The hypoactive delirium subtype is characterized by somnolence along with psychomotor slowing and is often confused with depression. Affected patients may appear uninterested or apathetic and often have difficulty maintaining attention and arousal. Patients with hypoactive delirium can be difficult for clinical staff to identify; unlike those with psychomotor agitation, they are quiet and do not demand attention from the staff. Maintaining a high index of suspicion and diligent direct examination are the best means to identify patients with these phenomena. The mixed subtype of delirium includes alternating states of agitation and hypoactivity [34]. Mixed delirium is most common (54.9 percent of cases), followed by the hypoactive subtype (43.5 percent), and pure hyperactive delirium (1.6 percent) [36]. Mixed delirium is more likely to feature agitation than other subgroups and may be misinterpreted as psychotic illness [32].

These specific symptoms can lead physicians to mistake delirium for other psychiatric illnesses. Because delirium can mimic almost any other psychiatric disorder, it is imperative that providers are careful not to base the premise of a new diagnosis on a delirious presentation. A thorough history with the use of a collateral informant is very important to assess baseline function; a lack of past psychiatric history with abrupt onset of attentional and other cognitive symptoms in the setting of medical illness is highly suggestive of delirium. Physicians must be cautious not to attribute symptoms of delirium to a patient's known chronic illness.

Etiology

Delirium is a direct physiological consequence of general medical illness that can be conceptualized as the brain's involvement in multi-organ system failure [12, 17, 34, 35, 37, 38]. Current hypotheses invoke excess dopamine transmission in the hyperactive subtype and insufficient cholinergic neuro-transmission in the hypoactive subtype [39–41]. Further details are beyond the intended scope of this chapter; Fricchione's 2008 article in the American Journal of Psychiatry details proposed pathways [40]. While the pathophysiology is not yet clear, there are established etiologies that are illustrated in the mnemonic I WATCH DEATH in Table 14.1 [42].

There are a number of risk factors that make a patient more likely to become delirious (see Table 14.2). Some factors are intrinsic to the patient, such as age, preexisting cognitive disorders, visual, hearing and functional impairment, smoking, and alcoholism or other substance use disorders. There are a number of factors that are associated with illness or are iatrogenic that can contribute to

Table 14.1 Etiology of delirium: I WATCH DEATH.

Disorder	Clinical examples
Infection	Systemic, sepsis, ARDS, CNS infection
Withdrawal	From alcohol or sedative/hypnotics such as benzodiazepines or barbiturates
Acute metabolic derangements	Acidosis; electrolyte abnormalities including hypercalcemia, hyponatremia; acute renal or hepatic failure
Trauma	To brain, or severe burns, hip fracture, or operations
Central nervous system	Infections, ischemic or hemorrhagic stroke, hematoma, tumor, seizure, vasculitis, hydrocephalus, paraneoplastic limbic encephalitis, meningeal carcinomatosis
Hypoxia	Anemia, hypotension, heart failure, respiratory failure
Deficiency	Vitamins such as B12, thiamine
Endocrinopathy	Hyper- or hypoglycemia, hyperparathyroidism, hypothyroidism, cortisol dysregulation
Acute vascular accident	Hypertensive encephalopathy, arrhythmia, shock
Toxins	Medications (esp. anticholinergic, GABA-ergic), organophosphates, solvents, illicit drug or alcohol, vitamin toxicity, carbon monoxide
Heavy metal	Lead, mercury

Adapted from Wise [42].

Table 14.2 Risk factors for delirium.

Host character	Illnesses associated and iatrogenic causes
Cognitive disorders	Physical restraints
Age	Bladder catheter or multiple IVs and central lines
Severe multisystem illness	Immobilization
Psychiatric illness	Malnutrition (can also be etiology)
Alcoholism	Two or more psychoactive medications
Hypertension	Three or more medications added during course
Smoking	Prolonged pain
Traumatic brain injury	Sleep disturbances (also a symptom)
ApoE4 polymorphisms	
Visual or hearing impaired	

Ely [43], Inouye and Charpentier [44], Inouye et al. [45], Morandi et al. [34], Van Rompaey et al. [46].

precipitation of delirium, including use of physical restraints, bladder catheters and intravenous catheter complications, immobilization, and malnutrition. The use of multiple psychoactive medications or the addition of three or more new medicines also present risk factors for delirium. Many medications are implicated in causing or worsening delirium, including anticholinergics, opioids, benzodiazepines, beta-blockers, antiemetics, antipsychotics, anticonvulsants, and other psychotropics [34, 43–46]. In delirious patients, especially those with pre-existing cognitive impairment, it is important to minimize exposure to medicines, particularly psychotropics and anticholinergics.

Approach to diagnosis

Detection is the most important step in the management of delirium, but it is often the most difficult. The evaluation of a delirious patient starts with a thorough history and physical examination. History from collateral sources should focus on tracking changes in cognition, perceptual experiences, and behavior and establishing pre-existing baseline function. History should be obtained with the known etiologies kept in mind. For example, prescription of deliriogenic medications and polypharmacy are common causes so a detailed medication list, including over-the-counter and alternative remedies, is imperative. A collateral informant such a as family member or care provider is required to establish onset, duration, and fluctuation of symptoms. Many features of delirium, including disorganization, affective lability, and waxing and waning of consciousness are more easily recognized by family members who know the patient better and nursing or support staff, who spend more time with the patient.

The mental status examination is a bedside assessment of a patient's appearance, affect, thought process, thought content, perceptions and cognition. As noted previously, the mental status examination in a delirious patient can mimic that of other syndromes because it may include illusions, hallucinations, delusions, or mood changes. Cognitive assessment of delirium may reveal fluctuation and clouding of consciousness, difficulty maintaining attention, disorientation, or impaired memory. Dysphasia and dysarthria are also common in this syndrome. While a screening tool such as the Mini-Mental State Exam (MMSE) or the Montreal Cognitive Assessment (MoCA) can be a helpful adjunct to systematically screen cognition, the bedside examination is the standard for diagnosis of delirium.

The thorough physical examination is important to elicit signs of pathology. For example, an exam may reveal racing pulse, delayed capillary refills, pallor, and poor skin turgor, indicating dehydration. Notably, a neurologic exam may indicate focal signs of stroke or other CNS disease. Frontal release signs such as the palmomental, grasp, snout, and glabellar reflexes are associated with brain pathology and may indicate delirium [47]. Given the vast potential etiologies, all organ systems must be evaluated for pathology. Initial laboratory investigation should include hematology, blood chemistry, thyroid function tests, vitamin levels, toxicology, urinalysis. EKG and chest x-ray are often done at this time as well to examine cardiac and respiratory status.

Consider the high-risk or life-threatening causes, including withdrawal reactions, hypoxia and brain hypo-perfusion, hypertensive encephalopathy, intracerebral hemorrhage, infection including meningitis and encephalitis, metabolic derangements including hypoglycemia and hyponatremia, and intoxicated states. These etiologies can be identified rapidly through physical examination including vital signs and the basic screening labs. While this list includes the most dangerous causes of delirium, the etiology in a given patient is often multifactorial, such as infection in combination with medication effects. Diligence is required to identify all potential risk factors and causes.

In the diligent pursuit of other medical etiologies of delirium, a second review of the medication list with a goal to minimizing the regimen and avoiding deliriogenic agents is warranted. Further testing may include HIV, brain MRI, heavy metal screening, and EEG. The EEG typically reveals slowing, peak power decrease, and sporadic delta waves (0–4 and 5–7 Hz respectively) in a diffuse, symmetric pattern particularly in the posterior basic rhythm in the case of delirium [48]. Other variants that may be seen in a patient with waxing and waning of consciousness are fast activity that is noted in delirium tremens, and discharges associated with nonconvulsive seizures. An EEG may support a diagnosis of delirium, but is not an indicated primary diagnostic tool given its limited sensitivity and specificity.

Differential diagnosis

The differential diagnosis for delirium is broad and includes primary cognitive, affective, and psychotic disorders. The keys to distinguishing these illnesses lie in a careful history and mental status examination. Findings from examination of a patient's level of consciousness, attention, and orientation will be telling in working through one's differential diagnosis.

Fluctuating level of consciousness is a feature of three psychiatric illnesses: delirium, catatonia, and advanced stages of dementia with Lewy bodies, or DLB. A history of onset over years, the presence of Parkinsonian motor symptoms, and falls will be the key to differentiate DLB from the first two. Delirium and catatonia are often hard to distinguish, particularly because both can present with hyperactive or excited states, but this distinction is important because their treatments are very different. An EEG can be most useful in this circumstance, as a delirious patient due to toxic or metabolic causes will have diffuse, symmetric slowing of the posterior basic rhythm with predominant delta or theta waves. Patients with catatonia due to a psychiatric disturbance such as bipolar disorder or schizophrenia generally have normal EEGs if it is a primary presentation. A patient can be delirious and catatonic simultaneously, with catatonia secondary to the delirium or delirium secondary to the decreased oral intake, or to medications used in the treatment of catatonia.

Distinguishing dementia from delirium is challenging, because they both prominently feature cognitive impairment. The distinctive features lie in the history; dementia is a global cognitive decline with onset over months or years. Delirium is rapid in onset, coming on over hours or days. Demented patients can and often do develop delirium, so providers must be aware of fluctuations of consciousness that would indicate delirium particularly in the setting of acute worsening in cognition. Some dementias have a baseline disrupted EEG pattern that can complicate EEG utility. Alzheimer's dementia features a reduction in wave power [49]. EEG tracing of patients with dementia with Lewy bodies can be especially problematic for interpretation because they feature reduced background activity and disrupted cortical reactivity patterns at baseline [50].

Affective disorders belong on the differential diagnosis for delirium. The hypoactive subtype of delirium resembles depression with its psychomotor slowing, social withdrawal, sleep disruption, and abulia. The primary way to differentiate depressive disorders from delirium is through history. Most primary affective disorders present in early adulthood, with the exception being some cases of depression. Delirium features abrupt onset of mood lability, whereas depressive disorders likely have a longer onset of weeks to months, and are often accompanied by a family history and a past psychiatric history. Key features of a depressive episode due to an affective disorder are low mood, poor self-attitude or lack of self-esteem and self-confidence, and associated physical symptoms including change in appetite, poor sleep, and low energy. Depression can also be marked by difficulty concentrating and remembering, referred to in some literature as pseudodementia or "dementia of depression," but this condition does not feature disorientation or alterations in levels of consciousness as delirium does.

Mania is often considered in cases of hyperactive delirium, which feature irritability and increased movements. Mania's core features are elated mood and elevated self-attitude, often to the point of grandiose self-esteem. The associated physical symptoms, or vital sense, of mania often oppose that of depression and feature increased energy and decreased need for sleep. As in the case of a depressive episode, a manic patient may appear cognitively impaired at times due to difficulty concentrating, but would not feature fluctuating consciousness. EEG tracings in a manic patient should be normal and may help to distinguish the two conditions.

Hallucinations and delusions are the symptoms most likely to cause a physician difficulty in the assessment of a delirious patient. Physicians frequently attribute this presentation to a psychotic illness, often schizophrenia, mania, or psychotic depression. Again, if these symptoms are present with disorientation or a fluctuating level of consciousness, and have been abrupt in onset with no previous history consistent with psychosis earlier in life, then delirium is the most likely diagnosis.

Conclusion

Delirium is a medical and psychiatric emergency with grave consequences. For patient safety and well-being, it must be identified early—a difficult task given its numerous different phenotypes that can mimic other psychiatric diseases. For optimal care, physicians must take a thorough history, diligently examine the patient, identify risk factors for delirium, be mindful of life-threatening etiologies, and pursue full medical and neurologic workup to identify cause, all the while minimizing illness-associated and iatrogenic factors that may contribute to confusion. Prompt detection and management of delirium may reduce patient morbidity, inpatient length of stay, long-term cognitive effects, and mortality. The following case illustrates this practice and highlights the complex presentation and phenotype of delirium.

Case study

The psychiatry consultation service was asked by the internal medicine team to evaluate Mrs. A, a 70-year-old African-American woman who was admitted for hypertensive encephalopathy, because of several days of bizarre behavior and hearing voices.

Her family history is notable for both of her parents dying of ischemic strokes in their 60s. Her mother was said to have a "nervous breakdown" at age 40 and took chlorpromazine or haloperidol thereafter. Her sisters have an alcohol use disorder. The patient's son had schizophrenia; he died 2 years ago of suicide at age 41. She has two daughters who are healthy.

Mrs. A was born and raised in Washington, DC. She met developmental milestones on time and had no behavioral issues as a child. She completed high school and worked as a receptionist until retirement at 65 years old. She lives with her husband of 47 years; he is a deacon. The patient has smoked one pack per day for almost 50 years. She last drank alcohol 3 years ago and previously would consume one or two drinks per month. She has never used illicit substances.

Past medical history includes hypertension, insulin-dependent diabetes mellitus (most recent hemoglobin A1c was 9.0%/75 mmol/mol), hyperlipidemia, and hypothyroidism. She has had two transient ischemic attacks in the past 3 years. She has bilateral cataracts, secondary to diabetes; she is scheduled to have lens removal and implantation in 1 month. She has no history of head trauma or seizures. She has never had major surgery. She reports no known drug allergies. A thirteen-point review of systems was notable for 1 week of dull, generalized headache.

Home medications include insulin glargine, insulin aspart sliding scale, lisinopril , nifedipine, levothyroxine, and multivitamin. She takes St John's Wort herbal supplements and noted taking more than directed on the pill bottle over the last week. She has not been adherent with her insulin regimen for the past 2 weeks.

The patient's personality is described by her husband as mild-mannered, reserved, organized, and future-oriented. However, the patient's husband has noticed some changes in her cognition over the past 4 years: she doesn't cook as she used to, is disorganized in her dressing, and has had difficulty with short-term memory and word finding. Over the past year, she started packing excessively to go out for the day and has had trouble remembering how to get home when they go on walks in their neighborhood together. She has gradually become more obstinate and argumentative over the past few months. She's become resistant to her husband helping with checking her blood sugar and giving her insulin.

Mrs. A has never seen a psychiatrist in the past. There is no evidence of syndromal depression, mania, or hypomania. She had an episode of confusion at age 50, during which she was first diagnosed with diabetes. She presented to the ER after 2 days of unusual behavior including burying nickels, dimes, and quarters in the front yard and making sexually bizarre and provocative statements. Her behavior and cognition returned to normal after correction of her glucose with insulin.

Over the past 6 months, the patient has had several unusual episodes. On three occasions she has woken up around 4 am and tried to leave the home. During Christmas shopping, she walked out of a store with a cart full of gifts, claiming the store owner owed her the contents. While out to dinner a few months ago, she exclaimed that their server was trying to poison her by bringing her cold food. These events were accompanied by some slight confusion and disorientation, but "nothing too alarming" according to her husband.

Two weeks prior to this presentation, the husband noticed that his wife had more significant memory problems and disorganization, particularly about her insulin regimen. The patient's husband took her for emergency assessment where her blood glucose was 575 mg/dl. She was treated with insulin but refused admission to the hospital and was discharged. She was agitated and slept less than 2 hours over the next 2 days. Mrs. A accused her husband of being an imposter and not her real husband. She repeatedly called him "the devil" and asked him to kill her when he refused to take her to see their deceased son. She was brought back to the ER, where her blood pressure was 215/125 mmHg. Blood chemistries were done and indicated a fasting glucose of 540 mg/dl, BUN 30 mg/dl, and creatinine of 2.1 mg/dl (baseline 0.9 mg/dl). Physical examination was notable for elevated jugular venous pulse and 2+ bilateral lower-extremity edema. Neurologic exam revealed bilateral papilledema, wide unsteady gait, and fine myoclonus in upper extremities. There were no signs of infection on examination. Urinalysis showed trace ketones but was otherwise negative. She was given lorazepam to sedate her for testing. Chest x-ray was normal. Brain MRI FLAIR showed lacunar infarcts, widening of sulci particularly in parietal lobes, and atrophy of hippocampus. EEG indicated diffuse and symmetric slowing of the posterior basic rhythm. Lumbar puncture was done because of headache but showed no signs of infection or intracranial process.

When not sedated by medications, the patient screamed at the demons she reports seeing in her room. She was agitated, and tried to remove her clothes, peripheral IVs, and urinary catheter. She continued to believe that her husband was replaced by an imposter and was fearful of him.

When evaluated by the psychiatry consultant, she was found lying in bed disheveled with both wrists in restraints. She appeared tired. Assessment of muscles revealed myoclonus. Gait was wide-based and unsteady. Speech was soft. Thought process was tangential. Mood was described as "scared." Affect was labile. There was no passive death wish, suicidal or homicidal ideation. She reported auditory and visual hallucinations of demons calling to her. The patient confirmed that she continues to doubt the identity of her husband and is paranoid of him as well as hospital staff, whom she has seen "conspiring" with him against her. She was oriented to the month and year, but not to date or day of week. She was not oriented to place, referring to the hospital as "where you come to rehearse." Registration was impaired with difficulty repeating words; short term memory was impaired (1/3 items) at 1 and 5 minutes. She had difficulty with attention, most evident by inability to perform repeated subtractions; she was unable to state the months of the year in reverse. Language naming was intact, able to follow instructions and able to write a sentence. Insight and judgment were assessed as poor.

The medical team was concerned by her agitation and hallucinosis and wished for evaluation and recommendation for possible new-onset psychotic illness. This patient has many risk factors for delirium. She is over age 65, smokes cigarettes, and has hypertension, a history of cerebrovascular disease, and visual impairment. A detailed history from her husband indicates several years of slow cognitive decline with amnesia, apraxia in dress, anomic aphasia, as well as perceptual disturbance evident in getting lost in their neighborhood. Possible etiologies of her altered mental status are hypertensive encephalopathy, likely contributed in part by taking St John's Wort, which induces metabolism of nifedipine. She also has associated acute renal failure and hyperglycemia. Iatrogenic factors in the course of her illness are the prescription of lorazepam (especially in light of her acute renal failure) and the use of physical restraints.

References

1 World Health Organization. Major depressive disorder. In International statistical classification of diseases and related health problems (10th ed.). 1990. Retrieved from http://apps.who.int/classifications/icd10/browse/2010/en#/F05.

2 Lipowski ZJ. *Delirium: Acute Confusional States.* Oxford University Press, New York, 1990, pp. 490.

3 Levkoff S, Cleary P, Liptzin B, Evans DA. Epidemiology of delirium: An overview of research issues and findings. *International Psychogeriatrics* 1991;3(2):149–167.

4 Siddiqi N, House AO, Holmes JD. Occurrence and outcome of delirium in medical in-patients: A systematic literature review. *Age Ageing* 2006;35:350–364.

5 Trzepacz PT. Delirium: Advances in diagnosis, pathophysiology, and treatment. *Psychiatric Clinics of North America* 1996;19(3):429–448.

6 Pun BT, Gordon SM, Peterson JF, Shintani AK, Jackson JC, Foss J, Harding SD, Bernard GR, Dittus RS, Ely EW. Large-scale implementation of sedation and delirium monitoring in the intensive care unit: A report from two medical centers. *Crit Care Med* 2005;33(6):1199–1205.

7 Elie M, Rousseau F, Cole M, Primeau F, McCusker J, Bellavance F. Prevalence and detection of delirium in elderly emergency department patients. *CMAJ Canadian Medical Association Journal* 2000;163(8):977–981.

8 Francis J, Kapoor WN. Delirium in hospitalized elderly. *Journal of General Internal Medicine* 1990;5(1):65–79.

9 Hustey FM, Meldon SW, Smith MD, Lex CK. The effect of mental status screening on the care of elderly emergency department patients. *Annals of Emergency Medicine* 2003; 41(5):678–684.

10 Ljubisavljevic V, Kelly B. Risk factors for development of delirium among oncology patients. *General Hospital Psychiatry* 2003;25(5):345–352.

11 Uldall KK, Berghuis JP. Delirium in AIDS patients: Recognition and medication factors. *AIDS Patient Care & Stds* 1997;11(6):435–441.

12 Ely EW, Shintani A, Truman B, Speroff T, Gordon SM, Harell FE. Delirium as a predictor of mortality in mechanically ventilated patients in the intensive care unit. *JAMA* 2004;291(14):1753–1762.

13 McCusker J, Cole M, Abrahamowicz M, Primeau F, Belzile E. Delirium predicts 12-month mortality. *Archives of Internal Medicine* 2002;162(4):457–463.

14 Pisani MA, Kong SYJ, Kasl SV, Murphy TE, Araujo KLB, Van Ness PH. Days of delirium are associated with 1-year mortality in an older intensive care unit population. *American Journal of Respiratory and Critical Care Medicine* 2009;180(11):1092–1097.

15 Shehabi Y, Riker RR, Bokesch BM, Wisemandle W, Shintani A, Ely EW. Delirium duration and mortality in lightly sedated, mechanically ventilated patients. *Critical Care Medicine* 2010;38(12):2311–2318.

16 Lin SM, Liu CY, Wang CH, Lin HC, Huang CD, Huang PY. The impact of delirium on the survival of mechanically ventilated patients. *Critical Care Medicine* 2004;32(11):2254–2259.

17 Thomason JWW, Shintani A, Peterson JF, Pun BT, Jackson JC, Ely EW. Intensive care unit delirium is an independent predictor of longer hospital stay: A prospective analysis of 261 non-ventilated patients. *Critical Care* 2005;9(4):375–381.

18 Ely EW, Gautam S, Margolin R, Francis J, May L, Speroff T. The impact of delirium in the intensive care unit on hospital length of stay. *Intensive Care Medicine* 2001;27(12):1892–1900.

19 McCusker J, Cole MG, Dendukuri N, Belzile E. Does delirium increase hospital stay? *Journal of the American Geriatrics Society* 2003;51(11):1539–1546.

20 Oimet S, Kavanagh BP, Gottfried SB, Skrobik Y. Incidence, risk factors and consequences of ICU delirium. *Intensive Care Medicine* 2007;33(1):66–73.

21 Stevens LE, de Moore GM, Simpson JM. Delirium in hospital: Does it increase length of stay? *Australian & New Zealand Journal of Psychiatry* 1998;32(6):805–808.

22 Rudolph JL, Marcantonio ER. Review articles: Postoperative delirium: Acute change with long-term implications. *Anesthesia and Analgesia* 2011;112:1202–1211.

23 Han JH, Eden S, Shintani A. Delirium in older emergency department patients is an independent predictor of hospital length of stay. *Academic Emergency Medicine* 2011;18: 451–457.

24 Inouye SK, Rushing JT, Foreman MD, Palmer RM, Pompei P. Does delirium contribute to poor hospital outcomes? A three-site epidemiologic study. *Journal of General Internal Medicine* 1998;13:234–242.

25 McAvay GJ, Van Ness PH, Bogardus ST. Older adults discharged from the hospital with delirium: 1-year outcomes. *Journal of the American Geriatrics Society* 2006;54:1245–1250.

26 Moller JT, Cluitmans P, Rasmussen LS, Houx P, Rasmussen H, Canet J. Long-term postoperative cognitive dysfunction in the elderly ISPOCD1 study. ISPOCD investigators. International Study of Post-Operative Cognitive Dysfunction. *Lancet* 1998;351(9106):857–861.

27 Girard TD, Jackson JC, Pandharipande PP. Delirium as a predictor of long-term cognitive impairment in survivors of critical illness. *Critical Care Medicine* 2010;38:1513–1520.

28 Saczynski JS, Marcantonio ER, Quach L. Cognitive trajectories after postoperative delirium. *The New England Journal of Medicine* 2012;367:30–39.

29 Breitbart W, Gibson C, Tremblay A. The delirium experience: Delirium recall and delirium-related distress in hospitalized patients with cancer, their spouses/caregivers, and their nurses. *Psychosomatics* 2002;43(3):183–194.

30 Leslie DL, Zhang Y, Bogardus ST, Holford TR, Leo-Summers LS, Inouye SK. Consequences of preventing delirium in hospitalized older adults on nursing home costs. *Journal of the American Geriatrics Society* 2005:53(3):405–409.

31 Collins N, Blanchard MR, Tookman A, Sampson EL. Detection of delirium in the acute hospital. *Age and Ageing* 2010;39(1):131e5. Epub 2009/11/18.

32 Meagher DJ, Leonard M, Donnelly S, Conroy M, Adamis D, Trzepacz PT. A longitudinal study of motor subtypes in delirium: Relationship with other phenomenology, etiology, medication exposure and prognosis. *Journal of Psychosomatic Research* 2011;71:395–403.

33 Margolis RL. Nonpsychiatrist house staff frequently misdiagnose psychiatric disorders in general hospital inpatients. *Psychosomatics* 1994;35(5):485–491.

34 Morandi A, Jackson JC, Ely EW. Delirium in the intensive care unit. *International Review of Psychiatry* 2009;21(1):43–58.

35 Maldonado JR. Delirium in the acute care setting: Characteristics, diagnosis and treatment. *Critical Care Clinics* 2008;24:657–722.

36 Peterson JF, Pun BT, Dittus RS, Thomason JWW, Jackson JC, Shintani AK, Ely EW. Delirium and its motoric subtypes: A study of 614 critically ill patients. *Journal of the American Geriatrics Society* 2006;54:479–484.

37 Griffiths RD, Jones C. Delirium, cognitive dysfunction and posttraumatic stress disorder. *Current Opinion in Anaesthesiology* 2007;20(2):124–129.

38 Pandharipande P, Jackson J, Ely EW. Delirium: Acute cognitive dysfunction in the critically ill. *Current Opinion in Critical Care* 2005;11(4):360–368.

39 Flacker JM, Lipsitz LA. Neural mechanisms of delirium: Current hypotheses and evolving concepts. *The Journals of Gerontology. Series A, Biological Sciences and Medical Sciences* 1999;54:B239–B246.

40 Fricchione GL, Nejad SH, Esses JA, Cummings TJ, Querques J, Cassem NJ, Murray GB. Postoperative delirium. *The American Journal of Psychiatry* 2008:165(7):803–812.

41 Steiner LA. Postoperative delirium. Part 1: Pathophysiology and risk factors. *European Journal of Anaesthesiology* 2011;28:628–636.

42 Wise MG, Brandt G. Delirium. In Hales RE, Yudofsky SC (eds.) *American Psychiatric Press Textbook of Neuropsychiatry,* 2nd ed. American Psychiatric Press, Washington, DC, 1992.

43 Ely EW, Girard TD, Shintani AK, Jackson JC, Gordon SM, Thomason JW, Pun BT, Canonico AE, Light RW, Pandharipande P, Laskowitz DT. Apolipoprotein E4 polymorphism as a genetic predisposition to delirium in critically ill patients. *Critical Care Medicine* 2007;35(1):112–117.

44 Inouye SK, Charpentier PA. Precipitating factors for delirium in hospitalized elderly persons. Predictive model and interrelationship with baseline vulnerability. *JAMA* 1996; 275:852–857.

45 Inouye SK, Bogardus ST Jr, Charpentier PA, et al. A multicomponent intervention to prevent delirium in hospitalized older patients. *The New England Journal of Medicine* 1999; 340:669–676.

46 Van Rompaey B, Elseviers MM, Schuurmans MJ, Shortridge-Baggett LM, Truijen S, Bossaert L. Risk factors for delirium in intensive care patients: A prospective cohort study. *Critical Care* 2009;13(3):R77.

47 Nicolson SE, Chabon B, Larsen KA, Kelly SE, Potter AW, Stern TA. Primitive reflexes associated with delirium: A prospective trial. *Psychosomatics* 2011;52(6):507–512.

48 Thomas C, Hestermann U, Kopitz J. Serum anticholinergic activity and cerebral cholinergic dysfunction: An EEG study in frail elderly with and without delirium. *BMC Neuroscience* 2008;9:86.

49 Adamis D, Sahu S, Treloar A. The utility of EEG in dementia: A clinical perspective. *International Journal of Geriatric Psychiatry* 2005;20:1038–1045.

50 Franciotti R, Iacono D, Della Penna S. Cortical rhythms reactivity in AD, LBD and normal subjects: A quantitative MEG study. *Neurobiology of Aging* 2006;27:1100–1109.

CHAPTER 15

Paraphilias and culture

Oyedeji Ayonrinde[1] and Dinesh Bhugra[2]

[1] *Consultant Psychiatrist, South London and Maudsley NHS Foundation Trust, London, UK*
[2] *Professor of Mental Health and Cultural Diversity, Institute of Psychiatry, King's College London, London, UK*

Introduction

Sexual activity is a universal phenomenon, strongly influenced by sexual orientation and fantasy. Attitudes to sex, sexuality, sexual orientation, and procreation are strongly influenced by individual cultures. Cultures also determine child-rearing patterns as well as our thought processes. Our cultural identities also influence our inner and external world views and it is inevitable that attitudes will be coloured by the manner in which we think and how our attitudes develop. Societies and cultures also decide what is seen as deviant and abnormal. In this chapter we propose to highlight some of the key issues related to diagnosis and management of paraphilias. Until relatively recently, paraphilias were known as sexual deviance or aberrations.

Definitions

The Diagnostic and Statistical Manual of the American Psychiatric Association (DSM-5) [1] defines paraphilia as:

> Any intense and persistent sexual interest other than sexual interest in genital stimulation or preparatory fondling with phenotypically normal, physically mature, consenting human partners. This interest is seen as any sexual interest greater than or equal to normophilic sexual interests.

Preferential sexual interests affect sexual activity and these can be seen as erotic activities as well as erotic targets. Paraphilias come to the attention of psychiatrists or other mental health professionals if there are legal complications. As long as two consenting adults in privacy of their home perform these acts they are not likely to be brought to clinical settings. Excess of distress or illegal nature of certain activities may lead to referral to legal or medical pathways.

Troublesome Disguises: Managing Challenging Disorders in Psychiatry, Second Edition.
Edited by Dinesh Bhugra and Gin S. Malhi.
© 2015 John Wiley & Sons, Ltd. Published 2015 by John Wiley & Sons, Ltd.

Paraphilic disorder

A paraphilic disorder is a paraphilia that is currently causing distress or impairment to the individual or a paraphilia whose satisfaction has entailed personal harm or risk of harm to others.

There are a large number and variety of paraphilic disorders and we do not propose a comprehensive list but only an illustrative one (see Table 15.1).

The DSM-5 stresses the importance of culture-related diagnostic issues: "knowledge of and appropriate consideration for normative aspects of sexual behaviour are important factors to explore to establish a clinical diagnosis and to distinguish a clinical diagnosis from socially acceptable behaviour" [1]. This highlights the need for an awareness of cultural context and cultural values of the group to which the individual belongs in the assessment and understanding of these patterns of behaviour. Individual patients' cultural identities and values will need to be explored and their significance confirmed with others from the same culture.

The role of sexual activity is fundamental to the preservation of the human race. However, the non-procreational role of sexual activity will be influenced by a range of factors such as available sexual partners, opportunities, and individual fantasies. These individual factors are set against a backdrop of culture, norms, taboos, religion, mores, and values of the society.

Table 15.1 Specific paraphilic disorders.

Type of paraphilia	Description
Voyeuristic Disorder	*Urge or practice of observing an unsuspecting person who is naked, undressing, or engaging in sexual activity, or in activity deemed to be private*
Exhibitionistic Disorder	*Exposing one's genitals to an unsuspecting person or performing sexual acts that can be observed by others*
Frotteuristic Disorder	*Touching or rubbing against a non-consenting person*
Sexual Masochism Disorder	*A desire to be humiliated, beaten, bound, or made to suffer for sexual pleasure*
Sexual Sadism Disorder	*Sexual pleasure through the infliction of pain or humiliation on another person*
Pedophilic Disorder	*Sexual preference for prepubescent children*
Fetishistic Disorder	*Use of inanimate objects to gain sexual excitement*
Transvestic Disorder	*Arousal from clothing associated with members of the opposite sex*

Other specified paraphilic disorders:
Zoophilia
Scatologia
Necrophilia
Urophilia

Society and culture have a significant impact on the recognition and acceptance of behaviours as normal or deviance. This relationship involves a complex interplay of factors, as culture determines "normality and abnormality" by defining norms of acceptable behaviour and permissible variants. In essence, the recognition of abnormal behaviour, the label ascribed, and explanatory model are culturally influenced.

Furthermore, the etiological role of culture in some disorders can be illustrated by considering the societal role and expectations of body image in anorexia nervosa, thereby influencing clinical presentation and its interpretation. The rates and distribution of disorders can also be culturally influenced, as is the case with culture-bound syndromes or alcohol-related health problems. It therefore stands to reason that culture influences the seeking, provision of treatment options, and care pathways within a society. Through these expectations of what constitutes treatment, culture influences the satisfaction or outcome of treatment interventions.

Within both normal and abnormal practice, a substantial range of behaviours exist. For instance, a man may dress in women's clothes for a fancy dress party, or may occasionally dress in such clothes for sexual pleasure and gratification, or actively pursue a change to the female gender role and the desire to wear women's clothes all the time. A snapshot of each situation would describe cross-dressing in a man, but the context is different in each scenario. The transitional role of uniforms as symbols that traverse fashion, fantasy, and fetish was highlighted by Bhugra and de Silva [2]

In some situations, the absence of opportunities for heterosexual activity may lead individuals to engage in homosexual activity, for example in prisons, boarding schools, and other settings where opportunities for heterosexual activity are limited. It is possible for a person with heterosexual orientation to maintain heterosexual fantasies while engaged in homosexual acts.

In light of this, it is worth emphasising that manifest sexual behaviour may not be a true measure of sexual preference or fantasy as circumstances determine. On the other hand, the perception of some deviant behaviour may be influenced by culturally determined norms such as the number of sexual partners and frequency of sexual activity in sexual addiction.

Help-seeking is likely to be determined by:

Societal acceptance of behaviours: how socially acceptable or rejected the behaviour is

Legalisation or criminalisation of the behaviour and whether disclosure may lead to serious consequences, such as imprisonment or death in some parts of the world.

The availability and type of therapeutic interventions for the behaviour

Medicalisation or disorder categorisation of the behaviour

While paraphilias are universal phenomena across all cultures, the prevalence, distribution, and legal status may vary in individual societies.

This chapter explores the impact and influence of culture on sexual behaviours and paraphilias. In addition, the controversies associated with defining these disorders and the range of sexual behaviour or deviance are considered.

Culture and the individual

Culture constitutes the symbolic and learned non-biological features of human society, including customs, conventions, and language, by which human behaviour can be distinguished. It influences the way individuals live, their values, and belief systems, as well as how they communicate. Culture may be explicit or implicit in presentation and is a non-static heterogeneous phenomenon with dynamic boundaries. In societies, there is an interplay between the community and the individual. Through acculturation, for instance, the individual may retain core values while adopting visible values such as clothing or dress code. The rate of growth or change of an individual within a culture is influenced by fluid differences between the individual and the overall societal values, duration in the culture, and individual and family factors, to mention a few.

Types of cultures

Cultures have been broadly described by Hofstede [3, 4] into sociocentric (collectivist) or egocentric (individualistic). Collectivist cultures believe in "we-ness" and the different stages of the lifecycle promote social cohesiveness and in-group loyalty. Sociocentrism promotes a collective identity, group solidarity, and emotional interdependence and shared obligations toward the wellbeing of the community. These cultures promote stable friendships and encourage decision making by kin or the group.

Individualistic cultures, on the other hand, believe in "I-ness" with loose ties between individuals and members of the society to promote the wellbeing of themselves and their immediate families. Egocentric cultures focus on emotional independence, individual initiative, autonomy, and the right to privacy. In addition, the "I-conscious" nature of these cultures encourages specific friendships and need for financial security.

Sociocentric and egocentric cultures have important differences. Cultural determinants of relationships influence social expectations as well as attitudes and behaviours. Personal relationships are salient in collectivist societies and trump some behaviours, such as seeking personal reward or pleasure-based sexual activity. Collective cultures have an influence on moral and sexual values and therefore on expression of sexuality, sex, and sexual behaviours.

Hofstede [3, 4] also described the dimensions of "masculinity-femininity." Gender roles vary in different cultures. In some societies men and women have equal rights and opportunities, while in others there is greater male dominance. In high masculinity societies women have restricted opportunities in vocation or societal hierarchy and there are higher degrees of individualism, financial reward, and limited support for the weaker in society. Conversely, feminine societies are relationship oriented and do not focus on emotional or social differentiation.

Other features of societies include *power distance* (a measure of interpersonal power or the degree of influence between a subordinate and his or her senior). Power distance reflects the degree of inequality. Uncertainty avoidance, on the other hand, is a measure of how tolerable the anxiety of the unknown plays in the society. Societies with low uncertainty avoidance tolerate challenges such as unemployment or work stress better because there are means of tapping on shared happiness. The final dimension is related to *long-versus short-term orientation*. Long-term orientation involves the preparation for the future and goals such as career planning.

These five dimensions rank differently in different societies and cultures. It has been suggested [5] that cultures that are masculine and individualistic, with low power distance and with low short-term orientation as well as low uncertainty avoidance, may have a greater expression of paraphilias. Cultural analysis and awareness of dimensions give insight into the variability of paraphilias and problem sexual behaviours.

Sociocultural aspects of human sexuality

Sexual practices are associated with the societal kinship structures and power gradients. Reiss [6] asserted that these sexual practices follow prescribed and shared cultural scripts, which both promote and discourage different types of sexual behaviour.

Sociocultural scripts of sexual behaviour may be innate (hence biological or nature) or may be learned (nurture and environmental) through cultural transmission. Culture may further define scripted roles on the basis of age, gender, social position, and religious faith. Such cultural transmission of sexual roles and behaviours may include folklore, song, dance, or depiction in artwork. Others may limit or promote behaviour through rites of passage into manhood or the expectation of blood-stained white sheets of the bride after the consummation of marriage to affirm the wife's virginity.

Kinship-based social roles promote long-term relationships between genders and with childrearing practice while providing support mechanisms. This may be more visible in Hofstede's sociocentric or collectivist cultures. Sexual scripts also determine gender roles, with the reinforced promotion of the often male position as being more dominant in many spheres of life—for example, head of the household, leading organisations, and the expectation to provide and ensure the wellbeing of others. Reiss's description of this bears some similarity to Hofstede's concepts and cultural dimensions of masculinity and femininity.

Arguing the role of nature (biology), Segall, Dasen, Berry, and Poortinga [7] indicate that the processes of sexual attraction and arousal are biological, for instance, in men involving a mental process, nerve transmission, and changes in blood supply to achieve penile erection. In essence, regardless of the culture and whether the underlying outlook is sociocentric or egocentric, these important biological mechanisms play a role in the process and manifestation of paraphilic behaviours.

Table 15.2 presents types of paraphilias on the strength of unusually sexually attracting stimuli for the purpose of sexual arousal.

Evidence supports the role of biological, cultural and individual factors in the development of paraphilias. The weight given to each component remains uncertain and will be explored further in this chapter.

Sexual behaviours, attitudes, and culture

Standards of what constitutes the normal range of sexually attractive, arousing experiences and behaviours are difficult to define. This may range from body size, skin tone, eye colour, hair, and fragrances, to mention but a few. These subjective individual experiences are influenced by yet transcend cultures and geographical borders

Table 15.2 Types of deviance and cultural-biological influences.

Deviance	Type	Cultural influences	Biological influences
Normal	Masturbation	+++	+
	Oral sex	+++	?
	Premarital sex	+++	?
Subcultural	Fetishism	+	?
	Sadomasochism	+	?
	Transsexualism	+	++
	Transvestism	++	?
Individual	Exhibitionist	+	?
	Rape	?	?
	Incest	?	?

Adapted from Bhugra et al. [5].
+ = positive correlation present.
? = unknown correlation.

Sex positive and negative cultures

Bullough [8] described societies and cultures as either sex-positive or sex-negative. Elaborating on this, it was viewed that sex-negative cultures see semen loss and even intercourse as a weakness and sexual asceticism is encouraged. Sex-positive cultures, on the other hand, emphasise the pleasurable, gratifying, rewarding, and non-reproductive aspects of sex.

A Western historical overview highlights the attitudinal changes over centuries as well as the changes in religious values. Early Greeks and Romans acknowledged and accepted alternative sexual behaviours with changes in attitudes toward sexuality. Religion and faith transmission of attitudes were promoted by religious doctrines and teaching. Procreation was essential to the sustenance of society and maintenance of a labour (farming) and military workforce. The non-procreative loss of semen was associated with loss of potent vital energy and the reproductive resource of the individual as well as the society.

Early Christianity generally disapproved of non-procreative sex. In addition, it condemned sex outside marriage, which was subsequently embedded into one of the Ten Commandments. Bullough [8] indicated that in the midst of competing and parallel religious systems, there were different interpretations to doctrines. Marriage did not automatically endorse the right to sexual activity and was expressed more as a duty and not a source of pleasure.

Islam, in contrast [8] (p. 205), appeared to lean more toward being sex-positive, with the historical understanding that the sexual traditions of pre-Islamic Arabs were more accommodating of sex. Women were sought for wedlock and not debauchery and reference is made to both transvestism and transexualism in historic documents (p. 234). However, a contradiction to the sex-positive view was that women were seen as inferior and subservient to men.

Hinduism, as a philosophy and religion, was seen as sex-positive, as illustrated in the carvings of sex acts in many temples and the Kama Sutra. The Kama Sutra extensively covers many aspects of courtship and sex acts, as do numerous erotic Hindu classics. While on the surface sexually liberal, the faith also contained a number of sexual restrictions. For instance, adultery was taboo, and intercaste relationships discouraged. However, transexualism and transvestitism, which would otherwise be termed deviance, were tolerated. Furthermore, there was an availability of penile appendages to alter shape and there was tolerance for bestiality under some conditions (p. 265). The culture permitted males to express their femininity and females their masculinity in particular contexts to promote understanding of the other sex [8] (p. 273). Loss of semen by the male, however, has a salience and may be associated with semen loss anxiety in many cultures.

Table 15.3 Interaction between individuals and cultures.

Variable	Sex-positive and non-procreative	Sex-negative and procreative
Sociocentric individual	–	++
Pleasure	+	?
Egocentric individual	++	?+
Pleasure	+++	++

Adapted from Bhugra et al. [5].
+ = positive correlation present.
– = negative correlation present.
? = unknown.

As societies have evolved, changed, and imbibed new customs, the values and attitudes regarding sexual activity and sexuality have changed. Religion has been a potent vehicle of these attitudes and practice with adaptation of views in regions of the world through evangelism (e.g., Africa). Interestingly, cultural differences may emerge within the same faith group such as the more "liberal" views being espoused by some churches, such as the Church of England regarding homosexual clergy, have been challenged by many African churches as deviating from original scripture and a sexual deviation.

Historical accounts and depictions of brothels and flagellation, homo-sexual prostitutes, pornographic media, and the industry in sex toys between 19th- and 21st-century England shed light on shifting values, attitudes, and tolerance of sexuality. While there has been a growing acceptance of female sexuality in some parts of the world, the expression or deviation from imposed roles may lead to the death penalty in other areas such as Taliban Afghanistan, where even female education is frowned upon (Table 15.3).

Prevalence of paraphilias

Sociodemographic risk factors

Exploring the prevalence of paraphilias and other sexual behaviours can be difficult even in the most liberal societies. Therefore, there is a dearth of empirical data regarding distribution and prevalence rates. Population studies into paraphilias face challenges such as embarrassment of individuals to acknowledge their behaviours and the illegal status of these sexual behav-iours in some societies. In addition, researchers are unlikely to be able to objectively verify findings. On the other hand, paraphilias in clinical settings are likely to be in the context of legal difficulties rather than self-referral. In less permissive societies (predominantly non-Western), research is sparse.

In light of the difficulties associated with investigating different paraphilias, indirect measures are often required. For instance, Dietz and Evans [9] explored the relative prevalence of some paraphilias by using the content of pornographic magazines. They suggested that alongside curiosity, pornography is likely to reflect the preexisting fantasies of the individual [10, 11]. They observed that the most common imagery was bondage and domination. Magazines often presented women wearing lingerie and high heels. This study is limited by the variable distribution of such material and inability to extrapolate this as a behaviour in subjects. The growth of diverse pornographic material on the Internet would confound such a study presently.

In Sweden in 1996 [12–14], a survey of sexuality and health was carried out with 2,450 randomly selected 18–60 year olds with questions regarding paraphilias and problem sexual behaviours. 3.1 percent of respondents experienced sexual arousal by exposing their genitals to a stranger on at least one occasion and 7.7 percent at least one incident of arousal spying on others having intercourse. Findings were associated with being male, more psychological problems, drug and alcohol use, and lower satisfaction with life. Men were nearly three times as likely to be involved in voyeuristic behaviour and twice as likely to expose than women, behaviours associated with pornography use and masturbation frequency. Researchers suggested no significant correlation between immigrant status and either of these paraphilic behaviours. It is not possible to make cultural extrapolations from these findings in the absence of specific information about these groups. The survey also noted a relationship between early childhood experience such as separation from parents and some paraphilias. Such activities may also reflect the notion of power that the exposer has. As mentioned above, childrearing and family environments vary across social class and cultures and may improve our understanding of paraphilias.

Langstrom and Zucker [14] observed 0.4 percent of women and about 2.8 percent men acknowledged at least one episode of transvestic fetishism. These individuals were more likely to have had childhood separation from parents, abuse, same-sex sexual experiences, high frequency masturbation, and sexual arousal with the use of pornography. They also reported higher rates of voyeurism and exhibitionism. Migrant groups in these Swedish surveys were less likely to report paraphilias. These findings should be interpreted with caution as immigrant groups may be hesitant to disclose paraphilic behaviours, may lack awareness of the status as a disorder, or may have genuinely lower rates. This study drew attention to similar associations as cited above such as separation from parents, childhood sexual abuse, same sex relationships, and general sexual arousability. A potential theory would be that cultures with lower rates of these events may have a different if not lower prevalence of paraphilias.

Further review of the sample [12] reported an association between hypersexuality and paraphilias. Men in this category were more likely to be young with early sexual activity, to have experienced separation from parents, and to reside in major cities. They were more likely to be involved in same-sex behaviour, sadomasochism, voyeurism, exhibitionism, and pay for sex. Paradoxically, while actively sexual, they were less satisfied with their sex lives and were involved in risk-taking behaviours such as substance misuse, gambling, and alcohol use. These findings suggest other behavioural and social associations with paraphilias. These may be tenuously contributory to or complement the paraphilia. A hypothesis would be that cultures with lower rates of these social and behavioural issues may reflect lower rates of paraphilic disorders. Cultures and societies that strongly proscribe sexual activity outside marriage may present fewer opportunities for these behaviours. An additional hypothesis would be that cultures that are more sexually liberal may have a higher threshold for satiety through conditioning of arousal stimuli and therefore manifestation of paraphilias.

Gender

Developmentally, boys explore genital pleasure more promptly and perhaps earlier than girls [15]. Childrearing and societal values are often more encouraging of boys toward sexuality while strongly discouraging girls. The pubertal girl may, for instance, learn about genitalia, menses, and sexuality with embarrassment while boys develop learning from peers, masturbation, and express less embarrassment with societal reinforcement. These gender roles and values regarding masturbation, the role of sex for procreation, and pleasure are culturally moulded.

Gender differences in the prevalence of different paraphilic disorders are well established. The interplay of biological and social factors has been proposed by Baldwin and Baldwin [16]. Men are on the whole more interested in sexual intimacy than women [17–21]. Men have more recurrent sexual thoughts [19] with an emphasis on physical pleasure [22], while women are less inclined to engage in sexual intimacy without an emotional bond [23].

Culture and the pedophilic disorder

In ancient Greece and Rome, adult-child sex was acceptable practice and permitted. There is evidence from other ancient populations and art that nubile children were part of the social culture. Furthermore, historical child molestation and safety concerns have been reported in some cultures in the past [24].

The age for consent for sex is influenced by the legislation of the land, the culture, and religious factors. In a similar vein, the acceptable age for marriage may be influenced by these factors. This may vary for heterosexual and homosexual activity.

In Western societies, pedophilia is socially and legally unacceptable and a lot of legislative, police, and psychological resources are being invested to identify and contain adults involved in such behaviour. The global reach of the Internet has complicated this further, given the absence of geographical and legal boundaries.

In Nigeria, for instance, all regions share the same national legislation; however, there are significant differences between the predominantly Muslim north and Christian south regarding culturally acceptable ages for sexual activity, marriage age, and family life. This is further influenced by the urban versus rural differences, with greater rural acceptance of female pubescent intimacy with an older male spouse. On the whole the cultures promote sexual activity after and not before a "marital" ceremony.

Social deficits have been described in some paraphilias. Pedophiles have, for instance, been found to be deficient in social skills, while Langevin [25] found them shy, lacking assertiveness, passive, and socially withdrawn [26, 27]. Developmental and family histories of pedophiles include disturbed childhoods, sexual abuse, inadequate parenting, and family dysfunction [28].

The bulk of research into pedophilia has been carried out in offender populations. A survey by Wilson and Cox [29] observed 71 percent of male paedophiles reported an attraction to boys aged 12–14 years and 12 percent a preference for girls aged 8–10 years, with about half with sexual fantasies. Seto, Cantor, and Blanchard [30] propose that child pornography may be a valid diagnostic indicator of pedophilia; however, this may relate to arousal and fantasy rather than actual behaviour with a child. It is very difficult to ascertain how representative these samples are given the significantly larger population of pedophiles outside the criminal justice system.

Fetishistic disorder

Kaplan [31] has written extensively about fetishes primarily from a psychoanalytic perspective suggesting the behaviours are underpinned by the need to transform something unfamiliar and intangible to something familiar and tangible (p. 1) as a feature of the fetishism strategy. The etymological and indeed non-sexual sense of the word is related to the excessive valuing of items such as wooden carvings, feathers or artificial objects. It is also related to false values, worship of useless objects, false, simulated, fictitious or artificial material (p. 2). Kaplan describes a fetishist as someone irrationally devoted to these worship practices. A number of substances such as leather, latex, and rubber have been associated with fetishism in different societies.

A psychoanalytic exploration by Kaplan [31] of exhibitionism opines that this is a form of narcissistic process that puts on show and empowers the exhibitionist while dehumanising or even commoditising the victim. In a sense also the fetishisation of the human body becomes sexualised by giving meaning to an ambiguous and unknown object. This reassuring external object is used to control the unconscious uncontrollable energies of the unknown. These theories are not society specific such as groups with non-sexual fetish objects.

The sexualisation of inanimate objects into fetishes may facilitate dealing with internal anxieties an ambiguity. This concept bears similarity to Hofstede's [4] cultural dimension of anxiety management through the mechanism of individual or societal uncertainty avoidance. It is difficult to generalise these models as different cultures provide different entry points and barriers to stimuli for sexual attraction and arousal. Interestingly, these may be determined by racial or phenotypic features, body build, and concepts of beauty, to mention a few.

Kaplan [31] proffers that "fetishism allows certain details into the foreground of experience . . . to mask and disguise other features that are thus cast into the shadows and margins and background" (p. 6). Hence, the purpose of the fetish is masked and the object of fetish becoming more obvious and dramatic. Illustrating with necrophilia, Kaplan states that the role of dead bodies as a fetish involves a transformation of the living body into the dead. In addition, "the more dangerous and unpredictable the threat of desire, the more deadened or distanced from human experience the fetish object must be" (p. 7). The sexual object's identity is endowed with a vast number of unpredictable realities and the dead object knowable and predictable. This reduces internal and external anxiety.

The feet and shoes

Kaplan [31] (pp. 35–50) gives a historical insight into the foot binding of Chinese females as a cultural fetish. Beginning in the 21st century BC, the practice was initially restricted to upper classes: the ruler's mistresses, concubines, and dancing girls in specific regions of the country. Over time, foot binding spread across China and has been attributed to a generalized anxiety about societal roles for women and male fear about competition and decline of the patriarchal structure [32]. Male control in such a manner can be considered fetishistic control over the object. The modern-day feet continue to draw attention with culturally reinforced female obsession with high-heel shoes and the admiration by men. Arguably a modern foot binding, these shoes predominantly designed by men based on or determining beauty commodify and fetishize the female body. These shoes invariably accentuate the legs while tilting the hips forward.

Clearly, the role of feet and shoes in the sexual fantasy or psyche has cultural variation. For instance, traditional cultures with less salience on footwear are unlikely to sexualise high-heel shoes but may find waist beads a source of intense sexual arousal. While some paraphilias may be recognisable across cultures, others may be virtually unknown or as illustrated above regarding stiletto heels, may have little sexual significance.

Kaplan [31] (p. 52) expressed that the female form was often used to demonstrate fetishistic emblem such as the vulnerable female figure and male gaze on her. Other practices such as body piercing, tattooing, and lacerating may be fetishistic in nature. These can be found in sexual, spiritual, and social rites in many cultures. It is asserted that fetishistic objects reflect their cultures of origin.

Procreation or pleasure

Fetishes may contribute to male potency by enhancing arousal. So why are behaviours that improve potency and potentially reproduction perceived problematic? A number of explanations may be possible. One is that they cause social and functional impairment and the other objectify female form. On the surface of it these should not be aberrations, especially in cultures that promote sexual intimacy for procreation.

In the absence of reliable data, it is hypothesised that in sociocentric cultures that promote sex for reproduction, the development or rates of sexual fetishes may be lower or less reported. On the other hand, egocentric cultures with a greater emphasis on pleasure for sex, the fetish contributes to commodification of the female form, thereby promoting erotic arousal.

As referred to earlier, psychoanalytically, the goal of sexual fetishism in these egocentric cultures may be the conquering and incorporation of the fetishistic object—a source of arousal and excitement. Kaplan [31] (p. 111) suggests the sexual fetishist uses the fetish to subdue and tame the unpredictable erotic vitalities of the sexual partner. The unpredictable nature of the erotic vitality may shift focus toward an inanimate object or near inanimate object, as in rape. The object of fetish may invariably be perceived as liberating for the individual.

Different cultures have different attitudes to sexual liberation based on value systems and the primary purpose of sexual activity: procreation or pleasure. In an increasingly globalised world, with rural to urban and international migration, changes may be experienced in sex-negative cultures toward greater levels of experimentation and changing expectations from sexual partners.

Cultural behaviour or paraphilia?

Some culturally acceptable behaviours may be perceived as paraphilic in other societies. For instance, in Papua and New Guinea, the Sambian boys perform fellatio on older men of the tribe, swallowing their semen to gain strength [33, 34]. After about a decade in homosexual relations, the young males imbibe fear about the polluting effects of women [35]. Once in heterosexual marriages, they disinvest in earlier same-sex experiences. These behaviours are limited to tribal rituals. After approximately 10 years of "heterosexual" childhood development, homosexual behaviour is developed as part of the rites of passage. The belief that semen is good for strength and growth makes such behaviour socially desirable. This homoerotic behaviour is not for pleasure but initiation rituals to assist with the development of masculinity [36]. The young men subsequently meet their potential spouses and heterosexual partners through rituals in which females are presented as sexually desirable, thereby promoting heterosexual and heterosocial behaviour.

Culture-modulated reorientation from homosexual to heterosexual practice illustrates how behaviour that erstwhile may be described as paraphilic can be normalised and subsequently reversed according to societal norms. While these Sambian men may maintain same-sex fantasies, the manifest sexual behaviour is heterosexual.

Technological advances with the Internet and camera devices have changed patterns of voyeuristic behaviour in some parts of the world such that physical proximity is no longer required to intimately observe another person.

In a similar vein, exhibitionism sometimes takes advantage of advances in visual technologies. The concept of "flashing" whereby an individual exposes genitals or breasts in public events is rare in non-Western parts of the world. Nudist colonies, on the other hand, should not be mistaken for a means of exposure for sexual gratification.

Frotteurism commonly occurs in crowded public places such as busy transport settings like crowded trains and large gatherings such as large concerts, where the frotteur is aware that their intentions cannot be easily identified. It stands to reason that distribution of this disorder is likely to be higher in urban than isolated rural settings.

Sexual masochism disorder

Sexual masochism is the intentional participation in an activity that involves being humiliated, beaten, bound, or otherwise abused to experience sexual excitement. Commonly associated with masochism, sexual sadism involves infliction of physical or mental suffering (e.g., pain, humiliation, terror) on the sex partner to stimulate sexual excitement and orgasm. These behaviours would be theoretically less in permissive cultures with high power distance or collectivist societies particularly since they encompass sexual activity involving the dominance of another (sadism) or being dominated (masochism).

The biology of sexual behaviours

Are sexual behaviours a product of nature, nurture, or a combination of both? The relationship is likely to be a complex one with a contribution of factors from both. Attempts shall be made to explore this further below. Intrauterine development of the human brain is partly modulated through the action of testosterone, male development through its presence and female development its absence [37]. With this in mind, how do intrauterine sexually differentiated identity, cognitive process, sexual orientation, and associated programmed behaviours interact with culture? If primarily a product of nature and biology, one would expect similar rates and distribution of paraphilias around the world, regardless of culture.

Berridge and Kringlebach [38] provide some biological and physiological insights. Stating that brain processes of emotion, motivation, and affect are significantly influenced by developmental experiences, they argue that the active mechanisms of the brain respond to stimuli, causing them reward. These rewards can be further divided into liking (a conscious cognitive process elaborated through brain mechanisms) and wanting (the motivation for reward involving conscious wanting and incentive salience) as well as explicit and implicit learning (p. 458). While pleasure and displeasure are common, pleasure is more than a mere sensation. It has been observed that pleasure is linked with hedonic processes in the brain that give it a "gloss" to make it liked, given that pleasure is associated with a reward sensation. That notwithstanding, different stimuli and experiences generate different levels of pleasure or displeasure. In the case of sexual pleasure, there is also a link to procreation and preservation of a species [39–41]. The displeasure associated with noxious stimuli and the pleasure from sexual activity and eating are intricately interwoven with human emotions. Cognitive and intellectual pleasures such as music, art, and altruistic activities are more likely to be products of learning and thereby culturally developed.

Individual cognitive schema are strongly influenced by culture and society, for instance, attractive body images and the use of fragrances and perfumes. This coding of pleasure involves neural activity in the brain. The behavioural and cognitive components of pleasure may be socially or individually derived.

Personal pleasure may be from the same source as social pleasure or alternative stimuli. In paraphilias, behavioural and cognitive processes work toward increasing personal pleasure with personal, social, or both personal and social rewards. In some situations, personal and social rewards may be at conflict with paraphilic dissonance in the society.

Neuroanatomical and neurophysiological issues: Mind (fantasy) Versus brain

Reward has been found to be mediated by various brain structures. The orbitofrontol cortex has been suggested to be the apex of pleasure representation [42] with the involvement of other subcortical structures and neurochemicals such as dopamine.

Lesions or disruption to these pathways have been associated with paraphilia [43], for instance, pathological changes in the hippocampus of subjects similar to those found after persistent stress or long-term glucocorticoid administration. It may be argued that these changes may have been associated with social childhood adversity discussed earlier in the chapter. Other researchers have observed different EEG recordings and anatomical differences in a number of specific frontal and temporal lobe areas among sex offenders with a diagnosis of paraphilia [44–48]. The neuroimaging, neurobiology, and neurochemistry of sexual activity present exciting areas of future research in light of advances in genetics and functional imaging. Current research [49] into the modulating role of the neurochemical oxytocin in the experience of pleasure and love sensations indicate further biological templates of emotion.

Pfaus and colleagues [50] propose that endogenous opioid activation in the brain forms the basis of sexual reward through the sensitization of hypothalamic and mesolimbic dopamine systems with cues that predict sexual reward. They hypothesise that a critical period exists during early sexual experience that creates a "love map" of features, feelings, movements, and interpersonal interactions associated with sexual reward. The role of oxytocin in the treatment of satiety-related difficulties is also being explored further [51].

There is also evidence of the impact of neurodevelopmental difficulties and head injuries in the presentation of paraphilias, for instance, learning disability, specific regional head injuries such as frontal lobe with impaired executive function and personality change. Childhood head injury has been reported by Blanchard and colleagues [52]. In another review, Blanchard and colleagues [53] suggested that some deviant sexual behaviours result from pathological or pathogenic developmental variables, which may impede normal sexual development. The evidence for this has been questioned by Rahman [54].

Conclusion

It appears that emotion, reward, and pleasure appear to be programmed to specific stimuli through experience and exposure. This programming involves certain brain structures as a neurodevelopmental process or in later life [55]. Paraphilias may emerge from these processes with disruption of normal psychosexual [56], social communication [57], and neural development [58, 59]. Research into these theories is limited and predominantly excludes a transcultural framework across geographical, faith, race, and ethnic boundaries.

Cross-cultural research would provide very helpful insights into the biological factors and their cultural interface in the development of paraphilias. So far, there is a dearth of literature on paraphilias and their presentation across different cultures, ethnic groups, and societies. Reaching diagnosis and looking at possible interventions in paraphilias must be seen in the context of cultures and also within the legal framework in that particular culture and society.

References

1 American Psychiatric Association. (2013). *Diagnostic and Statistical Manual of Mental Disorders*, 5th ed. (DSM-5). Washington, D.C.: American Psychiatric Association.

2 Bhugra D, De Silva P. (1996). Uniforms: Fact, fashion, fantasy or fetish. *Sexual and Marital Therapy*, 11, 393–406.

3 Hofstede G. (1980). *Culture's Consequences: International Differences in Work-Related Values*. Beverly Hills: Sage.

4 Hofstede G. (1984). *Culture's Consequences: International Differences in Work-Related Values* (abridged ed.). Beverly Hills: Sage.

5 Bhugra D, Popelyuk D, McMullen I. (2010). Paraphilias across cultures: Contexts and controversies. *Journal of Sex Research*, 47(2–3), 242–256.

6 Reiss IL. (1986). *Journey into Sexuality: An Exploratory Voyage*. Englewood Cliffs, NJ: Prentice Hill.

7 Segall MH, Dasen PR, Berry JW, Poortinga YH. (1990). *Human Behavior in Global Perspective*. Elmsford, NY: Pergamon.

8 Bullough VL. (1976). *Sexual Variance in Society and History*. Chicago: University of Chicago Press.

9 Dietz PE, Evans B. (1982). Pornographic imagery and prevalence of paraphilia. *American Journal of Psychology*, 139, 1493–1495.

10 Stoller RJ. (1975). *Perversion: The Erotic Form of Hatred*. New York: Pantheon.

11 Stoller RJ. (1979). *Sexual Excitement: Dynamics of Erotic Life*. New York: Pantheon.

12 Langstrom N, Hanson R. (2006). High rates of sexual behavior in general population; Correlates and predictors. *Archives of Sexual Behavior*, 35, 37–52.

13 Langstrom N, Seto MC. (2006). Exhibitionistic and voyeuristic behavior in a Swedish national population survey. *Archives of Sexual Behavior*, 35, 427–435.

14 Langstrom N, Zucker KJ. (2005). Transvestic fetishism in the general population: Prevalence and correlates. *Journal of Sex and Marital Therapy*, 31, 87–95.

15 Galenson E, Roiphe H. (1974). The emergence of genital awareness during the second year of life. In Friedman RC, Richart RM, Wiele RLV (eds.) *Sex Differences in Behavior: A Conference* (pp. 223–231). New York: Wiley.

16 Baldwin JD, Baldwin JI. (1997). Gender differences in sexual interest. *Archives of Sexual Behavior,* 26(2), 181–210.

17 Blumstein P, Schwartz R. (1983). *American Couples: Money, Work, Sex.* New York: Pocket Books.

18 Greer A, Buss D. (1994). Tactics for promoting sexual encounters. *Journal of Sex Research,* 31, 185–201.

19 Laumann EO, Gagnon JH, Michael RT, Michaels S. (1994). *The Social Organisation of Sexuality: Sexual Practices in the United States.* Chicago: University of Chicago Press.

20 Sprecher S. (1989). Premarital sexual standards for different categories of individuals. *Journal of Sex Research,* 26, 232–248.

21 Sprecher S, McKinney K. (1993). *Sexuality.* Newbury Park, CA: Sage.

22 Frazier PA, Esterly E. (1990). Correlates of relationship beliefs: Gender, relationship experience and relationship satisfaction. *Journal of Social and Personal Relationships,* 7(3), 331–352.

23 Carroll JL, Volk K, Hyde J. (1985). Differences between males and females in motives for engaging in sexual intercourse. *Archives of Sexual Behavior,* 14, 131–139.

24 Green R. (2002). Is pedophilia a mental disorder? *Archives of Sexual Behavior,* 31, 467–471.

25 Langevin R. (1983). *Sexual Strands: Understanding and Treating Sexual Anomalies in Men.* Hillsdale, NJ: Lawrence Erlbaum Associates.

26 Bard LA, Carter DL, Cerce DD, Knight RA, Rosenberg R. Schneider B. (1987 Spring) A descriptive study of rapists and child molesters: Developmental, clinical, and criminal characteristics. *Behavioral Sciences and the Law,* 5(2), 203–220.

27 Langevin R. (1985). *Erotic Preference, Gender Identity, and Aggression in Men: New Research Studies.* Hillsdale, NJ: Erlbaum Associates.

28 McAnulty RD. (2006). Paedophilia. In McAnulty RD, Burnette, MM (eds.) *Sex and Sexuality* (Vol. 3, pp. 81–96). Westport, CT: Praeger.

29 Wilson G, Cox N. (1983). *The Child-Lovers: A Study of Paedophiles in Society.* London: Peter Owen.

30 Seto MC, Cantor JM, Blanchard R. (2006). Child pornography offenses are a valid diagnostic indicator of pedophilia. *Journal of Abnormal Psychology,* 115, 610–615.

31 Kaplan LJ. (2006). *Cultures of Fetishism.* New York: Palgrave Macmillan.

32 Ping W. (2000). *Aching for Beauty: Foot Binding in China.* Minneapolis: University of Minnesota Press.

33 Herdt GH. (1981). *Guardians of the Flute: Idioms of Masculinity.* New York: McGraw-Hill.

34 Herdt GH. (ed.) (1984). *Ritualized Homosexuality in Melanesia.* Berkley: University of California Press.

35 Stoller RJ, Herdt G. (1985) Theories of origin of male homosexuality: A cross-cultural look. *Archives of General Psychiatry,* 42, 399–404.

36 Baldwin JD, Baldwin JI. (1989). The socialization of homosexuality and heterosexuality in a non-Western society. *Archives of Sexual Behavior,* 18(1), 13–29.

37 Swaab DF. (2007). Sexual differentiation of the brain and behavior: Best practice and research. *Clinical Endocrinology & Metabolism,* 21, 431–444.

38 Berridge KC, Kringelbach ML. (2008) Affective neuroscience of pleasure: Reward in humans and animals. *Psychopharmacology,* 199(3), 457–480.

39 Kringlebach ML. (2008). The hedonic brain: A functional neuroanatomy of human pleasure. In Kringlebach ML, Berridge KC (eds.) *Pleasure of the Brain* (pp. 202–221). Oxford, England: Oxford University Press.

40 Panksepp J. (1998) *Affective Neuroscience: The Foundations of Human and Animal Emotions.* Oxford, England. Oxford University Press.

41 Rolls ET. (2005). *Emotion Explained.* Oxford, England: Oxford University Press.

42 Kringlebach ML. (2005). The human orbitofrontal cortex: Linking reward to hedonic experience. *Nature Reviews Neuroscience,* 6, 691–702.

43 Casanova MH, Mannheim G, Kruesi M. (2002). Hippocampal pathology in two mentally ill paraphiliacs. *Psychiatry Research: Neuroimaging,* 115, 79–89.

44 Flor-Henry P, Lang RA, Frenzel RR. (1988). Quantitative EEG investigation of genital exhibitionism. *Sexual Abuse: A Journal of Research and Treatment,* 1, 49.

45 Flor-Henry P, Lang RA, Koles ZJ, Frenzel RR. (1991). Quantitative EEG studies of paedophilia. *International Journal of Psychophysiology,* 10, 253–258.

46 Hucker S, Langevin R, Dickey R, Handy L, Chambers J, Wright S. (1988). Cerebral damage and dysfunction in sexually aggressive men. *Annals of Sex Research,* 1(1), 32–48.

47 Hucker S, Langevin R, Wortzman G, Bain J, Handy L, Chambers J, Wright S. (1986). Neuropsychological impairment in pedophiles. *Canadian Journal of Behavioural Science,* 18(4), 440–448.

48 Kirenskaya-Berus AV, Tkachenko AA. (2003). Characteristic features of EEG spectral characteristics in persons with deviant sexual behaviour. *Human Physiology,* 29, 273–287.

49 Schneiderman I, Zagoory-Sharon O, Leckman JF, Feldman R. (2012). Oxytocin during the initial stages of romantic attachment: Relations to couples' interactive reciprocity. *Psychoneuroendocrinology,* 37(8), 1277–1285.

50 Pfaus JG, Kippin TE, Coria-Avila GA, Gelez H, Afonso VM, Ismail N, Parada M. (2012). Who, what, where, when (and maybe even why)? How the experience of sexual reward connects sexual desire, preference, and performance. *Archives of Sexual Behavior,* 41(1), 31–62.

51 Wudarczyk OA, Earp BD, Guastella A, Savulescu J. (2013). Could intranasal oxytocin be used to enhance relationships? Research imperatives, clinical policy, and ethical considerations. *Current Opinion Psychiatry,* 26(5), 474–484.

52 Blanchard R, Kolla NJ, Cantor J, Klassen PE, Dickey R, Kuban ME, Blak M. (2007). Handedness and pedophilia in adult male patients stratified by referral source. *Sexual Abuse: Journal of Research and Treatment,* 19, 285–309.

53 Blanchard R, Kuban ME, Blak T, Cantor JM, Klassen P, Dickey R. (2006). Phallometric comparison of pedophilic interest in nonadmitting sexual offenders against stepdaughters, biological daughters, other biologically related girls and unrelated girls. *Sexual Abuse: Journal of Research and Treatment,* 18, 1–14.

54 Rahman Q. (2005). The neurodevelopment of human sexual orientation. *Neuroscience and Behavioral Reviews,* 29, 1057–1066.

55 Rahman Q, Symeonides DJ. (2008). Neurodevelopmental correlates of paraphilic sexual interests in men. *Archives of Sexual Behavior,* 37, 166–172.

56 Castillo RJ. (1995). Culture, trance and the mind-brain. *Anthropology of Consciousness,* 6(1), 17–34.

57 Emmers-Sommer TM, Allen M, Bourhis J, Sahlstein E, Laskowski K, et al. (2004). A meta-analysis of the relationship between social skills and sexual offenders. *Communication Reports,* 17(1), 1–10.

58 Garnett ES, Nahmias C, Wortzman G, Langevin R. Dickey R. (1988). Positron emission tomography and sexual arousal in a sadist and two controls. *Sexual Abuse: A Journal of Research and Treatment,* 1(3), 387–399.

59 Hendricks S, Fitzpatrick D, Hartmann K, Qauife MA, Stratbucker RA, Graber B. (1988). Brain structure and function in sexual molesters of children and adolescents. *Journal of Clinical Psychiatry,* 49, 108–112.

CHAPTER 16

Pseudodementia: History, mystery and positivity

Alistair Burns[1] and David Jolley[2]

[1] Professor of Old Age Psychiatry, Vice Dean for the Faculty of Medical and Human Sciences, National Clinical Director for Dementia in England, University of Manchester, Manchester, UK

[2] Honorary Reader in Psychiatry of Old Age, Personal Social Services Research Unit, University of Manchester, UK

Dementia

Dementia has become hot property. From a place in the shadows, a condition hardly daring to speak its name it has become high profile, the subject of interest to national and international leaders: a necessary reference for every informed and caring individual and organisation [1–3].

Logic has been pressing for this for decades as the epidemiology of dementia and the changing age profile of the world population determines that its incidence, prevalence, and cost implications, both personal and economic rise higher and higher [4, 5]. Somehow a threshold was passed within recent years as individuals, including well-known celebrities and their families, have come to experience dementia and began to share their experiences openly [6]. Lobbying by care organisations, including the Alzheimer's societies of individual countries and at international level, have gathered information, encouraged research, and demanded better care and prospects for treatment [7, 8]. The pharmaceutical industry and research community have fanned the flames to encourage investment to improve understanding and knowledge, which can inform strategies that might reduce incidence, ameliorate symptoms, and improve care [9].

There are two strands to the campaigners' message:
Dementia can be a dreadful condition to live with and die with.
There are things that can be done to make it less of a threat. This includes careful assessment to identify treatable or reversible components of the condition.

We have come to know dementia as a syndrome defined by Lishman [10] as "an acquired global impairment of intellect, memory and personality, but

Troublesome Disguises: Managing Challenging Disorders in Psychiatry, Second Edition.
Edited by Dinesh Bhugra and Gin S. Malhi.

without impairment of consciousness. As such it is almost always of long duration, usually progressive and often irreversible, but these features are not included as part of the definition" (p. 9).

Thus dementia as a syndrome is a clinical concept, not one defined by neuropathology. It carries the possibility of "causation" by a number of underlying conditions and additional factors that may occur singly or in combination. Detailed symptomatology, experience, and outcome are thence a function of the individual's constitution, the natural history, and interactions of the underlying and associated conditions, and of the interventions proffered: physical, psychological, and social interventions.

While Lishman caricatures the specific dementias of Alzheimer's disease, Pick's disease, and others as "progressive and widespread brain degeneration with, at the moment, a hopeless prognosis" (pp. 8–9). The same is not true of the syndrome. Careful assessment may identify reversible or ameliorable factors.

Berrios [11, 12] has traced the international and historical story of dementia, the usage of the word, and the concept being captured. The Latin word *demens* was used by Celsus in his writings in early Roman texts [13] and variations on this appeared in several medical traditions from then onward. The concept of dementia had a legal aspect: "those who are in this state are incapable of informed consent, cannot enter into contracts, write their wills or be members of a jury" (D'Argis, quoted by Berrios [12], p. 832) and a clinical aspect: "those affected by this condition exhibit foolish behaviour and cannot understand what they are told, cannot remember anything, have no judgement" (D'Aumont, quoted by Berrios [12], p. 832).

Differentiation from what we now look on as delirium when prolonged or sub-acute was not clear, nor was differentiation from life-long difficulty with learning. The term *amentia* was sometimes preferred and included all these states (Cullen, 1827, quoted by Berrios [12]). The belief developed that true dementia (amentia) was always irreversible and usually associated with progressive degeneration of the faculties and functions. Post-mortem examinations revealed shrunken and altered brains (Willis, 1684, quoted by Berrios [14]).

Pseudodementia

It was known that some people who presented with clinical features of dementia did not deteriorate and some might recover. This phenomenon of reversibility was accommodated by the term *vesanic* dementia (Ball and Chambard, 1882, quoted by Berrios, 1985 [14], p. 394) and later by *pseudodementia*, which is attributed to Wernicke [15] by Bleuler [16].

Pseudo is a descriptive term with origins in Greek and translates as "false," "sham," "spurious," or "deceptively resembling" [17]. It is widely applied in medicine to capture conditions that have similarities to a well-known syndrome or diagnostic entity but that on closer inspection do not fulfil all its criteria: thus pseudo-hypoparathyroidism, pseudo-pseudo-hypoparathyroidism [18]. At the time that "General Paralysis of the Insane" was a common mental disorder and cause of hospitalisation, there was the concept of "Pseudo General Paralysis" [12].

Within a world that has been seized with terror and fascination with the prospects of inevitable deterioration to dependency and death by Alzheimer's (now more feared than cancer among older people [19], the concept of pseudodementia with the possibility of recovery has real attractions.

Lishman devoted 14 pages to the topic of "The Pseudodementias" [10] (pp, 561–575) and identified four main varieties: the Ganser syndrome [20], hysterical pseudodementia, simulated dementia, and depressive pseudodementia. He pointed out that these are not mutually exclusive and that individuals are encountered whose condition does not fit into any of these categories.

The Ganser syndrome was originally described in prisoners. It includes the phenomenon of approximate answers. Answers are often absurd and may be accompanied by disturbance of consciousness, hallucinations, or other abnormal mental phenomena. There is often evidence of coarse brain disease.

Hysterical pseudodementia occurs in situations of psychological conflict or ambivalence. The relationship of its onset and course to stresses is often easily seen by an objective observer. It is more common in people with a learning disability or otherwise evidenced immaturity of emotional development or personality. Yet it can occur in anyone under great stress and is facilitated by coexistent brain damage or other illness.

Simulated dementia is probably rare. Such a diagnosis requires that an individual is knowingly falsifying symptoms and behaviour for a calculated gain.

Jaspers [21] had applied the label *pseudodementia* to patients with the Ganser Syndrome of Hysterical Amnesia, including "talking past the point" (Vorbeireden, pp. 194, 220, 391). He did not identify a depressive subtype.

Yet depressive pseudodementia must surely be the variant that demands the greatest attention. The presentation of severe depression often includes cognitive change with reduced concentration, slowness of thought, difficulty in registering current events, and a subjective feeling that the brain is not working as it should. This picture may appear in successive relapses. In middle-aged and older people the picture may be very suggestive of dementia, with slowness of movement, loss of confidence, weight-loss, and an appearance of a stooped, wrinkled persona much older than their chronological age [22].

Other causes of pseudodementia include the major psychoses: hypomania and schizophrenia, or other neurotic disorders.

Kiloh

Kiloh described ten cases of pseudo-dementia [23] in what has become a key and influential paper. He was writing just a short time after the publication of Roth's studies, which made clear the differentiation in symptoms and outcomes for old people admitted to mental hospitals with depression, dementia, or delirium [24]. Kiloh's cases illustrated the importance of careful clinical assessment and awareness that depression could sometimes mimic dementia and that it is treatable, especially with electroconvulsive therapy. This is a wonderful message and holds true.

The late Tony Whitehead [25], a great pioneer of services for old people, enthused to the paradox: "Where there is depression, there is hope."

In his review of pseudodementia and tribute to Leslie Kiloh on the 50th anniversary of the 1961 publication, John Snowdon [26] chose to entitle his paper "Pseudodementia: A Term for Its Time."

It was certainly an important corrective to any slackness of thought that might have taken Roth's work to mean that dementia is always of hopeless prognosis. The implication that the term was useful then, but redundant now [27, 28], is surely incorrect.

Caine [29] certainly saw pseudodementia as an important and relevant concept, though he suggested a kinship with sub-cortical dementia.

Berrios, writing with Bulbena [30], accepted that pseudodementia was a phenomenon worthy of consideration. They noted at least 30 publications in scholarly journals but found most to be characterised by "anecdotal reporting, skewed series and speculation."

Berrios concluded that they were describing, "A collection of clinical states rather than a process . . . the common denominator is an ability to impair cognition or to disable the mechanisms by which cognition is expressed" (p. 87).

The paper reviewed 61 cases from the literature and added 22 new cases. It was felt that most could be accommodated by a tripartite sub-classification: essentially hysterical pseudo-dementia after Madden [31], reversible dementia Kiloh [23] (after Wernicke), and delirium – reversible, symptomatic organic psycho-syndromes.

As in Kiloh's series, Berrios's 61 cases from the literature were relatively young (average age in their late 50s). Women outnumbered men. More than half had a history of previous mental illness, usually depression and more than half, where information was given, had evidence of a neurological deficit. Impaired memory was evident in two-thirds, depression in more than half, delusions, hallucinations, confusion, lability of mood, or admixture of elevated mood present in significant minorities. Twenty-six patients received

ECT and all recovered. The additional 22 patients from Fulbourn Hospital were older, more likely to be female, but otherwise similar in symptom profile and outcomes.

In the previous edition of this Troublesome Disguises, Pitt [32] updated the review of the literature and considered the mechanisms which contribute to real or apparent memory disorder in association with depression. In these he included: poor motivation in tasks, negativism (taking against testing), response bias ("I don't know"), over-caution, learned helplessness, anergy and retardation, preoccupation, agitated inattentions, iatrogenic factors (including medication), altered brain function and language impairment.

In addition he drew from a paper by Wells [33] a list of features favouring a diagnosis of depressive pseudodementia and anticipating good prognosis: short history, previous or family history of affective illness, definite time of onset, misery or lack of joy, disparity between subjective and objective assessment (with the patient feeling their memory is much worse than testing reveals), drawing attention to the disability, moderate (rather than severe) cognitive impairment, absence of confabulation (after Post [34]), 'Don't know' answers, no 'cortical' features such as dyspraxia or dysphasia, no progression to disability, and good response to antidepressants or ECT. These fit well with Kiloh's descriptions.

Pitt added four case histories to make particular important points:

A 50-year-old man presented with depression associated with ill health, a diagnosis of glaucoma, and learning of the unfaithfulness of his wife. Despite treatment in a psychiatric unit with antidepressants and ECT, he remained withdrawn, frail, and became incontinent of urine. A brain scan showed cortical atrophy and a diagnosis of presenile dementia was made and he was place in long-term care. Three years later there had been no further deterioration. Treatment with antidepressants resulted in recovery, discharge home, and return to work.

An edgy old man had become bleak in his outlook and constantly fussing, to the irritation of his wife. Psychological testing reported findings diagnostic of moderate dementia. In view of his low mood a trial of six ECT treatments was given. His mood and cognitive function improved.

A 40-year-old man whose business had failed took on work selling ice cream. He became irritable and irascible. A brain scan demonstrated cortical atrophy and psychological tests confirmed dementia. Three years later he had not deteriorated; treatment with antidepressants produced a complete recovery

A 67-year-old dentist had become convinced that he was suffering from Alzheimer's disease because his memory had become unreliable. He had seen a similar development in his mother-in-law. Brain scans showed no changes but clinical psychology showed a pattern consistent with dementia. Treatment with an antidepressant saw resolution of his symptoms.

Fisman [35] had reported two similarly successive rescues of patients where determined treatment of depression reversed a long-held diagnosis of dementia.

The moral of all these stories is that in the presence of depression a diagnosis of dementia should be provisional even when structural brain change is demonstrated by a brain scan and/or psychological tests give results that fall within the range usually associated with a degenerative dementia.

As Kiloh had urged from 1961 and Tony Whitehead throughout his career: Where there is depression there is hope. A trial of antidepressants and maybe ECT should always be considered and hope not dismissed.

More recent contributions to understanding: While Bulbena and Berrios counted 30 or more publications prior to their 1986 paper, a simple review of Medline identifies 50 more recent articles.

Clinical series and response to treatment

Pitt and his colleagues [36] took their interest further and, from an analysis of symptoms among 128 patients with a differential diagnosis of pseudodementia, produced an 18-item questionnaire that differentiates between organic dementia and pseudodementia with 98 percent sensitivity and 95 percent specificity. In addition they proposed a subdivision of pseudodementia into Type I and Type II, with predominantly subjective or objective dysmnesia respectively.

Reports of improved cognitive function when depression is effectively treated with ECT continue to appear [37, 38].

Jason Hepple [39] contributed a personal series of 10 patients collected over 12 years. This equates to the "hysterical" syndrome described by Lishman [10], Madden [31], Jaspers [21] and others. Hepple's cases are characterised by chronic, progressive deterioration of mental, physical, and social functioning but appeared to remain cognitively preserved. Many had histories of previous depression, abnormal personalities, and additional stresses. You are left wondering if a more aggressive attempt to treat mood might have been rewarding.

Follow-Up studies

Saez-Fonseca and colleagues [40] provide a potentially influential paper in which they followed up older people admitted to a psychiatric unit during a 3-year period and given an ICD-10 diagnosis of moderate to severe depression. Sixty-seven patients were identified out of an original 182 after consideration of exclusion factors. Twenty-one patients were designated "Reversible Cognitive Impairment (RCI)," defined as having an MMSE score of less than 24/30 on admission and 26 or greater after treatment of their depression. They are looked on as the pseudodementia cohort. The remaining patients who had

MMSEs greater than 24/30 on admission were designated "Not Cognitively Impaired (NCI)." Follow up at 5–7 years found that 71.4 percent of the RCI carried a diagnosis of dementia. This was so in 18.2 percent of the NCI group. Kral and colleagues [41] had reported even more spectacular conversion rates in patients diagnosed with pseudodementia: of 44 patients followed up for 8–18 years, 39 (89 percent) became demented.

These gloomy prophets would equate pseudodementia with a harbinger of inevitable true and degenerative dementia not long delayed. Their operational criteria may have drawn them to a more easily collected cohort of patients with the symptom of depression in early dementia, rather than the much less common cases of true pseudodementia.

Their conclusions are countered by the straightforward 12-year follow up of 19 patients in Sydney [42], where only one patient certainly and a second possibly had developed dementia, and by the smaller case collections from the classical papers and Pitt's chapter.

The Australian follow-up echoed the findings from Johns Hopkins [43], where a careful study of 15 people with pseudodementia, 13 patients with probable Alzheimer's disease, and 11 with depression without cognitive impairment were contrasted. People with pseudodementia clustered close to those with probable Alzheimer's disease in terms of CT scan and neuropsychological evaluations. But 2 years on only one from the pseudodementia group showed cognitive decline while all those with Alzheimer's disease had deteriorated further.

Interestingly, it is the reports of poor outcome which have been cited most often. It seems that pessimism and nihilism are difficult to eradicate from people's prejudices about life and health in old age.

Neuropsychology, brain imaging, and other investigations

Updating neuropsychological testing and brain structure findings using brain scans, the Maudsley group [44] demonstrated reduced memory and prolonged latency in 70 percent of older people with depression. The memory impairment in depression was of a different pattern to that seen among people with Alzheimer's disease and improved in most patients when their depression lifted. Ventricular brain ration computed from scans showed changes among depressives with the greatest cognitive changes.

Azorin and colleagues [45] found that neither MMSE scores, CT scans, Dexamethasone Suppression Test, nor Well's criteria separated six people with pseudodementia from four with organic dementia. They did differ, however, with the pseudodementia patients having higher plasma levels of 3-methoxy-4-hydroxyphenylglycol and by changes in EEG measures of sleep.

Buysse and colleagues [46] had previously reported higher Rapid Eye Movement (REM) sleep amongst people with pseudodementia and greater REM rebound after sleep deprivation when compared with people with primary degenerative dementia.

Cho and colleagues [47] reported significant decreases in cerebral blood flow in the right temporal region and both parietal lobes of seven patients with pseudodementia when compared with patients with depression and normal people when studied using SPECT scans. Patients with Alzheimer's disease showed more widespread reductions of blood flow. These findings place pseudodementia between normality or pure mood disorder and degenerative brain disease, reflecting entirely the clinical picture and probably "state-dependent." Similar but not identical findings had been reported using PET scans [48].

Gottlieb and colleagues [49] demonstrated that while patients with depressive pseudodementia could be reliably differentiated from normals and people with dementia using the "odd-ball" paradigm, the P300 wave form produced in the Passive Listening condition did not distinguish between these groups.

False positive errors differentiate pseudodementia from Alzheimer's disease [50]. Cognitive complaint scores, not surprisingly, differentiate between people with depression and people with pseudodementia [51].

Conclusion

What are we to make of all this? Poon [28] writing from Athens reviewed aspects of the literature and recent analyses of patterns of altered cognition in depression and dementia and concluded that there is no room nor need for a term or concept of pseudodementia and recommended it be abandoned. The follow-up studies, which show high conversion rates from pseudodementia to degenerative dementia, encourage a nihilism that many people seem to feel is essential when considering any aspect of later life.

Donnet and colleagues [52] had reviewed the concept sympathetically and positively from the perspective of the French tradition, a view which most experienced clinicians will own.

The more we learn the more we know about the detailed changes in function and structure associated with age.

Depression, which is clearly a functional disorder, has been shown to be associated in some patients with altered vascular supply and other changes in the brain [53]. Some of these can be identified in blood vessels in more easily biopsied locations [54]. Such changes are more common among people whose depressive illnesses become prolonged and are resistant to treatment. That does not mean they have transformed to cases of dementia. Nor does it mean that attempts to treat the mood disorder should be given up as futile. Quite often symptoms do ameliorate after sustained therapy and expectant management [55].

It is accepted that some people with Alzheimer's disease, vascular dementia, or other forms of dementia experience symptoms of anxiety and depression [56]. In the presence of dementia, response of the mood disorder to therapy may not be encouraging [57], but every individual must receive a thorough assessment and tailored treatment plan with a realistic hope that the mood components of their difficulties can be resolved.

The coming of memory clinics [58] and medication that is modestly effective in the treatment of Alzheimer's disease and perhaps other dementias [59, 60] has encouraged people to present early in the course of dementia. People who have become anxious or have degrees of depression may present when there is little or no objective evidence of serious cognitive decline. Some will be found to show minor changes and these may be associated with structural changes demonstrable by brain scans. There is an increasing collection of individuals who have received a diagnosis of dementia "well-made" by a memory clinic or similar who show little or no deterioration that would place them within Lishman's definition of the clinical concept. There are celebrated instances of people who have received a diagnosis of dementia, only to recover when stresses upon them pass or their mood otherwise resolves [61–63] and younger people clinging to "dementia" as an explanation for their difficulties [64]. In their various ways these may be said to represent current versions of pseudodementia.

Sadly, some people who present with symptoms that include depression will go on to deteriorate and to be proven cases of a degenerative dementia. Instances where this has happened and families have become bewildered and frustrated by apparent misdiagnosis are sometimes used as criticism of the treating clinicians [65]. Whilet it is always important to determine the true underlying condition, as illustrated by case histories described briefly by Brice Pitt and others in their clinical series, treating the mood component of a presentation determinedly despite the sure evidence of organic brain disorder is the right way to proceed. Some patients will do well and few will be disadvantaged.

While attempts to capture pseudodementia by checklists such as those of Wells [33] and Yousef and colleagues [36] have much to commend them, this is not a disorder that falls easily into a checklist/tick-box discipline. There is a real hazard, as demonstrated by some follow-up series, that the essence will be lost by attempts to make the rare and atypical more common and less extraordinary through operational criteria that deny its subtlety.

Each story is unique. Being aware of the possibility and potential for resolution requires close and sensitive clinical involvement with the patient, knowledge of the history as well as detailed examination of the mental state. It is likely that the most worthwhile accounts and analyses will continue to include: anecdotal reporting, skewed series, and speculation, for this is the nature of the phenomenon.

There is a sense of romance and mystery in the concept. We should not lose that. Medicine is greatly helped by science, but sometimes it can be confounded and mislead by it. Clinical diagnosis remains an art form.

Acknowledgments

Thanks to Professor Brice Pitt and Drs Susan Jolley, Claire Hilton, and Richard Atkinson for comments on drafts.

References

1 Department of Health. *Living Well with Dementia: A National Dementia Strategy. Accessible Summary.* London: Department of Health, 2009.

2 Department of Health. *The Prime Minister's Challenge on Dementia. Delivering Major Improvements in Dementia Care and Research by 2015: A Report on Progress.* London: Department of Health, 2009.

3 World Health Organisation. Dementia: A public health priority. www.who.int/mental_health/publications/dementia_report_2012/en/ (accessed 23.8.2013).

4 Ferri C, Prince M, Brayne C, et al. Global prevalence of dementia: A Delphi consensus study. *Lancet* 2005; 366 (9503): 2112–2117.

5 Knapp M, Prince M. *Dementia UK.* London: Alzheimer's Society, 2007.

6 Practical Alzheimers. 25 famous people with Alzheimer's. http://practicalalzheimers.com/25-famous-people-with-dementia/ (accessed 23.8.2013).

7 Alzheimer's Society. Leading the fight against dementia. http://alzheimers.org.uk/ (accessed 23.8.2013).

8 Alzheimer's Disease International. The global voice on dementia. http://www.alz.co.uk/, 2013 (accessed 23.8.2013).

9 Ballenger J, Whitehouse P, Lyketsos C, Rabins P, Karlawish J. *Treating Dementia: Do We Have a Pill for It?* Baltimore: John Hopkins University Press, 2009.

10 Lishman WA. *Organic Psychiatry.* Oxford: Blackwell Science, 1978.

11 Berrios G. Descriptive psychopathology: Conceptual and historical aspects. *Psychological Medicine* 1984; 14: 303–313.

12 Berrios G. Dementia during the seventeenth and eighteenth centuries: A conceptual history. *Psychological Medicine* 1987; 17 (4): 829–838.

13 *Celsus De Medicina* (English Translation by W. G Spencer) Loeb Collection. London: Heinemann, 1971.

14 Berrios G. Depressive pseudodementia of melancholic dementia: A 19th century view. *Journal of Neurology, Neurosurgery and Psychiatry* 1985; 48: 393–400.

15 Wernicke C. *Grundriss der Psychiatrie in Klinischen Vorlesungen.* Leipzig: Thieme, 1900.

16 Bleuler E. *Textbook of Psychiatry.* New York: MacMillan, 1934.

17 Chambers Dictionary. Edinburgh: Chambers Harrap Publishers, 1998.

18 Dorland's *Medical Dictionary for Health Consumers.* Saunders, Amsterdam: Elsevier, 2007.

19 NHS Choices. Alzheimer's in the news: Fear and fascination 2011. www.nhs.uk/news/2011/08August/Documents/Alzheimer's%20in%20the%20press.pdf (accessed 10.8.2013).

20 Ganser S. A peculiar hysterical state. In Hirsch S, Shepherd M (eds.) *Themes and Variations in European Psychiatry.* John Wright and Sons Bristol, 1974, pp. 67–77. Translation by CE Schorer, previously published: British Journal of Criminology 5: 120–126 from the original lecture delivered in 1897 at the Central Psychiatric and Neurological convention in Halle. This version accompanied by a commentary from PD Scott.

21 Jaspers K. *General Psychopathology.* Published as Allgemeine Pathologie, 1923 Springer Verlag, Berlin, Gottingen and Heidelberg. Translated by Hoenig J and Hamilton M 1963, Manchester University Press, Manchester, 1923.

22 Post F. *The Clinical Psychiatry of Late Life.* Oxford: Pergamon, 1965.

23 Kiloh L. *Pseudo-dementia. Acta Psychiatrica Scandinavica* 1961; 37: 336–351.

24 Roth M. The natural history of mental disorders of old age. *Journal of Mental Science* 1955; 101: 281–301.

25 Whitehead T. *In Service of Old Age: The Welfare of Psychogeriatric Patients.* John Wiley, 1978.

26 Snowdon J. Pseudodementia, a term for its time: The impact of Leslie Kiloh's 1961 paper. *Australasian Psychiatry* 2011; 19 (5): 391–397.

27 Mahendra B. Pseudo-dementia: Abandon the term? *American Journal of Psychiatry* 1984; 141: 471–472.

28 Poon L. Toward an understanding of cognitive functioning in geriatric depression. *International Psychogeriatrics* 1992; (4) Supplement 2: 241–266

29 Caine E. Pseudodementia: Current concepts and future directions. *Archives of General Psychiatry* 1981; 38 (12): 1359–1364.

30 Bulbena A, Berrios G. Pseudodementia: Facts and figures. *British Journal of Psychiatry* 1986; 148: 87–94.

31 Madden J, Luhan J, Kaplan L, et al. Non-dementing psychoses in older persons. *JAMA* 1952; 150: 1567–1570.

32 Pitt B. Pseudodementia. In Bhugra D, Munro A (eds.) *Troublesome Disguises: Under-Diagnosed Psychiatric Syndromes.* Oxford: Blackwell Sciences, 1997, pp. 195–205.

33 Wells C. Pseudodementia. *American Journal of Psychiatry* 1979; 136 (7): 89–90.

34 Post F. Dementia, depression and pseudodementia. In Benson F, Blumer D (eds.) *Psychiatric Aspects of Neurological Disease.* New York: Grune and Stratton, 1975.

35 Fisman M. Intractable depression and pseudodementia: A report of two cases. *Canadian Journal of Psychiatry* 1988; 33 (7): 628–630.

36 Yousef G, Ryan W, Lambert T, Pitt B, Kellett J. A preliminary report: A new scale to identify the pseudodementia syndrome. *International Journal of Geriatric Psychiatry* 1998; 13: 389–399.

37 Allen R. Pseudodementia and ECT. *Biological Psychiatry* 1982; 17 (12): 1435–1443.

38 Stoudemire A, Hill C, Morris R, Dalton S. Improvement in depression-related cognitive dysfunction following ECT. *Journal of Neuropsychiatry and Neuroscience* 1995; 7 (1): 31–34.

39 Hepple J. Conversion pseudodementia in older people: A descriptive case series. *International Journal of Geriatric Psychiatry* 2004; 19: 961–967.

40 Saez-Fonseca J, Lee L, Walker Z. Long-term outcomes of depressive pseudodementia in the elderly. *Journal of Affective Disorders* 2007; 101 (1–3): 123–129.

41 Kral V, Emery O. Long-term follow up of depressive pseudodementia of the aged. *Canadian Journal of Psychiatry* 1989; 34: 445–446.

42 Sachdev P, Smith J, Angus-Lepan H, Rodriguez P. Pseudodementia twelve years on. *Journal of Neurology, Neurosurgery and Psychiatry* 1990; 53 (3): 254–259.

43 Pearson G, et al. Structural brain CT changes and cognitive deficits in elderly depressives with and without reversible dementia ('pseudodementia'). *Psychological Medicine* 1989; 19 (3): 573–584.

44 Abas M, Sahakian B, Levy R. Neuropsychological deficits and CT changes in elderly depressives. *Psychological Medicine* 1990; 20 (3): 507–520.

45 Azorin J, Donnet A, Habib M, Regis H. Diagnostic criteria of depressive pseudodementia. *Encephale* 1990; 16 (1): 31–34.

46 Buysse D, et al. Electroencephalographic sleep in depressive pseudodementia. *Archives of General Psychiatry* 1988; 45 (6): 568–575.

47 Cho M, et al. Brain single photon emission tomography findings in depressive pseudodementia patients. *Journal of Affective Disorders* 2002; 69 (1–3): 159–166.

48 Dolan R, et al. Regional cerebral blood flow abnormalities in depressed patients with cognitive impairment. *Journal of Neurology, Neurosurgery and Psychiatry* 1992; 55 (9): 768–773.

49 Gottlieb D, Weetman E, Bentin S. Passive listening and task related P300 measurement for the evaluation of dementia and pseudodementia. *Clinical Electroencephalography* 1991; 22 (2): 102–107.

50 Gainotti G, Marra C. Some aspects of memory disorders clearly distinguish dementia of the Alzheimer type from depressive pseudodementia. *Journal of Clinical and Experimental Neuropsychology* 1994; 16 (1): 65–78.

51 O'Boyle M, Amadeo M, Self D. Cognitive complaints in elderly depressed and pseudodemented patients. *Psychology of Ageing* 1990; 5 (3): 467–468.

52 Donnet A, Habib M, Azorin J. Current concept of pseudodementia. *La Revue de medecine interne* 1990; 11 (2): 133–141.

53 Simpson S, Jackson A, Baldwin R, Burns A. Subcortical hypersensitivities in late life depression. *International Psychogeriatrics* 1997; 9 (3): 257–273.

54 Paranthaman R, et al. Relationship of endothelial function and atherosclerosis to treatment response in late life depression. *International Journal of Geriatric Psychiatry* 2012; 27 (9): 967–973.

55 Baldwin R, Simpson S. Treatment resistant depression in the elderly: A review of its conceptualisation, management and relationship to organic brain disease. *Journal of Affective Disorders* 1997; 46 (3): 163–173.

56 Burns A, Jacoby R, Levy R. Psychiatric phenomena in Alzheimer's disease: iii Disorders of Mood. *British Journal of Psychiatry* 1990; 157: 81–86 and 92–94.

57 Banerjee S, et al. Sertraline or Mirtazepine for depression in dementia (HTA-SADD): A randomised, multi-centre, double-blind, placebo-controlled trial. *Lancet* 2011; 378 (9789): 403–411.

58 Jolley D, Moniz-Cook E. Memory clinics in context. *Indian Journal of Psychiatry* 2009; 51, S70–S76.

59 National Institute for Health and Social Care Excellence. Clinical Guideline 42. Dementia: Supporting people with dementia and their carers in health and social care. 2006.

60 National Institute for Health and Care Excellence. Alzheimer's Disease: Donepezil, galantamine, rivastigmine and memantine (TA217) 2011.

61 Warner J. Ronson: Ernest's Alzheimer's was my idea, 2009. www.independent.co.uk/news/business/comment/jeremy-warner/jeremy-warner-ronson-ndash-ernests-alzheimers-was-my-idea-1698217.html (accessed 23.8.2013).

62 Hennigan T. 'Lucid' Pinochet charged with murder, 2006. http://martinfrost.ws/htmlfiles/nov2006/pinochet_charged.html.

63 Blank L. *Alzheimer's Challenged and Conquered?* London: Foulsham, 1995.

64 Adeyemo Y. I want to have dementia. Old Age Psychiatrist, 2013; 57. www.rcpsych.ac.uk/pdf/I_want_to_have_dementia.pdf (accessed 3.9.2013).

65 Whitman L. *Telling Tales about Dementia*. London: Jessica Kingsley, 2010.

CHAPTER 17

Culture-bound syndromes

Oyedeji Ayonrinde[1] and Dinesh Bhugra[2]

[1] Consultant Psychiatrist, South London and Maudsley NHS Foundation Trust, London, UK
[2] Professor of Mental Health and Cultural Diversity, Institute of Psychiatry, King's College London, London, UK

Introduction

Mental disorders and mental illness have been reported from across cultures even though rates of different illnesses vary due to a number of factors. Cultures influence the way distress is expressed and thus notions of culture-bound emerged, arguing that certain conditions were confined to certain specific cultures only. As a consequence of colonialism, psychiatrists as well as anthropologists from Europe and America have had a significant influence on the early descriptions of unfamiliar presentations of mental distress in other cultures. Their research interests led to the dissemination of descriptions of exotic manifestations of mental disorders in indigenous or native groups around the world. Descriptions of these indigenous health systems, idioms of distress and therapeutic interventions were found appealing and led to the emergence of "cultural" diagnoses. Over the years, the medicalisation of social expression of distress has led to the evolution of "new syndromes" and disorders in scientific literature.

Yap [1] described culture-bound psychogenic psychoses as a way of harmonising a wide range of disorders with a complex socio-cultural influence on their presentation. In 1969 he subsequently abbreviated this terminology to culture-bound syndromes [2].

Elaborating on this, Bhugra and Jacob [3] observed that these syndromes described "rare, exotic unpredictable and chaotic behaviours at their core among uncivilised people." These authors asserted that these behaviours were described in the context and against a backdrop of Western diagnostic systems with little appreciation of socio-environmental influences and the tolerance of symptoms within the culture. This Western medicalisation was felt to lead to Eurocentric labelling of culturally acceptable behaviour in non-Western populations.

Troublesome Disguises: Managing Challenging Disorders in Psychiatry, Second Edition.
Edited by Dinesh Bhugra and Gin S. Malhi.
© 2015 John Wiley & Sons, Ltd. Published 2015 by John Wiley & Sons, Ltd.

In a similar vein, Hughes and Wintrob [4] emphasised the need for a contextual frame of reference for the full appreciation of unfamiliar clinical presentations.

Initial descriptions of these syndromes were predominantly from Far East Asia; however, Western culture-bound syndromes such as Type A behaviour patterns and bulimia have been suggested by Hughes [5] and Littlewood [6] respectively. Type A personality is based on the cultural salience of goal pursuance, working against time pressure, and the frustration experienced at not achieving these goals. Explored in cultural context, this may reflect the "individualistic" or egocentric nature of the society with a greater emphasis on "I-ness." In such societies kinship or family links may be weaker, compared with collectivist or "sociocentric" societies, which promote group relationships and kinship sharing of resources [7]. Such societal values may influence individuals and the normalisation of behaviours.

This chapter reviews the historical and current status of culture bound syndromes in contemporary clinical practice by exploring the development of two well documented syndromes and their current relevance. Focusing on brain fag syndrome and on dhat highlights historical evolution and questions the nosological, diagnostic and therapeutic relevance of these concepts.

Society and illness

Societal differences in economic, political, and social functioning influence healthcare, and the rates and distribution of common mental disorders in the population [8]. Culture within each society also determines what counts as aberrant behavior, such as a crime or mental disorder, as well as what is acceptable. The interplay between culture and mental wellbeing can be observed in all spheres of life, such as attitudes to diet, body image, relationships, vocation, and study.

Over the last half century, there has been an evolution in the names used to describe unfamiliar or unique cultural phenomena (see Figure 17.1):
Ethnic or exotic psychosis
Culture-reactive (ICD 10) [9]
Culture-Bound Syndromes
Culture Specific Disorders (ICD-10)
Cultural Concepts of Distress (DSM-5)

Nosological definitions of culture-bound syndromes have not been static over the decades. The core features, syndrome features, and labels have been inconsistent.

Bound: The concept of boundedness has been a controversial one, as it is uncommon for a particular set of symptoms within a syndrome to be bound to a specific culture. This presents a further challenge in that cultures seldom have

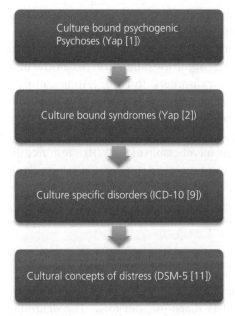

Figure 17.1 Nosological timeline.

clearly defined boundaries of their own. Hughes [12] observed that labels suggesting exotic syndromes and atypical psychoses are grounded on the premise that these disorders deviate from recognised and perhaps standard Western diagnoses.

Exotic indicates something unusual, foreign, not indigenous, alien, and different. However, differences do not imply psychopathology and would require an awareness from within the culture before considering labelling with a diagnosis. Failure of the clinician to put an unfamiliar behaviour in the true cultural context may lead to the pathologisation of normal or acceptable behaviour.

Culture-bound syndromes in the diagnostic manuals (DSM and ICD)

ICD-10

The International Classification of Diseases (ICD-10) [9] recognises a number of culturally uncommon symptom patterns and presentations referred to as culture-specific disorders. While they were felt to have diverse characteristics, they shared two key features:

Not being easily accommodated in established and international diagnostic categories

Initial description in a particular population or cultural area and subsequent association with this community or culture

Systematic study of culture specific disorders faces additional challenges of the frequently acute and transient as well as rare.

The ICD-10 indicates the status of culture specific disorders is controversial in that researchers argue the differences of cultural disorders are in degree from existing familiar disorders, thus suggesting cultural disorders are only local variations of established disorders such as depression. In light of this, only tentative associations were made by the ICD-10 between cultural syndromes and recognised psychiatric categories pending a stronger evidence base. Given the large membership of the WHO, resource differences, research, and health priorities of member countries, it is no surprise caution is being exercised with endorsing specific symptom clusters. It is anticipated that the salience given to cultural issues and specific syndromes will shift in the ICD-11, as has been the case with the DSM classificatory system.

DSM-IV-TR [10]

The term *culture-bound syndrome* "denotes recurrent, locality-specific patterns of aberrant behaviour and troubling experience that may or may not be linked to a particular DSM-IV diagnostic category." This definition was based on the premise that culture-bound syndromes had the following characteristics:

Characteristics of culture-bound syndromes [10]

Indigenously considered illness or afflictions, therefore a recognition within the society as a deviation from normal or healthy presentation

Local names: the ascription of a specific local name to the experience of mental distress; often in the indigenous or key language of communication and may be components of folk diagnostic categories

Symptoms, course, and social response often influenced by local cultural factors; for instance, the folk healing systems for the symptoms based on the explanatory model of the experiences

Limited to specific societies or cultural areas: may be a geographical region, areas with shared ethnic history or identity; for instance, some cultural practice and artefacts of the Yoruba culture of western Nigeria may also be found in Brazil

Localised: therefore experiences that are not globally recognised or span different regions

DSM-5 changes, 2013

The DSM-5 [11] discarded the concept of culture-bound syndromes with a preference for the term *cultural concepts of distress*. This was defined as "ways cultural groups experience, understand, and communicate suffering, behavioural problems, or troubling thoughts and emotions."

Introducing this change, DSM-5 elaborates on three cultural concepts:

Syndromes: clusters of symptoms and attributions occurring among individuals in specific cultures

Idioms of distress: shared ways of communicating, expressing or sharing distress

Explanations: labels, attributions suggesting causation of symptoms or distress

Controversy regarding the concept of culture-bound syndromes has received wide recognition. The DSM-5 contends that the terminology ignores the influence of culture on more specific experience and expression of distress. This questions the validity of culturally circumscribed collections of symptoms as had been the case previously. Reinforcing this view, the DSM-5 stresses all mental distress is culturally framed and different populations have culturally determined ways of communicating distress, explanations of causality, coping methods, and help-seeking behaviour.

These World Health Organisation and American Psychiatric Association diagnostic classificatory systems have had continuous reviews and amendments to incorporate new anthropological, psychiatric, and social research findings, and recognise societal changes in idioms of distress, illness awareness, and explanatory models.

These views highlight the nosological challenges of using a term when it can be argued that all psychiatric disorders are culture bound.

Culture bound syndromes in the diagnostic manuals (DSM and ICD)

While a large number of culture-bound syndromes have been described over the years, the enduring nature of each varies. For instance, the DSM-IV-TR described 25 syndromes; however, the DSM-5, published in 2013, reduced the number of detailed cultural concepts of distress (culture-bound syndromes) to 9 in light of the current research evidence base (see Tables 17.1 and 17.2).

Interested readers are referred to Simon and Hughes [12, 13] and the DSM (DSM-IV and DSM-5 glossaries [10, 11] for more detail on different culture-bound syndromes and concepts of distress.

Table 17.1 Various culture-bound syndromes.

	Culture bound syndrome	Country/region	ICD-10 (12 syndromes) - described	DSM IV-TR (25 syndromes) - described	DSM 5 (9 syndromes) - described
1.	Amok	Malaysia	x	x	
2.	Ataque de nervios	Latin America/ Latino Caribbean		x	x
3.	Bilis and colera	Latino		x	
4.	Boufee delirante	West Africa, Haiti		x	
5.	Brain fag	West Africa		x	
6.	Dhat	India	x	x	x
7.	Falling-out (blacking out)	South USA, Caribbean		x	
8.	Ghost sickness	American Indian (Native American)		x	
9.	Hwa-byung	Korea		x	
10.	Koro	Malaysia	x	x	
11.	Khyâl cap	Cambodia			x
12.	Kufungisisa	Zimbabwe			x
13.	Latah	Malaysia, Indonesia	x	x	
14.	Locura	Latino, USA, Latin America		x	
15.	Mal de ojo	Mediterranean		x	
16.	Maladi moun	Haiti			x
17.	Nervios	Latino, Latin America	x	x	x
18.	Pibloktoq	Artic Circle	x	x	
19.	Qi-gong psychotic reaction	China		x	
20.	Rootwork	Southern USA, Caribbean		x	
21.	Sangue dormido	Portuguese Cape Verde		x	
22.	Shenjing shuairuo	China		x	x
23.	Shen-k'uei	China	x	x	
24.	Shin-byung	Korea		x	
25.	Spell	Southern USA		x	
26.	Susto	Latino/ South America	x	x	x
27.	Taijin kyofusho	Japan	x	x	x
28.	Zar	Ethiopia, Somalia, Egypt, Sudan. North Africa, Middle East		x	
29.	Others				
	Pa-leng	China	x		
	Ufufuyane, saka	Southern Africa	x		
	Uqamairineq	Arctic Circle	x		
	Windigo	N.E. North America	x		

x indicates description of the syndrome in the different diagnostic manuals.

Specific culture-bound syndromes

Brain fag syndrome: A case study of the stability of a culture-bound syndrome [15]

Brain fag syndrome has been embedded in anthropological, social science and psychiatric literature as a West African culture-bound syndrome for many years. In 1960, Raymond Prince, a Canadian psychiatrist and anthropologist working in Nigeria, published some observations made during his clinical practice in the country. He described a cluster of symptoms unfamiliar to him as the brain fag syndrome, characterised by somatic, affective, anxiety, and cognitive complaints in African individuals engaged in educational pursuit [16].

Ever since his original report, descriptions of brain fag syndrome have achieved wide acclaim in peer-reviewed psychiatric journals, textbooks, and classificatory volumes such as the ICD-10 and DSM-IV-TR.

It is not uncommon to read flamboyant descriptions in contemporary textbooks of this exotic "African syndrome" and the need to give careful consideration when presented with an African student manifesting somatic, affective, or anxiety symptoms. This is usually illustrated by accounts of African immigrant students presenting to college or university health centres with burning or crawling sensations, difficulty with recall, and anxiety. The texts reinforce the notion that these students from an unfamiliar culture may be particularly vulnerable when studying and may also apply faulty study techniques with detrimental effects on their mental wellbeing.

In these contemporary texts, brain fag syndrome was initially coined and described in Nigeria and the etymology of the phrase "brain fag" rooted in a form of pidgin Nigerian-English, colloquially referring to forms of mental exhaustion.

Interestingly, this version of the history of "brain fag" has been a source of pride in some quarters as a unique manifestation of a specific mental disorder discovered in West Africa, hence putting the region on the nosological map of psychiatric literature. There remain some serious questions. For example, was the phrase "brain fag" coined in West Africa? Are some West African individuals particularly vulnerable to education and study? Is this presentation unique or do similar presentations exist in other regions of the world? In essence, is the brain fag syndrome truly culture bound?

An etymological exploration of the term "brain fag"

Contrary to the popular belief that its origins were in 1960s Africa, the concept of brain fag was initially described in Britain in the early 1800s and subsequently disseminated around the British Empire with the colonial spread of the English language in the same way semen-loss anxiety was used and treated both in Britain and the U.S. [17].

In 19th-century Britain, concern about the impact of study on education started manifesting during the post-industrial revolution when increasing emphasis was laid on non-manual vocations and their contribution to society. Apprenticeships, while important, were not felt to be sufficient for the nation's development leading to the rise of "brain workers." Brain workers were individuals whose vocations required more mental than manual effort, such as lawyers, book-keepers, writers, and students. This stage of British history may be referred to as the "Educational Revolution" with the promulgation of education acts and the drive for the establishment of more schools and institutions. Compulsory education was to become the order of the day. This inadvertently served to heighten concern of the more educated classes of society about the impact this may have on working class groups. At the time, structured study at a national level was alien and uncertainties abound regarding the appropriate age, gender, social class, and activity level for schools. Furthermore, there was no template for the number of hours, breaks, and methods required for knowledge acquisition and education.

Hysteria about the health risks of faulty study spread widely and media reports on suicides, nervous diseases, insanity, and lethargy from "overstudy" received prominent acclaim. Mental disorders in schools and colleges were not infrequently labelled a consequence of "overstudy," which later became a diagnostic category and grounds for admission asylums.

The time was ripe for the emergence of the phrase "brain fag," the scourge of "brain workers." In 19th-century English, to be "fagged" meant to be tired and the word "fag" referred to fatigue, exhaustion, or tiredness.

Anxiety about the impact of brain fag was fuelled by headlines with the proliferation of quack remedies and adverts in the British press while the medical profession sought to answer the question of what was causing this new disease. Charlatans advised the use of stimulants, rest, hydrotherapy, vibrators, alcohol, and sexual abstinence, among other things. Trade in spectacles also thrived.

In the late 1800s and early 1900s the American media raised the alarm that there was an illness called "brain fag" in England that was taking a toll on British "brain workers" and rapidly on its way across the Atlantic. Brain fag was feared to be a serious threat to developing civilisation at the turn of the 19th century and some proponents suggested reverting to traditional ways.

A historical review of medical and social science literature yielded interesting attitudes regarding study and mental wellbeing. Presenting a paper titled "Intemperance in Study" to the British Medical Association in 1879, Tuke [18] stated, "having met from time to time with cases of *brain-fag* and also actual insanity, arising from excessive mental work . . . I regard it as a serious evil . . . still I fear it is in schools and colleges . . . and among students." Intemperance (an old English term for the lack of self-control or excessive indulgence) in study and educational pursuit was opined as a cause of insanity. These themes later evolved with "overstudy" being classified as a sub-type of "moral insanity."

Alongside its role in clinical parlance, idiomatic use of brain fag in the early 20th century was evident in medical dictionaries, as seen in these sample definitions:

Brain fag: exhaustion due to overwork with the brain [19]

Brain fag: the effects on the brain of mental overwork [20]

Concern about the harmful consequences of study was observed in a number of peer reviewed scientific journals as well. In 1926, the *Journal of Neurology and Psychopathology* published an article describing "The fatigue syndrome to which the name 'neurasthenia' has been characteristically applied, included the following symptoms and physical signs: 'brain-fag' with sensations of pressure in the head; poor memory, lack of concentration, irritability of temper, increased reflexes, poor sleep, anorexia and various aches and pains. This syndrome is rarely met with alone . . . and illustrates the occurrence of fatigue and its significance in a wide variety of conditions [21]." It is noteworthy that these somatic symptoms closely mirror brain fag described three decades later on another continent. A few years later, (1933) in London, Gillespie published his clinical observations in the *Lancet* on the psychoneuroses and brain fag [22]. Describing categories of curable functional nervous conditions, he reported "the curable disorders include many cases included in the purely symptomatic categories" such as " Nervous exhaustion, in which, in addition to feeling exhausted, the patient often complains of *brain-fag*, poor memory, excessive fatigue, irritability, or insomnia." Elucidating with a vignette, he wrote:

> This was a man of middle-age who complained of "brain-fag" which took the form of inability to read for more than about 40 minutes at a time. He then had to rest for half an hour before he could resume. This had handicapped him considerably in his work for examinations which had been essential to his scientific career. We investigated the history of the symptom in a straightforward, chronological way. It had first appeared 30 years or more ago, when the patient was about 13. At that time he was taking some of his work in classes from the headmaster of his school, whom he disliked very much. The headmaster remarked to his mother that the boy had an under-developed brain, and the mother had injudiciously communicated this to the boy. The latter, although doing well in his other subjects, believed this, and noted anxiously that he gained weight in the summer and lost it in the winter. He concluded that this was the result of overstrain of his "under-developed brain," and so he became afraid to read for more than a certain period of time. In his fear he automatically assumed that he would become fatigued after this period and it had become a habitual fear producing the effect long after the reason for it had been forgotten [22].

This rich descriptive account from a London hospital vividly illustrates how patients presented with specific use of the term "brain fag" during consultations as well as the psychosomatic aspects of their distress. Through history we are given a rich insight into the role of culture in the emergence of a mental illness.

The new "brain fag": Africa

Over one and a half centuries after the early British accounts of brain fag, a very similar (possibly identical) account emerged on the west coast of Africa. As Nigeria achieved independence in 1960, Prince's seminal paper was published and the "African" brain fag was born [16]. It shared not only the same name as the previously described idiom of distress, but also symptom clusters and core etiological models.

The original report of brain fag syndrome that subsequently evolved in Western literature and nosology as an African culture bound syndrome stated:

> The distinctive symptoms of the syndrome are intellectual impairment, sensory impairment (chiefly visual), and somatic complaints most commonly of pain or burning in the head and neck. In addition there are a variety of other complaints that often militate against the student's ability to study. The patients have an unhappy, tense facial expression and a characteristic gesture is frequently noted—that of passing the hand over the surface of the scalp or rubbing the vertex of the skull, especially when discussing a question that requires concentration [16].

Prince observed an incidence of symptoms "during periods of intensive reading and study prior to examinations or sometimes just following periods of intensive study." Here lay the key explanatory model of causation for this cluster of symptoms, study. He elaborated that patients attribute their illness to fatigue of the brain due to excessive "brain work." It was on the basis of the use of this idiom of distress that Prince gave the designation *brain fag syndrome*. In his opinion, this expression seemed to be used by Nigerians generally to describe any psychiatric disturbance occurring in "brain workers." From this historical perspective, the roots of brain fag were diagnostically heterogeneous and based on a perceived association between study, administrative or paperwork roles, and mental distress.

The cultural salience of symptoms suggested the transmission of an infective agent (in this case study) on the minds of the host with the development of a disorder—brain fag.

The early literature on brain fag in Nigeria based its explanatory model on a psychosocial explanation: "It is clear that the syndrome is related to 'westernization', for prior to the 19th century when significant European influence commenced, the written word and the student life, which are so intimately bound up with the syndrome, symptoms were unknown to the inhabitants of Southern Nigeria." It was further stated: "the syndrome is rarely seen in the European." History, however, shows us that concern about the impact of study had been a major theme in 19th-century Britain. "It would appear then that the illness is related in some way to the fusion of European learning techniques with Nigerian personality" [16].

Table 17.2 Nosological interplay between psychiatric disorders and culture-bound syndromes [14].

Psychiatric disorder	Diagnostic category	Associated culture-bound syndrome
"Neurosis"	Anxiety	Koro
		Dhat
		Brain fag
	Depersonalisation	Amok
		Latah
	Personality disorder	Ataque de nervios
Psychosis	Affective	Brain fag
		Koro
	Schizophrenia	Amok
		Susto
Others	Eating disorders	Anorexia nervosa
		Bulimia

Textbook of Cultural Psychiatry, edited by Dinesh Bhugra and Kamaldeep Bhui, Cambridge University Press, 2007.

Prince suggested that "European learning techniques emphasize isolated endeavour, individual responsibility and orderliness—activities and traits which are foreign to the Nigerian by reason of the collectivistic society from which he derives." At first, this may appear to be critical of African culture; however, the concept of "individualist" and "collectivist" cultures was developed further by Hofstede over two decades later and remains relevant to the understanding of other societies [7].

While the views expressed above are dated, there is a relative dearth of contemporary evidence based literature on brain fag. In the era of evidence-based medicine, what support is there for brain fag syndrome in the 21st century? Did idiomatic use of the colonial phrase "brain fag" become syndromised, and how reflective is this of 21st-century Nigeria?

A media database exploration observed significant decline in the use of the term *brain fag* after its peak use in the late 19th and early 20th centuries [17, 23] (see Figure 17.2).

1980s to date

It could be argued that the description of brain fag syndrome by a non-native psychiatrist may have over-emphasised the exotic nature of the presentation; however, a number of indigenous psychiatrists have supported or challenged the validity and relevance of this "culture-bound syndrome") [24]. Morakinyo,

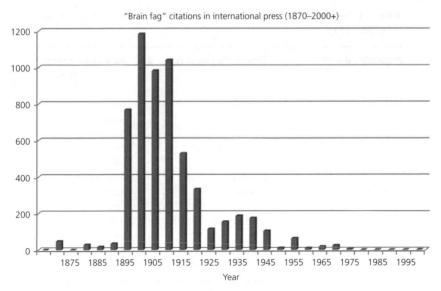

Figure 17.2 Number of publications on Brain Fag citations.

an indigenous Nigerian psychiatrist, explored several features of brain fag syndrome, hypothesizing the psychophysiology and cognitive processing of mental disorders in African students and apprentices [25]. Jegede (also a Nigerian psychiatrist), however, questioned the validity of the syndrome, asserting that it was a nosological misnomer and should be more accurately categorised as a depressive or anxiety neurosis [26]. On the other hand, Ola and colleagues [27] describe brain fag as a tetrad of somatic complaints, cognitive impairments, sleep-related complaints, and other somatic impairments while acknowledging that there have been questions relating to the nosological status of the syndrome as an objective or subjective phenomenon. They conclude that the conceptual history is divided into four major perspectives: traditional medicine, psychoanalysis, biopsychological, and transcultural psychiatry. They [27] assert brain fag as a phenomenon is subjectively real and is best classified with the framework of psychiatry, psychology, and or sociology. An area of agreement among authors was that the course, management, and outcome remain unclear.

Despite this debate about the validity of brain fag as a specific disorder, further dissemination about its existence occurred in the DSM as a specific culture-bound syndrome. The DSM-IV-TR describes it as a culture-bound syndrome affecting West African students which is attributed to overwork. It is reported to be characterised by a loss of ability to concentrate, learn, remember, or think and usually accompanied by sensations of pain, pressure, or tightness around the head or neck and blurred vision [10].

The strength of evidence behind this is unclear and this has been reflected in the DSM-5, which has withdrawn the section for this disorder with only a small reference to the association with anxiety disorders [11].

Is brain fag a syndrome?

A syndrome is a combination of signs and/or symptoms that forms a distinct clinical picture indicative of a particular disorder. While the individual symptoms in the cluster may be well recognised by clinicians, it is doubtful they actually constitute a circumscribed syndrome. The symptoms of Brain Fag include symptoms of depression, somatisation disorder, and anxiety disorder with notable areas of overlap. With such levels of heterogeneity and absence of pathognomonic symptoms and signs, diagnostic stability is not assured.

Is it culture bound?

The concept of boundedness in this context suggests that presentation is limited to or predominantly identified with a specific culture or peoples. Modern literature on brain fag has been associated with a very culturally diverse Nigerian population, and other West African, North, South, and East African countries [28, 29]. The undiscerning reader may naively assume Africa shares a homogenous population. With such a geographical, historical, social, and cultural spread, this is not culture bound. The issue here is that as cultures and societies progress the symptoms change too. With industrialisation both semen loss and brain fag started to disappear in Britain.

In conclusion, brain fag syndrome has been described as a culture-bound syndrome associated with mental exertion and study in West Africans. Furthermore, modern psychiatric, social science, and anthropological literature over the last half century describe the emanation of the term and its idiomatic use as a reference to mental distress as rooted in Nigeria. Brain fag was subsequently described as a syndrome characterised by somatic, affective, anxiety, and cognitive features.

The nosological validity of brain fag as a culture-bound syndrome is questionable however.

An etymological exploration, however, discovered that "brain fag" was actually a well-established phrase used in 19th-century British society [17, 24]. Furthermore, the historic use of the term presented with similar clinical features to descriptions in contemporary scientific literature, such as an association with "overstudy" and nervous exhaustion in "brainworkers."

In essence, the term "brain fag" does not emanate from West Africa but had actually been a well-established term in Britain about 150 years earlier. In addition, the symptom cluster is not culture bound or unique to any region of the world.

The DSM-5 pays significantly less prominence to brain fag than the DSM-IV-TR with the recognition that "thinking too much" is a common idiom of distress across many cultures and geographical regions. It elaborates further that this may be related to conditions such as depressive disorder, generalised anxiety disorder, obsessive-compulsive disorder, and post-traumatic stress disorder [11].

Dhat or semen-loss anxiety syndrome
Etymology
This syndrome was derived from the Sanskrit word *dhatu,* which means "metal." *Dhat* is a colloquial term for semen. Early description in 1960 by Wig reported dhat syndrome as composed of vague somatic complaints of weakness, fatigue, anxiety, loss of appetite, guilt, and sexual dysfunction attributed to semen loss following masturbation, nocturnal emissions, or micturition [30].

Ancient Indian Ayurvedic texts describe symptoms of semen-loss anxiety. Between 5000 BC and the seventh century, semen production was described as "food converts to blood which converts to flesh which converts to marrow and ultimately to semen." This process is reported to take 40 days for 40 drops of food to convert to a drop of blood and 40 drops of blood convert to a drop of flesh [31]. The depth of this historical narrative heightens the salience of semen in the cultural psyche. In light of this, somatic symptoms of anxiety and depression manifest as physical symptoms. The symptom cluster is widely recognised across the Indian subcontinent with treatments advertised in a range of public media such as TV, walls. and newspapers. Clinical studies show somewhat different aspects (see Table 17.3).

About 40 years ago, a study of dhat in Chandigarh, North India [32], explored 175 individuals aged 30–50 years in the community with a vignette looking at perceptions of semen loss, causal factors, and management. Responses were influenced by social class, with a third not favouring any intervention and a greater perception of abnormality with the experience of nocturnal emissions in social-class IV respondents. Marriage and diet were felt to be helpful management strategies, while avoiding masturbation, bad company, and exotic literature. Described as the "sex neurosis of the Orient," vulnerability was associated with belief systems regarding semen loss. Patterns of help seeking varied from alternative therapists to Western medical interventions [32].

Studies in clinical groups vary among physical, urological, and psychiatric diagnoses. A study by Chadda and Ahuja of 52 patients presenting primarily with complaints of dhat in their urine found 80 percent of subjects had "hypochondriacal" symptoms. An alternative interpretation of the findings is that dhat is a form of hypochondriasis [33]. In a sexual dysfunction clinic, Bhatia and Malik [34] reported 93 out of 144 consecutive attendees

Table 17.3 Findings of studies conducted in clinical settings (originally published in *Textbook of Cultural Psychiatry*, Bhugra D, Bhui K (eds.) [14]).

Study	Setting	No	Inclusion criteria	Presenting symptom	Attributes to semen loss	Duration of semen loss	Mode of loss (one or more)					
							In sleep	With urine	Masturbation	Sex heter	Sex homo	Other
Behere and Natraj [35]	Psychiatric outpatient clinic at psychiatry dept., Institute of Med. Sci., India	50	Consecutive referrals. Main complaint of dhat discharge	Associated symptoms: impotence, marital probs. premature ejaculation, weakness, others??	No, this was the presenting symptom itself	Less than 3 months to more than 1 year.	? Yes unclear	? Yes unclear	? Unclear as given it a cause	? Unclear		
Singh G [36]	Psychiatric outpatient clinic, Ptia. India	50	50 consecutive patients of male potency disorder and complaint of dhat (N=30)	Primary complaint of loss of semen but accompanied by mental and physical symptoms	Unclear. No reference attribution.	Not reported	No? NR?	Yes	No? NR?	No? NR?	No? NR?	No NR?
De Silva Dissanayeke [37] Descriptive study	Referrals to a university psychiatric clinic in Sri Lanka	38	Clear (see next column). They belonged to 4 different clinical presentation.	Four different groups: 1. Excessive loss of semen 2. Specific sexual dysfunction 3. Anxiety about present or future sexual function 4. Multiple phys/psych. symptoms	The presenting complaint. Yes Yes Yes	6 months–20 years	Yes	Yes	Yes	Yes	Yes	Yes
Chadda and Ajuha [33] Descriptive study	University psychiatric clinic in India/Delhi	52	Passage of dhat in urine was presenting feature but has elicited somatic symptoms		Yes (all)	1–12 months			Yes	Yes	Yes	Yes

*Indicated seen in majority/common NR–not reported.

presented with dhat. Further exploration with Hamilton rating scales and ICD-9 diagnostic criteria found somatic complaints (physical weakness), sexual difficulties, and caseness for depression in half of the patients.

Janaki and colleagues [38] studied sexual attitudes and misconceptions in 12 35-year-old attendees in a psychiatric outpatient clinic. They found the most common misconceptions among the patients were that masturbation was wrong and may lead to loss of potency. Prevalence was found to be 24 percent, approximately double the rates found in the general population (11.2 percent). Debunking the myth that dhat occurred only in the Indian subcontinent or among Indian diaspora, Jadhav [39] explored symptoms of dhat syndrome among 47 white Britons in London, presenting for the first time with a clinic diagnosis of ICD-9, depressive neurosis (dysthymic disorder, ICD-11). A specific question within the British study enquired whether subjects considered semen loss or retention was causative to their personal suffering. In addition, they were asked if this might cause psychological problems.

By obtaining narrative accounts from patients and analysis of quantitative scores on the Hamilton Depression Rating Scale, Jadhav observed that 48 percent linked semen retention with psychological problems. Content analysis of responses by white British subjects diagnosed with dysthymic disorder suggested a psychological variation of a local white British somatisation phenomena previously unrecognized, semen retention syndrome. Key symptoms were loss of energy, diminished libido, multiple somatic symptoms (tension, twitching, bloating), depression, anxiety, and the attribution of symptoms to retention of semen. Core to this finding was that anxiety and depressive symptoms experienced were primarily through cognitive biases, namely, a core irrational belief and a cognitive error focused on a misconception of semen physiology. Jadhav hypothesized that an ethnocentric focus on familiar mood idioms by white British patients and health professionals leads to a preferred diagnosis of mood disorder, and therefore treatment interventions focused on this. Cultural validity in the understanding of phenomena was felt to be critical to reducing diagnosis category errors and influence international diagnostic classificatory systems [39]. It can be deduced from this study that concern regarding semen in anxious and depressed men is not restricted to Asian groups or the Asian subcontinent.

The diagnostic heterogeneity of dhat was highlighted by a systematic review of literature on dhat syndrome by Udina and colleagues [40]. The majority of original studies were from the Indian subcontinent. Studies reviewed showed high rates of heterogeneity, with dhat syndrome more common in younger men. Depressive and anxiety symptoms were common with key symptoms of fatigue, sleepiness, and sexual dysfunction. Social support, sexual education, and clinical engagement were found beneficial in some cases. They concluded that dhat was probably a manifestation of depression or anxiety disorders in some cultures.

Prakash [41] described symptom duration varying from less than 3 months up to 1 year even up to 20 years in extreme cases. Individuals reported loss of semen in sleep, with urine, masturbation, and both heterosexual and homosexual sex.

Not surprisingly, both sexual dysfunction and common mental disorders accompany semen-loss anxiety. Psychosexual dysfunctions associated with dhat were predominantly erectile dysfunction (22–62 percent) and premature ejaculation (22–44 percent), while depressive neurosis (40–42 percent), anxiety neurosis (21–38 percent), and somatoform/hypochondriasis (32–40 percent) were the most frequently reported psychiatric disorders in these groups. The review observed that individuals with dhat syndrome showed significantly different illness-related beliefs and behaviors compared to controls. Presentation had similarities with recognized somatic syndromes. In this sample, about two-thirds recovered (66 percent), 22 percent showed improvement, and 12 percent had no symptom change. It is worth noting that the majority of individuals identified did not attend follow-up treatment or reviews, suggesting a dissatisfaction with medical explanations proffered [41].

Dhat, or semen-loss anxiety, reflects attitudes to masculinity, sex role, procreation, and the role semen plays in confirming virility. Any loss reflects weakness. It is entirely possible that in a sex-negative society, where the function of sex is purely procreative, it is inevitable that loss of semen due to masturbation, nocturnal emission, or other means will carry with it serious anxieties. When semen-loss anxiety was much more prevalent in Britain and the U.S., treatments such as dietary additions including corn flakes and crackers recommended by Kellogg and Graham, respectively, were common panacea. Similarly, at the present time in India many traditional healers offer dietary supplements and herbal preparations offering virility and return to masculinity. Whether this semen-loss anxiety has entirely disappeared from the West is an open question that needs exploration. It must also be remembered that using dhat as an idiom of distress may allow individuals to seek help, whereas having erectile dysfunction or depression may well carry more stigma and prevent seeing a health practitioner. Cultural influences are more relevant in understanding what is needed and what expressions are acceptable.

The future of culture-bound syndromes

The future of culture-bound syndromes or culture-specific manifestations of distress as a range of disorders is uncertain. While dhat has endured centuries of societal and cultural change in the Indian subcontinent, brain fag has gone through substantial nosological decline. In fact, only very few Nigerian students in modern times would have ever heard the idiom of distress "brain fag," given the colonial legacy of the term.

Effect of globalisation

Globalisation has led to the cross fertilisation of cultures and belief systems. Real-time use of social media such as Facebook and Twitter has led to the open discussion of ideas and values in different geographical and cultural regions. In the less technologically developed world, this is limited to urban areas with power and Internet resources. In addition, the penetration of global corporations such as McDonalds and Coca-Cola into different cultures merges the experience of some younger generations. However, it is inevitable that with increased compression of time and fast transmission of ideas as a result of globalization, cultural values and attitudes will change. If that leads to further acculturation and changes in idioms of distress, then the culture-boundedness too will change. Furthermore, current migration trends for economic reasons or fleeing conflict would suggest that groups of individuals may well carry their idioms of distress and folk illness categories with them but in the new country may face challenges seeking help or being understood by practitioners they present to.

Urbanisation

Within the same country or geographical region, additional differences may present between urban and rural areas. Folk illness and explanatory models are more likely to be preserved in rural areas than in urban cities with some forms of distress. Conversely, the waves of panic and hysteria associated with Koro or "disappearing penises" are more pronounced in densely populated cities than villages in Nigeria.

Globalisation and migration contribute to the rapid industrialisation of some parts of the world with observable social evolution in countries such as Brazil, China, India, and South Africa. For example, a new syndrome, *hikiko-mori*, is being described from Japan, where teenagers become withdrawn socially. Whether this is a genuine response to changing pressures related to social media remains to be seen, but this reflects the likelihood that newer syndromes may well continue to develop and emerge.

Conclusion

Idioms of distress and certain psychiatric syndromes are very strongly influenced by cultural attitudes and values. Contents of delusions on the one hand will be affected by personal, social, and cultural experiences, and as cultures progress and evolve the terms used to explain distress will also change. It is inevitable that culture-bound syndromes will be no longer culturally bound but culturally influenced. We anticipate some previously described culture-bound or specific disorders will decline over time and may well go extinct, whereas new ones may well emerge. Other syndromes may become more prominent as societal value systems shift, for instance, attitudes to body mass and the relationship with eating disorders. The alternative prediction is that with better understanding of other societies, there may eventually be a less Western diagnostic weight given to the appreciation of mental distress in less familiar settings or individuals.

Acknowledgments

Thanks to Cambridge University Press for permission to reproduce Tables 17.2 and Table 17.3 from *Textbook of Cultural Psychiatry*, edited by Dinesh Bhugra and Kamaldeep Bhui, Cambridge University Press, 2007.

References

1 Yap PM. (1962). Words and things in comparative psychiatry with special reference to exotic psychosis. *Acta Psychiatrica Scandinavia* 38, 157–82.
2 Yap PM. (1969). The culture bound syndromes. In *Mental Health Research in Asia and the Pacific*, Cahil W, Lin TY (eds.), pp. 33–53. Honolulu: East-West Centre Press.
3 Bhugra D, Jacob KS. (1997). Culture bound syndromes. In *Troublesome Disguises*, Bhugra D, Monro A (eds.), pp. 296–334. Oxford: Blackwell.
4 Hughes CC, Wintrob RM. (1995). Culture bound syndromes and the cultural context of clinical psychiatry. In *Review of Psychiatry*, Oldham JM, Riba M (eds.), pp. 565–97. Washington, DC: APA.
5 Hughes CC. (1996). The culture bound syndromes and psychiatric diagnosis. In *Culture and Psychiatric Diagnosis: A DSM IV Perspective*, Mezzich J, Kleinman A, Fabrega H, et al., pp. 298–308. Washington, DC: APA.
6 Littlewood R. (1996). Cultural comments on culture bound syndromes: I. In *Culture and Psychiatric Diagnosis: A DSM IV Perspective*, Mezzich J, Kleinman A, Fabrega H, et al., pp. 309–12. Washington, DC: APA.
7 Hofstede G. (1980). *Culture's Consequences: International Differences in Work-Related Values.* Beverly Hills: Sage.
8 Maercker A. (2001). Association of cross-cultural differences in psychiatric morbidity with cultural values: A secondary data analysis. *German Journal of Psychiatry* 4, 17–23.
9 World Health Organisation. (1992). ICD 10, *International Classification of Diseases: Classifications of Mental and Behavioural Disorder.* Geneva.
10 American Psychiatric Association. (2000). *Diagnostic and Statistical Manual of Mental Disorders*, 4th ed. (DSM-IV-TR). Washington, DC.
11 American Psychiatric Association. (2013). *Diagnostic and Statistical Manual of Mental Disorders*, 5th ed. (DSM-5). Washington, DC.

12 Hughes CC. (1985). Glossary. In *Culture Bound Syndromes,* Simons RC, Hughes CC (eds.), pp. 465–505. Dordrecht: Reidel.

13 Simons RC, Hughes CC. (1985). *Culture Bound Syndromes,* pp. 465–505. Dordrecht: Reidel.

14 Bhugra D, Sumathipala A, Siribaddana S. (2007). Culture-bound syndromes: A re-evaluation. In *Textbook of Cultural Psychiatry,* Bhugra D, Bhui K (eds.), pp. 141–56. Cambridge: Cambridge University Press.

15 Ayonrinde O. (2008). Brain fag syndrome: New wines in old bottles or old wine in new bottles. *Nigerian Journal of Psychiatry* 6(2), 47–50.

16 Prince R. (1960). The "brain fag" syndrome in Nigerian students. *Journal of Mental Science* 106, 559–70.

17 Ayonrinde O. (2009). *A History of "Brain Fag" in the 19th and 20th Century.* Thesis. Society of Apothecaries, London.

18 Tuke DH. (1880). Intemperance in study. *Journal of Mental Science* 25, 495–504.

19 *American Illustrated Medical Dictionary.* (1901). Philadelphia and London: W.B. Saunders and Co. 2nd ed.

20 *Lippincott's New Medical Dictionary.* (1910). Philadelphia and London: J. P. Lippincott Co.

21 Gillespie RD. (1926). Fatigue: A clinical study. *Journal of Neurology and Psychopathology* 7, 26.

22 Gillespie RD. (1933). Psychotherapy in general practice. *Lancet* 221, 5706, 7, 1–8.

23 Ayonrinde O, Obuaya C. (2008). *Brain Fag Syndrome: The extinction of a culture bound syndrome? Abstracts of 161st Meeting of the American Psychiatric Association,* Washington DC, May.

24 Ayonrinde O, Obuaya C. (2008). *"Brain Fag": A British culture bound syndrome. Abstracts of Annual General Meeting of the Royal College of Psychiatrists.* London, July.

25 Morakinyo O. (1980). A psychophysiological theory of a psychiatric illness (the brain fag syndrome) associated with study among Africans. *Journal of Nervous and Mental Disorders* 168(2), 84–9.

26 Jegede RO. (1983). Psychiatric illness in African students: "Brain fag" syndrome revisited. *Canadian Journal of Psychiatry* 28(3), 188–92.

27 Ola BA, Morakinyo O, Adewuya AO. (2009). Brain fag syndrome: A myth or a reality. *African Journal of Psychiatry* 12(2), 135–43, 199.

28 Harris B. (1981). A case of brain fag in East Africa. *The British Journal of Psychiatry* 139, 162–63.

29 Peltzer K, Cherian VI, Cherian L. (1998). Brain fag symptoms in rural South African secondary school pupils. *Psychololgy Reports* 83(3 Pt 2), 1187–96.

30 Wig NN. (1960). Problems of the mental health in India. *Journal of Clinical & Social Psychiatry* (India) 17, 48–53.

31 Bhugra D, Buchanan A. (1989). Impotence in ancient Indian texts. *Sexual and Marital Therapy* 4, 87–92.

32 Malhotra HK, Wig NN. (1975). A culture bound sex neurosis in the Orient. *Archives of Sexual Behaviour* 4, 519–28.

33 Chadda RK, Ahuja N. (1990). Dhat syndrome: A sex neurosis in India Subcontinent. *British Journal of Psychiatry* 156, 577–79.

34 Bhatia MS, Malik SC. (1991). Dhat syndrome: A useful diagnostic entity in Indian culture. *British Journal of Psychiatry* 159, 691–95.

35 Behere PB, Natraj GS. (1984) Dhat syndrome: The phenomenology of a culture bound sex neurosis of the orient. *Indian Journal of Psychiatry* 26(1), 76–8.

36 Singh G. (1985) Dhat syndrome revisited. *Indian Journal of Psychiatry* 27(2), 119–22.

37 De Silva P, Dissanayake SAW. (1989) The loss of semen syndrome in Sri Lanka. A clinical study. *Sexual and Marital Therapy,* 4, 195–204.

38 Janaki R, Vikhram R, Thiruvikraman S, Naveen S, Anjana R, Srinivasan B, Ramasubramanian C. (2012). A study of sexual misconceptions and prevalence of Dhat syndrome in adolescents and young males presenting to psychiatry outpatient department. *Indian Journal of Psychiatry* 54/(S88).

39 Jadhav, S. (2007). Dhis and Dhat: Evidence of semen retention syndrome amongst white Britons. *Anthropology & Medicine* 14(3), 229–39.

40 Udina M, Foulon H, Valdes M, Bhattacharyya S, Martin-Santos R. (2013). Dhat syndrome: A systematic review. *Psychosomatics: Journal of Consultation and Liaison Psychiatry* 54(3), 212–18.

41 Prakash O. (2007). Lessons for postgraduate trainees about Dhat syndrome. *Indian Journal of Psychiatry* 49(3), 208–10.

CHAPTER 18

Delusional infestations

Julio Torales

Professor of Psychiatry and Medical Psychology and Head of the Psychodermatology Unit,
Department of Psychiatry, School of Medical Sciences, National University of Asunción, Paraguay

Introduction

Delusional infestation (DI), sometimes known as delusion of parasitosis, is a clinical entity classified in the Koblenzer's "strictly psychiatric skin conditions" group. It is characterized by patients' fixed belief that their body, mainly their skin, is infested by small, vivid or non-vivid pathogens in the absence of any dermatological or microbiological evidence [1–3]. The delusion can lead to abnormal cutaneous symptoms such as itching, biting, or crawling sensations. Patients often show self-destructive behavior in an effort to rid the pathogens from under their skin, leading to excoriations, ulcerations, and serious secondary infections [3, 4]. The patients are reluctant to seek help from psychiatrists, and are likely to consult family and general physicians, dermatologists, and even microbiologists first [5]. These treatment approaches may lead to problems in the patient's care due to difficulties in accurate diagnosis and inappropriate use of treatment programs.

In most cases, the prognosis is generally good, as long as the affected patients are adequately treated in a multidisciplinary way by dermatologists and psychiatrists with expertise in the disease [5].

This chapter presents information about how these patients may present and how psychiatrists, dermatologists, and general physicians in various settings can diagnose and manage this challenging group of patients. An illustrated case will be presented to highlight key clinical features, current diagnosis, management, and treatment of patients with DI.

Troublesome Disguises: Managing Challenging Disorders in Psychiatry, Second Edition.
Edited by Dinesh Bhugra and Gin S. Malhi.

Historical context

In 1938, Ekbom provided detailed description of the clinical picture, deepened its psychopathology, and called the syndrome by a German term, *Dermatozoenwahn* (from the ancient Greek "derma"=skin, "zoon"=living being/animal, and German "Wahn"=delusion). Because the original term was found somewhat difficult to use in different countries, the condition was called Ekbom's syndrome. However, several authors considered this eponym ambiguous and recommended not using it, because this term is also used to refer to restless legs syndrome [1], but often the term and its use persist.

Some other terms such as *dermatophobia, acarophobia,* and *parasiticphobia* have been used, but from a psychopathological standpoint, these terms are not entirely suitable because the patient experiences are not phobia or secondary avoidance behaviors but delusions. Similarly, the term *illusion of parasitosis* is not correct, since the entity is not characterized by the presence of illusions, but by delusions. In 1946, Wilson and Miller introduced the term *delusions of parasitosis* [5–7] and it has become one of the most used and recognized names for the condition.

However, patients may report various forms of infestation, thus the name has the disadvantage of covering only one type of pathogens [1]. Therefore, the broader term *delusional infestation* should be preferred because it has two main advantages: It highlights the psychopathological aspect (a thought expressing delusional disorder), and it covers all varieties of imaginary pathogens by referring to the delusional theme "infestation" and not to a single species.

Strictly, DI is not a diagnosis per se and has no category of its own in the DSM-5 or ICD-10; however, it is included both in the ICD-10 and DSM-5 in the "delusional disorders" section, in the case of primary DI [8].

Case presentation

Written informed consent was obtained from the patient for publication of this case presentation. A copy of the written consent is available from the author.

Mr. A, a 48-year-old Caucasian male, divorced, a bus driver, with 2 years of history of multiple excoriations and ulcers widely distributed over his chest, back, and lower limbs (see Figure 18.1) and no previous psychiatric history, presented with his 67-year-old mother to the psychodermatology outpatient unit. He had been previously seen and assessed by a general dermatologist, who decided to refer the patient to this unit.

The initial dermatology assessment led to the diagnosis of DI as the patient believed that his skin injuries had been produced by "black bugs and white

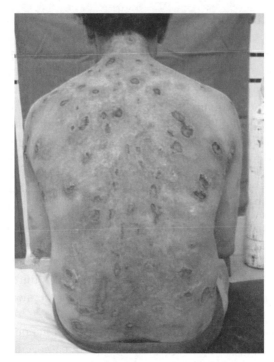

Figure 18.1 Multiple excoriations and ulcers widely distributed in patient's back.

worms that are in his skin and eat his flesh." He added that "these bugs and worms forced him to scratch his skin with his fingers, rocks, stones, and other elements to scrape them out of his flesh. His mother helped him in this task." The patient's past medical history was not significant. Dermatology assessment ruled out parasitic infestation. The patient's mother confirmed her son's history and she asked for help in order to cure his son. She also explained that she had been helping her son "using a little rock to scratch her son's back."

On evaluation in the psychodermatology unit, the patient was oriented to place and time. His sensorium was clear. His affect was euthymic and there were no other abnormal behaviours, thoughts, or delusions. At work, he was able to function normally. At the first assessment his insight and judgment were judged to be poor. All these features favored a diagnosis of DI in Mr. A. Main differential diagnosis with DI was schizophrenia, other delusional disorders, dermatitis artifacta, and excoriation (skin picking) disorder [2].

Due to the multiple excoriations and large ulcerations, treatment with colloidal solution to be applied over the cutaneous lesions was initiated in Mr. A. Also, it was decided to commence the patient on risperidone 3 mg/day in a single nocturnal dose.

After 2 weeks of treatment, the skin injuries began to heal and the delusional state of Mr. A improved and at the same time his mother's mental state

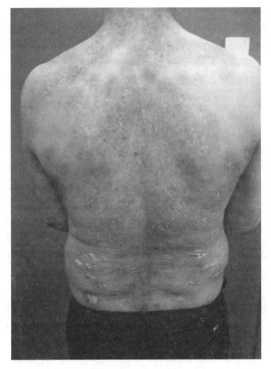

Figure 18.2 Appearance of cutaneous lesions after healing.

changed and she became more amenable to the idea that the condition was psychiatric. Fourteen days after starting risperidone, the patient started to question the presence of bugs and worms in his skin. After 8 weeks, there were no evidence of excoriations and ulcers in the patient's skin (see Figure 18.2), and the delusions had disappeared. Antipsychotic treatment was continued for 6 months and the patient remained symptom-free. Mr. A. remains symptom-free at the time of this writing.

Clinical features

The typical patient

The typical DI patient is generally a middle-aged or elderly female with limited social contacts, generally no previous psychiatric history, and normal cognitive function [9]. DI can occur in people with any type of personality, but it is said to be more frequent in those with obsessive or paranoid characters [4, 10].

The affected body sites can include: skin, hair, various parts of the body, or natural orifices. The DI onset may be sudden or slow, and it is often accompanied by itching, which is followed by intense scratching [5, 10, 11].

When patients are able to "catch some of the pathogens," they are taken to the physician as proof of infestation. These specimens are usually presented in a small bin, vessel, bag, piece of paper, or plastic foil to protect them. The "proof" usually consists of dull and uncritical material, such as dander, crusts, scabs from healing skin lesions, hair, threads, and other particles from clothes, fibers, dirt, or sand [12]. Increasingly patients present movies or digital photos of the sites said to be infected [1]. This peculiar behavior was named the "matchbox sign" in the *Lancet* [13]. However, Freudenmann and Lepping have proposed the name specimen sign, because it seems more appropriate to point to the "pathogen" rather than the receptacle. This term is preferable as this is comprehensive and covers all kinds of delivered material, including digital photos [2].

Not surprisingly the more the patients try in vain to free themselves from the infestation, the more distressed and desperate they become [2]. The literature describes dangerous actions such as burning one's "infested" furniture or clothes or running away from home [14] to avoid further infestations. Furthermore, some patients have burned their own skin using abrasive detergents to "kill the pathogens" [4]. Sometimes patients go on to develop secondary depressive symptoms within the context of the delusional disorder. Occasional cases of attempted suicide and suicide have been reported [15].

From a clinical perspective, DI is a delusional disorder, of somatic type, with dermatological specific content. Le and Gonski [16] classify DI as follows:

Primary DI, when the disease is the only psychiatric disorder present

Secondary DI (functional), when there is an underlying psychiatric disorder, such as major depressive disorder, anxiety disorder, or others that may lead to delusion

Secondary DI (organic or substance-induced), when there is an underlying medical disorder that may cause the delusion or the delusion is substance-induced

The clinical course of DI is quite variable and depends mainly on the type of DI. Primary DI has an insidious onset and a chronic course. This kind of chronic course is also seen in patients with DI secondary to medical illnesses (most of the patients in this category are likely to be elderly). In contrast, substance-induced DI has an acute onset and its symptoms last only for hours, days, or weeks.

Epidemiology

There is a relative deficiency of reliable data on the epidemiology of DI for most countries [2]. Trabert, in a meta-analysis, found higher prevalence of the disease in women (with a ratio of 2–6:1 in comparison with males), especially among those 50–55 years old. This difference increases proportionally with age [17]. Ekbom attributed this to aging and deterioration of brain functions. No relationship has been reported with economic or social factors [11]. DI is usually a disorder of middle-aged and elderly patients [2, 4, 5]. According to

Table 18.1 Minimal criteria for DI.

Minimal criteria for DI

1. Conviction of being infested by pathogens (small, vivid, inanimate [rare], often "new to science") without any medical or microbiological evidence for this, ranging from overvalued ideas to a fixed, unshakable belief.
2. Abnormal sensations in the skin explained by the first criterion (usually meeting criteria of qualitatively abnormal sensations).

Additional symptoms	Additional facultative psychotic and nonpsychotic symptoms (e.g., visual illusions or hallucinations) may be present.
Location	Skin (on, in, or under), but all parts of the body may be infested.
Duration	Typically months or years (chronic), ranging from minutes (if secondary to toxic psychosis or delirium) to years.

Trabert's meta-analysis [17], the mean age at clinical presentation was 57.02 (±14.6) years. Men and patients with schizophrenia were significantly younger than the average patient [18].

Diagnosis

Freudenmann and Lepping [2] have proposed a set of minimal criteria for the diagnosis of DI, taking into account that the disease is not classified as an independent entity in the ICD-10 or DSM-5 (see Table 18.1):

Differential diagnosis

In trying to understand DI, the first step is to check whether this is primary or secondary. Thus it needs to be differentiated from other psychiatric conditions, such as schizophrenia, obsessive compulsive disorder, major depressive disorder (with psychotic symptoms), excoriation (skin picking) disorder, and dermatitis artifacta (see Table 18.2); from organic or substance-induced conditions (general medical conditions, brain disorders, prescribed medication, and illicit substances [e.g., "cocaine bugs"]); and from formication [2, 4, 5].

Treatment

The therapeutic approach to DI depends primarily on etiology [19]. In cases of primary DI and those secondary to schizophrenia, the main intervention is antipsychotic medication (usually given orally; less frequently intramuscular depot formulations may be used when patients' adherence and compliance to treatment is problematic). Cases secondary to depression must focus on treating depression treated as any other major depressive episode with psychotic symptoms, with antidepressants plus antipsychotics [9]. Occasionally major depressive disorder with concomitant DI symptoms may respond to antidepressant therapy alone without the need for antipsychotic treatment. For both primary and secondary DI, decisive clinical trials are still missing [1, 4, 5].

Table 18.2 Main differential diagnosis of DI.

Diagnosis	Main difference
Schizophrenia	Delusions and behaviors in schizophrenia are often bizarre, in contrast to delusions in delusional disorders such as primary DI [4].
Major depressive disorder (with psychotic symptoms)	Patients with a major depressive disorder (with psychotic symptoms) usually present with delusions of guilt or hypochondriacal ideas, while psychotic symptoms from the spectrum of DI are rare complications.
Excoriation (skin picking) disorder	The skin manipulations and lesions seen on the excoriation (skin picking) disorder can be similar to those seen in DI, but they are not based on an imaginary presence of pathogens in the skin.
Dermatitis artifacta	This entity represents a form of factitious disorder [5].
Formication	The symptom of "feeling ants crawling on the skin" (from Latin "formica" = ant) is very frequent and unspecific and does not justify a diagnosis of DI. The absence of a fixed belief of being infested would indicate that DI is absent [2].

The first-line antipsychotics to be used are the atypical ones, such as risperidone. Older studies have shown good results following the use of pimozide [4, 5]. although it has been suggested that this drug is no longer the treatment of choice for reasons of drug safety [1, 2]. The initial dose should be as low as possible with gradual build-up if needed, in order to avoid the occurrence of adverse effects, which would be responsible for the discontinuation of the medication. With treatment, the improvement of the condition is about 50–75 percent [5].

Delusions may also respond and change considerably with adjunctive psychological approach. In all cases it is necessary to conduct a comprehensive psychiatric diagnosis. Secondary injuries to scratching, secondary infection, or ulceration should be treated with appropriate dermatological therapy.

Management problems and potential solutions

Mind the skin

In 2002, Revelli and colleagues adapted the original Koblenzer's classification of 1983 and distinguished three types of connections between the psyche and the skin [20]:

Strictly psychiatric skin conditions, which include dermatitis artifacta, excoriation (skin picking) disorder, and DI.

Dermatoses connected with psychological factors, where we would find neurodermatitis, lichen planus, and some chronic hives.

Skin disorders modified by stress, which include psoriasis, atopic dermatitis, and seborrheic dermatitis, among others.

Patients with any of these diseases initially consult a dermatologist (or a general physician), who has responsibility to discover whether the skin condition is related to psychological or psychiatric factors. If so, the professional can then refer the patient to a psychiatrist. However, in reality this situation is hindered in practice for the patients' reluctance to seek consultation with a mental health specialist, because they may not accept that their skin condition is the product of a psychiatric disorder. An ingenious solution, often practiced in Europe and now in use at the National University of Asunción (Paraguay), is conducting a psychodermatology assessment. This is a multidisciplinary consultation, in which a dermatologist and a liaison psychiatrist are closely involved in joint assessments. The consultation usually takes place in the dermatology facility. The simultaneous presence of two doctors, one who looks and touches and another one who listens, improves the link between the skin and psyche and allows the patient to feel considered as a whole. This helps obviate the patient's reluctance to undergo a psychiatric evaluation and forms an effective and accurate therapeutic alliance, which ensures the success of treatment [4, 5, 20].

Approaching a patient with DI

To better prepare the treating physician, some approaches have been proposed [1, 2, 4, 5, 21–23]. Although some of the suggestions listed below (see Table 18.3) have a low level of evidence, they are helpful tips for clinical management of patients with DI [2].

Table 18.3 Some suggestions for approaching a patient with DI.

Approaching a patient with DI

Take the necessary time to take a careful history.

Perform the diagnostic investigations needed (even if you are sure that the patient has no infection). Examine all "specimens" carefully.

Acknowledge the patient's suffering.

Paraphrase the symptoms ("you are itching," "the sensations," "the crawling," etc.) instead of reinforcing or questioning them.

Answer that you did not find any pathogens so far, but you are sure that the patient really suffers from his perceptions.

Try to introduce antipsychotics as the only substances helpful against these processes, as suggested by current research.

Use the names "unexplained dermopathy" or "Ekbom's syndrome" if the patient asks for the diagnosis.

Do not try to convince the patient or question the patient's beliefs.

Do not use words like "delusion(al)," "psychotic," "psychological," "psychiatric," etc.

Do not prescribe antibiotics or any other anti-infective without a real infection (thus avoiding further reinforcing the delusion).

Do not forget to ask patients with despair and signs of manifest depression about suicidal ideation and to evaluate any risk to others.

Conclusions

DI is a strictly psychiatric skin condition, sometimes difficult to diagnose and treat. The condition can occur as a delusional disorder of somatic type (primary DI) or secondary to numerous other conditions. Patients with DI pose a truly interdisciplinary problem to the medical system.

DI prognosis lies in how quickly the diagnosis and the treatment are established and how the condition is assessed by both dermatologists and psychiatrists. Dermatologists should be aware of the possibility of finding skin conditions strongly linked to psychological/psychiatric factors and should seek the assistance of a mental health specialist in order to establish a psychodermatology approach, which is crucial for therapeutic success.

In primary DI, antipsychotics are the treatment of choice. If adequately treated, the DI prognosis is good, with improvements in 50–75 percent of cases. Worse prognosis is noted in patients with concomitant organic disease and those with a chronic course of the illness.

Future research should focus on the neural basis, pathogenesis, and psychobiology of DI, as well as on conclusive clinical trials, which are still lacking. In order to do so, there will be a need for creative, patient-oriented, and psychodermatology approaches, since otherwise patients are unlikely to adhere to any study protocol.

References

1 Heller MM, Wong JW, Lee ES, Ladizinski B, Grau M, Howard JL, Berger TG, Koo JY, Murase JE. Delusional infestations: Clinical presentation, diagnosis and treatment. *Int J Dermatol* 2013; 52(7):775–83.

2 Freudenmann R, Lepping P. Delusional infestation. *Clin Microbiol Rev* 2009; 22(4):690–732.

3 Revelli C, Pichon M, Cambazard F, Pellet J, Misery L. Consultation dermato-psychiatrique. *Annales de Dermatologie et de Vénéréologie* 2002; 129:742–45.

4 Torales J, Arce, A, Bolla L, González L, Di Martino, Rodríguez M, Knopfelmacher O. Delirio parasitario dermatozoico: Reporte de un caso. *An Fac Cienc Méd* (Asunción) 2011; 44 (2):81–7.

5 González L, Torales J, Arce A, Di Martino B, Valdovinos G, Rodríguez M, Knopfelmacher O, Bolla L. Síndrome de Ekbom: A propósito de un caso. *Art Terap Dermatol* 2010; 33:140–45.

6 Musalek M, Bach M, Passweg V, Jaeger S. The position of delusional parasitosis in psychiatric nosology and classification. *Psychopathology* 1990; 23:115–24.

7 Wilson JW, Miller HE. Delusions of parasitosis (acarophobia). *Arch Dermatol* 1946; 54:39–56.

8 American Psychiatric Association. *Diagnostic and Statistical Manual of Mental Disorders*, 4th ed. Arlington, VA. American Psychiatric Association, 2013.

9 Freudenmann RW, Schönfeldt-Lecuona C, Lepping P. Primary delusional parasitosis treated with olanzapine. *Int Psychogeriatr* 2007; 19:1161–68.

10 Chuleung K, Jinmi K, Mounghoon L. Delusional parasitosis as "folie a deux." *J Korean Med Sci* 2002; 18:462–65.

11 Lyell A. Delusions of parasitosis. *Br J Dermatol* 1983; 108:485–89.

12 Wykoff RF. Delusions of parasitosis: A review. *Rev Infect Dis* 1987; 9:433–37.

13 Lee WR. Matchbox sign. *Lancet* 1983; ii:457–58. (Letter)

14 Goddard J. Analysis of 11 cases of delusions of parasitosis reported to the Mississippi Department of Health. *South Med J* 1995; 88:837–39.

15 Monk BE, Rao YJ. Delusions of parasitosis with fatal outcome. *Clin Exp Dermatol* 1994; 19:341–42.

16 Le L, Gonski PN. Delusional parasitosis mimicking cutaneous infestation in elderly patients. *Med J Aust* 2003; 179:209–14.

17 Trabert W. 100 years of delusional parasitosis: Metaánalysis of 1223 case reports. *Psychopathology* 1995; 25:238–46.

18 Trabert W. Epidemiology of delusional ectoparasitic infestation. *Nervenarzt* 1991; 62:165–69.

19 Freudenmann RW. Delusions of parasitosis: An up-to-date review. *Fortschr Neurol Psychiatr* 2002; 70:531–41.

20 Revelli C, Pichon M, Cambazard F, Pellet J, Misery L. Consultation dermato-psychiatrique. *Annales de Dermatologie et de Vénéréologie* 2002; 129:742–45.

21 Slaughter JR, Zanol K, Rezvani H, Flax J. Psychogenic parasitosis. A case series and literature review. *Psychosomatics* 1998; 39:491–500.

22 Zanol K, Slaughter J, Hall R. An approach to the treatment of psychogenic parasitosis. *Int J Dermatol* 1998; 37:56–63.

23 Zomer SF, De Wit RF, Van Bronswijk JE, Nabarro G, Van Vloten WA. Delusions of parasitosis: A psychiatric disorder to be treated by dermatologists? An analysis of 33 patients. *Br J Dermatol* 1998; 138:1030–32.

CHAPTER 19

Baffling clinical encounters: Navigating a pain and psychiatric Quichua syndrome

Sioui Maldonado-Bouchard[1], Lise Bouchard[2], and Mario Incayawar[3]

[1] Research Associate, Runajambi Institute for the Study of Quichua Culture and Health, Otavalo, Ecuador
[2] Director of Research, Runajambi Institute for the Study of Quichua Culture and Health, Otavalo, Ecuador
[3] Director, Runajambi Institute for the Study of Quichua Culture and Health, Otavalo, Ecuador

A puzzling encounter

Mrs. Lema's daughter, Miss Farinango (fictitious names), was feeling helpless. Concerned by her mother's health the past several months, Miss Farinango had decided, as a last resort, to seek the help of a doctor in Quito, the capital of Ecuador. This had been an effort in money, time, and energy, traveling to the city from their village; long hours walking to the nearest road with her ill mother, and then several bus rides to the capital. Once in Quito, they had consulted a doctor, but he had dismissed the illness, labeling the symptoms as the result of Quichua superstition and nothing more. Mrs. Lema and Miss Farinango had returned to their home in the mountains feeling that the entire trip had been in vain. Mrs. Lema continued to feel ill, and nothing seemed to help. It had begun suddenly, shortly after a family quarrel over land. She began losing her appetite, and soon felt weak for hours at a time. It was usually worse during the evenings. She would complain that her mouth felt dry, and she felt light headed. Often she would wrap herself in blankets, complaining of cold. At first, Mrs. Lema thought that this would pass, but with time her symptoms only became more severe, until she began feeling as though she did not have a reason to live. She was certain one of her neighbors, who had been part of the quarrel over land, had put a curse on her. She felt powerless and betrayed, and could not understand how they could have taken such terrible action. Worried that she was suffering from *llaqui*, Mrs. Lema and her daughter went to see several *yachactaitas* (Quichua traditional healers). Mrs. Lema would feel better after the *yachactaitas'* treatments, but the symptoms would eventually come back. She ultimately returned to see a doctor, who said her loss of appetite could be due to a problem with her gall bladder. Using up an important part of their life savings, Mrs. Lema underwent surgery for removal of her gall bladder. Yet her symptoms persisted after the surgery. In despair Mrs. Lema and Miss Farinango contacted Dr. Incayawar, after hearing about one of his articles on Andean syndromes, published in a local newspaper. A transcultural psychiatrist and pain specialist from the Runajambi Institute diagnosed Mrs. Lema as suffering from *llaqui*, a Quichua pain and psychiatric syndrome.

The two solitudes

The western view

The clinical encounter with a Quichua patient suffering from *llaqui* is challenging for a biomedically trained doctor or health professional. The syndrome appears relatively simple yet at the same time impenetrable; the doctor is faced with the same feelings someone experiences when dealing with the unknown and strange.

The symptoms presented by the Quichua patient suffering from *llaqui* are the ones we commonly encounter in general medical practice in any society. Patients will primarily present a wide array of somatic symptoms to their doctors, including headaches, fatigue, nausea, vomiting, minor fever, migratory pain, and stomach pain. This is followed by some psychological symptoms such as worries, easy weeping, sadness, and the like. However, the doctor never gets a profile of symptoms that would allow a proper diagnosis. After close examination of a series of *llaqui* patients, it may look as though any symptom could be present in any patient. For this reason, researchers suggest that the identification of this culture-bound syndrome should not be based on symptoms configuration but rather on the local causes attributed to it [1].

The sources of this challenging medical encounter lie in at least in two factors: (1) lack of knowledge regarding the nature of *llaqui*, despite it being a highly prevalent condition among the Quichuas of the Andes, and (2) physicians' ethnic or racial bias.

Lack of knowledge about the nature of llaqui

Typically, the *mishu*[1] doctor (as the mestizos or Latinos are called in Quichua) will focus on the most familiar somatic symptoms and will figure out a diagnosis such as "lack of vitamins," malnutrition, pain, and parasitic disease, among others. Consequently, the treatment is polypharmacy based on vitamins, aspirin, or combination of analgesics, and occasionally medicines against helminths. As a result of this quick, simplistic approach, doubts remain concerning the accuracy of the diagnosis performed and appropriateness of the treatment plan adopted. Some patients will return again and again complaining of the same symptoms that led the doctor to dismiss a patient or to declare that nothing is wrong and "all is in your head" in the first place. On occasion, especially when patients claim having *llaqui*, which is a local culture-bound syndrome, physicians conclude that it is not a real illness; that it is rather an ailment resulting from superstition, and therefore lacking in any clinical importance. This misunderstanding reinforces the deeply held belief among the Quichuas that the *mishu* doctor knows little about *llaqui*, or is not qualified to treat it. Understandably, some patients will not return, realizing that the doctor does not give credit to their complaints and the treatment offered does not work. The poor-quality medical care frequently does not translate to relief for patients, but rather results in their deterioration or, even worse, in their death. For this reason, almost all Quichua patients are fearful of seeking care from biomedically trained doctors and some are so mistrustful that they believe that the doctors' mission is to kill Quichua patients. The doctors' lack of knowledge about *llaqui* clearly contributes to their disgraceful image within the Quichua society in the Andes.

Physicians' ethnic or racial bias

Despite the fact that the *mishu* doctors live surrounded by millions of Quichua people in the Andes, they globally disregard the Quichuas and therefore create a social space where two solitudes co-exist. For a population of five and a half million Quichuas in Ecuador, there are only five Quichua physicians [2]. Physicians in the Andes are almost exclusively unilingual Spanish speakers. Therefore they do not speak the Quichua language; they rarely interact with the Quichua people outside the clinical field; and they do not receive any course on cultural competence during medical training, so they are not skilled to provide services that are culturally sensitive. Appallingly, a report from the World Health Organization reported that the indigenous people are racially discriminated against, and treated as second-class citizens and as inferiors [3]. These massive cultural and linguistic barriers, lack of training in cultural dimensions of illness, plus racism and ethnic discrimination, makes the Quichua patients feel they are not welcomed in a *mishu* medical setting. In addition, the history of brutal colonialism of the last five centuries in the Americas makes the Quichua patients suspicious and fearful that they will not be helped or treated respectfully but rather humiliated, attacked, or even killed by *mishu* health professionals [4].

Racial profiling and ostracism in medical care

The indigenous peoples of the Americas, including the Quichuas of the Andes, are viewed in the Western imagery as savages, dangerous, violent, and stoic. In this biased colonialist view, Quichuas are dirty, backward people, illiterate, a barrier to progress, a nuisance in the medical encounter and good public health. It is not surprising to find that in many countries in the Americas, not only the military but also health policy makers will whisper that the "best Indian is a dead Indian."

With such deeply entrenched and generalized prejudices in the mainstream *mishu* society, it comes as no surprise that expressions of racism, bigotry, ostracism, bias, and discrimination against the Americas' first inhabitants are used in the medical arena. The most dramatic manifestation occurred recently when an entire population was blamed for the outbreak of epidemics that threatened the public health of an entire nation.

For nearly a decade, in the 90s, a particularly deadly epidemic of cholera surged in the Andes, including Ecuador. Thousands died, and entire communities were in panic. Public health officials and health services in the country were overwhelmed. Shamefully, health professionals, health officials, and the lay *mishu* population blamed the Quichuas for this crisis. Soon, on the streets, in public places, and in hospitals, *mishu* (Latinos) were attributing the cholera epidemic in Ecuador to the Quichuas' bad customs, hygiene, habits, values, and culture. They literally blamed the victims of this deadly disease for the epidemic and deflected the responsibility of the outbreaks from the public health institutions and health officials to the Quichua victims. For example, educated *mishus* and health professionals deplored the "detestable" Quichua tradition of washing the body of the dead before burial, because they thought the bacterium Vibrio cholera contaminated waters and spread the disease.

This phenomenon of blaming an entire group for an epidemic affected not only Ecuador but other countries in the region such as Venezuela [5]. Many *mishu* doctors and health policy makers concluded, "If they are not able to help themselves, why should we help them?" Throughout history in Ecuador, other diseases that ravaged the Quichua people, such as malnutrition, goiter, tuberculosis, and others, were attributed to their bad cultural traits and behavior rather than to the outrageous poverty, slavery, systematic blatant racism, and marginalization to which they were subjected.

The racist ideology in the Andes is equivalent to that which existed in North America in the 19th century. It was believed that the "savages," including Native Americans and African-Americans, were incapable of feeling pain; only civilized Whites, particularly of European origin, were highly sensitive to pain. Physicians and intellectuals described a disease called

"Dysaesthesia aethiopsis" or "obtuse sensibility of body" as being present among African-Americans. This disease was thought to render them insensitive to pain when subjected to punishment [6, 7]. Even during the time of the American Enlightenment, physicians and the priest Samuel Stanhope Smith of Princeton University, who was granted honorific degrees from Yale and Harvard, held the conviction that Native American people were insensitive to pain. He said, "We know that among Indians the squaws do not suffer in childbirth. Among your red Indian and other uncivilized tribes, the parturient female does not suffer the same amount of pain during labor as the female of the white race" [6, p. 154].

The clinical encounter between the biomedically trained *mishu* physician and Quichua patients suffering from *llaqui* is not only challenging in medical terms. The troubled medical encounter in the Andes is charged with massive barriers imposed by doctors' bigotry, lack of knowledge, racism, prejudice, discrimination, and a history of five centuries of colonization.

The Quichua view

One of the first steps that physicians should take in a medical encounter with patients from cultural backgrounds other than their own is to learn the basics of their patients' health belief system. This will help them improve communication bidirectionally, both by improving their understanding of their patients' illness and symptom descriptions, and by improving their ability to negotiate and explain appropriate treatment options to the patients. The goal of the physician in this context is to become aware of cultural differences and gain some grasp of the theory of illness of patients, not to become an anthropological expert in a variety of cultures.

Llaqui and the Quichua theory of illness

Llaqui is a highly prevalent syndrome among the Quichua people of the Andes. It is a complex illness category composed of four subtypes. Contrary to Western biomedicine, the subtypes of *llaqui* are differentiated mainly by their causes rather than their symptoms. Moreover, each of the subtypes of *llaqui* requires a specific treatment strategy. According to the Quichuas' theory of illness, *llaqui* is divided into four classes: *mancharishca-huairashca* (victim of evil spirits, for brevity these two classes are merged into one category), *shungu nanai* (heart pain), and *rurashca* (sorcery) [1].

Mancharishca-huairashca (victim of evil spirits)

When someone experiences intense fright and fear, that person can develop *mancharishca-huairashca*. This fright results in the temporary separation of the person's spirit from the body, after which evil spirits from nature (*cucucuna*) can take possession of the person's spirit. In the case of *huairashca*, evil winds or particles of misfortune can enter the person's body, causing illness.

In *mancharishca*, the patient's spirit leaves the body as a result of experiencing an intense fright. It is thought that at that moment, *cucucuna*, present everywhere in nature, can sequester the person's spirit and hold it captive. The separation of the spirit from the body is thought to cause the symptoms. The treatment is aimed at negotiating with the spirits and liberating the patient's captive spirit and reintroducing it into the body. In the case of *huairashca*, evil winds (*huaira*) or particles of misfortune (*chiqui*) suddenly enter the frightened person's body. A variety of signs and symptoms will follow the exposure to those evil winds or particles of misfortune.

There are many potential sources of fright. Fright can be triggered by humans, animals, plants, and inanimate objects. Some of the most severe causes of fright are inanimate objects such as waterfalls, water springs, and ditches. Once a person suffers from *mancharishca*, the illness can last from 1 week to several months. *Huairashca*, on the other hand, is usually an acute illness, lasting about a week, when treated. Without treatment, however, *huairashca* can become chronic, last months or years, and become resistant to treatment. The symptoms of *mancharishca-huairashca* include a wide range of psychological and somatic symptoms such as sadness, irritability, insomnia, diarrhea, back pain, fever, thirst, and tremors, among others.

Shungu nanai (heart pain)

Shungu nanai is an illness that can result from experiences of hardship and sorcery. A series of negative life events can lead to *shungu nanai*. Common examples of negative life events include land disputes, the death of a relative or a valued animal, family plights or conflicts with *mishus* (Latinos), poverty, illness, lost harvests, marital conflicts, social exclusion, and lack of social support, among others. At first, a person may experience *pinsamintu*, a complex emotional state composed of sadness, anxiety, and anger. *Pinsamintu* can then transform into *shungu nanai*. It can take up to 1 year for the symptoms of *shungu nanai* to become noticeable, and the illness usually lasts from 1 month to several years. Many symptoms are experienced by patients suffering from *shungu nanai*. However, there are two specific symptoms attributed specifically to *shungu nanai*: pain to the *shungu* (epigastrium) and convulsions.

Yachactaitas' treatment aims first to ensure that evil winds (*huaira*) are not present and that the person's spirit is safe. Secondly, the treatment seeks to improve the emotional state of the patient. Therapies include *ñacchachi*, in which the head of the patient is rubbed systematically, from the forehead to the occipital region, or the *yachactaita's* preparation of an infusion composed of 12 medicinal herbs used specifically for the treatment of *shungu nanai*.

Interestingly, according to the Quichuas, *shungu nanai* is the only *llaqui* sub-category for which physicians' treatment can also be sought.

Rurashca (sorcery)

Rurashca is the illness resulting from being the victim of sorcery. *Rurashca* occurs when a *yachactaita* (Quichua healer) puts a curse on a patient by request of an envious enemy. Individuals at risk for *rurashca* are those who are well-off and enjoy privileges, such as having successful harvests, a house, connections with influential mishu people, or many friends, for they may spur envy in the people around them. Having a cheating spouse, conflicts with neighbors, or lawsuits can also increase one's risk of *rurashca*. Patients suffering from *rurashca* experience the same symptoms already described for the other forms of *llaqui*. A person suffering from *rurashca* must be treated by a *yachactaita*. *Rurashca* is considered a severe illness, and if left untreated, can lead to death. The *yachactaita*'s treatment is multidimensional, and includes the expulsion of evil spirits from the patient's body, the release of the person's spirit from the evil spirits, and care to relieve the patient from the intense emotional state.

Llaqui as a culture-bound syndrome in the Andes

There are virtually no studies on *llaqui* in the Quichua population of around 28 million. The studies that do exist were done among the Latinos and focus on concepts of *susto, espanto,* or *colerín* [8–11]. These syndromes share some traits with *llaqui*, because centuries of interactions with the Quichua culture shaped the mishu's theory of illness, but deviates from it as it is also influenced by 17th-century European, Persian, and Arab theories of illness and worldviews [12].

We recommend that when Quichua patients present symptoms such as those listed above, physicians seriously consider the possibility of *llaqui*, in Quichua terms.

Bridging the two solitudes

Using western diagnostic tools

In a unique study conducted in Ecuador [1], it was shown that contrary to the common belief among Ecuador's physicians, *llaqui* is not merely a primitive superstition. It is a real illness; a syndrome with depressive, somatoform, and anxiety features. Using Western medicine instruments such as the DSM-III-R criteria and a Quichua version of the Zung Depression Scale with proper cultural adaption, Incayawar [1] was able to identify multiple psychiatric disorders among *llaqui* patients. Eighty-two percent of the 50 patients suffering from *llaqui* who participated in the study met the DSM-III-R criteria for depression and scored high on the Zung Depression Scale. In addition, 44 percent of the patients presented somatoform disorders and 40 percent had anxiety disorders (see Table 19.1).

Furthermore, the patients with *llaqui* were suffering from various types of pain (see Table 19.2).

These findings are particularly important for Andean countries with a large Quichua population. In Ecuador, for instance, Quichua people make up over 40 percent of the population. These results can also be useful for physicians in other countries around the world where Quichua immigrants are present, such as Canada, the United States, and many European countries. Physicians working with Latino immigrants from South America, who are strongly influenced by the Quichua culture, may also find this information valuable. It is important to keep in mind that with appropriate culturally adapted psychometric tools, cultural sensitivity, and input from Quichua traditional medicine, the *llaqui* syndrome of the Andean region could be successfully managed by Western trained physicians.

Clinical recommendations

In order to be able to diagnose a patient with *llaqui*, physicians should pay attention to the following cultural and linguistic issues during the medical encounter.

First, they should become aware of patients' health beliefs and theories of illness, as recommended by Kleinman [13]. This will help them reach a better understanding of the patients' conditions, expectations, and culture.

Table 19.1 Psychiatric diagnoses (more than one diagnosis per patient), $N=50$.

Psychiatric diagnoses	% of patients	Zung (mean)
Depressive disorders	82	65
Somatoform disorders	44	63
Anxiety disorders	40	59

Table 19.2 Pain somatic symptoms detected during the medical interview (more than one diagnosis per patient), $N=50$.

Type of pain	Number of patients	% of patients
Multiple migratory pain	26	52
Stomachache	25	50
Cephalalgia	24	48
Dysuria	7	14

Second, physicians should demonstrate linguistic sensitivity by recognizing the expressions that patients use to convey their suffering. For instance, in the first moments of the clinical encounter, *llaqui* Quichua patients express solely physical symptoms to the physician. They abstain from talking about psychological distress altogether, even when asked to do so. The Quichua people categorize illnesses in two broad categories: the "Quichua illnesses," which are treatable by a *yachactaita* (Quichua healer), and the rest, such as serious injuries and a variety of chronic or acute diseases, which are treatable by a physician. Depending on the type of illness from which they believe to be suffering, the Quichua patients will choose to consult either a healer or a physician. Because they consider the physician to be specialized in treating physical ailments, talking about emotional problems with a doctor is perceived as inappropriate and to be avoided. Hence, Quichua patients will only report physical symptoms to physicians [14]. Given these beliefs, how can we prime Quichua patients to share emotional symptoms with a physician? *Llaqui* is frequently accompanied by complaints of physical pain. The physicians treating a Quichua patient should thus keep in mind that pain could be a psychological marker for *llaqui* and hence for depressive, somatoform, and anxiety disorders among the Quichuas of the Andes. A health professional working among Quichua patients should ask the patients to express their feelings and emotions by using a very specific phrase: "*Pinsamintuta charingui-chu?*" (Do you have sad thoughts, worries?) This will trigger an abundant expression of worries and concerns, if they are present.

Third, within a cross-cultural medical encounter, physicians should seek to improve mutual understanding. When conducting their interview, physicians could phrase their questions in various ways to ensure that their message is accurately transmitted to the patient. They should also avoid using highly technical jargon. In addition, to verify that they have in turn clearly understood their interlocutor, it could be useful for physicians to paraphrase their patient's statements.

Finally, physicians should be aware that information obtained from ad-lib interpreters without any formal training in medical terminology may not always be reliable [15].

Llaqui is a complex and multi-dimensional illness. To improve clinical success, we suggest physicians who suspect that a patient is suffering from *llaqui* to rely on both the Quichua and Western medical systems for designing a treatment plan. Whenever possible, physicians should seek to work in collaboration with a *yachactaita* (Quichua healer) in the making of a diagnosis as well as in the preparation of a treatment plan, which could include, for example, anti-depressants and *yachactaita*'s interventions. Such collaboration, in our experience, results in better patient satisfaction and clinical outcomes.

Lastly, when treating Quichua patients, it is essential to be cognizant of the history of oppression and colonization that indigenous peoples have endured, as these experiences pervasively influence indigenous patients' worldview, their attitude toward biomedically trained doctors, and responses to their clinical interventions.

The basics reviewed here regarding Quichua theory of illness will be vital to physicians working with Quichua populations in order to provide culturally appropriate medical care. Furthermore, the Quichua theory of illness regarding *llaqui* can serve as a model for the physicians, elsewhere in the world, wishing to provide more culturally appropriate care to patients in a multicultural setting. It is an example of how patients from different cultural origins may report and view illnesses in very different terms than those learned by the physician, whose medical approach is in turn also influenced by his or her own culture.

Final remarks

Mrs. Lema finally met a transcultural psychiatrist and pain specialist from the Runajambi Institute. To come to a final diagnosis, he combined both the *yachactaita's* and his Western medicine diagnosis. Mrs. Lema was diagnosed as suffering from *llaqui* (Quichua diagnosis) and exhibiting comorbid depression-anxiety and chronic pain (Western diagnosis). Her treatment plan included a *yachactaita* intervention based on healing ceremonies and infusion of medicinal plants and an anti-depressant medication prescribed by the psychiatrist. Four months after beginning the treatment, Mrs. Lema was free of symptoms, including pain, and had returned to her normal daily activities.

Note

1. Mishu is the Quichua term that refers to the dominant Spanish-speaking group in Latin America. They are individuals of partial indigenous descent, but seek to identify themselves as Whites and as being of European descent only, rejecting their indigenous roots. They are also known in Spanish as mestizos or Latinos.

References

1 Maldonado MG. (a.k.a. Mario Incayawar). Llaqui et dépression; une étude exploratoire chez les Quichuas (Équateur). (Master's thesis). McGill University, Montreal; 1992.
2 Incayawar M. Indigenous peoples of South America: Inequalities in mental health care. In: Bhui K, Bhugra D (eds.), *Textbook of Culture and Mental Health Disorder*. London: Arnold Publishing; 2007, pp. 185–190.

3 Cohen A. *The Mental Health of Indigenous Peoples: An International Overview*. Geneva: Nations for Mental Health, Department of Mental Health, World Health Organization; 1999.

4 Incayawar M, Maldonado-Bouchard S. The forsaken mental health of the Indigenous Peoples: A moral case of outrageous exclusion in Latin America. *BMC Int Health Hum Rights*. 2009;9(1):27.

5 Briggs CL, Mantini-Briggs C. *Stories in the Time of Cholera: Racial Profiling during a Medical Nightmare*. Berkeley: University of California Press; 2003.

6 Pernick MS. "They don't feel it like we do": Social politics and the perception of pain. In *A Calculus of Suffering: Pain, Professionalism, and Anesthesia in Nineteenth-Century America*. New York: Columbia University Press; 1985.

7 Clark EB. "The sacred rights of the weak": Pain, sympathy, and the culture of individual rights in antebellum America. *J Am Hist*. 1995;82(2):463–493.

8 Gillin J. Magical fright. *Psychiatry*. 1948;11(4):387–400.

9 Rubel AJ. The epidemiology of a folk illness: Susto in Hispanic America. *Ethnology*. 1969;3:268–283.

10 Sal y Rosas F. The disease of fright. *Psychiatr Commun*. 1960;3:37–46.

11 Sal y Rosas F. El mal de corazón (sonko-nanay) del folklore psiquiátrico del Perú. *Acta Psiquiatr Psicol Am Lat*. 1967;13:31–37.

12 Foster GM. Relationships between Spanish and Spanish-American folk medicine. *J Am Folk*. 1953;66(261):201–217.

13 Kleinman AM. *Patients and Healers in the Context of Culture: An Exploration of the Borderland between Anthropology, Medicine, and Psychiatry*. Berkley: University of California Press;1980.

14 Bouchard L. A linguistic approach for understanding pain in the medical encounter. In Incayawar M, Todd L (eds.) *Culture, Brain and Analgesia: Understanding and Managing Pain in Diverse Populations*. London: Oxford University Press; 2013, p. 9–19.

15 Bouchard L. Using a linguistic approach in pain medicine: Advances in doctor-patient communication. *J Pain*. 2013;14(4):S7.

Index

Note: Page numbers in *italics* refer to Figures; those in **bold** to Tables